The Modification of Language Behavior

The Modification of Language Behavior

Edited by

BENJAMIN B. LAHEY

Florida Technological University
Orlando, Florida

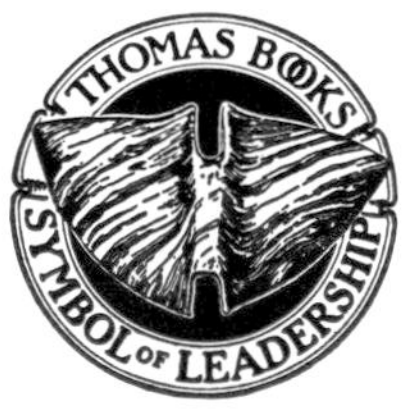

CHARLES C THOMAS · PUBLISHER

Springfield · Illinois · U.S.A.

Published and Distributed Throughout the World by

CHARLES C THOMAS • PUBLISHER
BANNERSTONE HOUSE
301-327 East Lawrence Avenue, Springfield, Illinois, U.S.A.

ISBN 0-398-02692-0- (cloth)
ISBN 0-398-02759-5- (paper)

Library of Congress Catalog Card Number: 72-88482

With THOMAS BOOKS *careful attention is given to all details of manufacturing and design. It is the Publisher's desire to present books that are satisfactory as to their physical qualities and artistic possibilities and appropriate for their particular use.* THOMAS BOOKS *will be true to those laws of quality that assure a good name and good will.*

Printed in the United States of America
F-1

CONTRIBUTORS

DONALD M. BAER
Department of Human Development
University of Kansas

LEONARD DILLER
Chief, Behavioral Science Department
Institute of Rehabilitation Medicine
New York University Medical Center

JAMES L. FITCH
Department of Speech
New Mexico State University

ROBERT GOODKIN
Behavioral Science Department
Institute of Rehabilitation Medicine
New York University Medical Center

DOUG GUESS
Kansas Neurological Institute

JURGEN R. HARTUNG
Department of Psychology
University of Houston

ROGER INGHAM
Department of Psychology
University of New South Wales

BENJAMIN LAHEY
Department of Psychology
Florida Technological University

RICHARD R. MARTIN
Department of Speech Science, Pathology and Audiology
University of Minnesota

SHEILA MCKENNA-HARTUNG
Department of Psychology
University of Houston

NANDINI SHAH
Department of Behavioral Sciences
Institute of Rehabilitation Medicine
New York University Medical Center

LAWRENCE SIMKINS
Head, Department of Psychology
University of Missouri at Kansas City

PREFACE

THE PURPOSE of this book is to provide an up-to-date summary of the recent advances in the application of behavior modification techniques to problems of language. It was compiled to serve the needs of teachers, researchers and practitioners of communication disorders, special education and psychology. The strategy employed was to select leaders in several areas of language problems and to ask them to contribute a chapter on their specialty. Each author or authors has written an original chapter on their work. I wish to thank those authors again for their outstanding contributions. I would also like to thank the Department of Psychology of Florida Technological University for their support of this project. This book was compiled because of B. F. Skinner, J. R. Kantor and W. S. Verplanck, and for Susan and Megan.

INTRODUCTION

IT HAS BEEN only a recent development in the history of man's study of man that his own behavior has been treated as a natural phenomenon. The systematic relationships between behavior and antecedent and consequent stimulus conditions outlined by Pavlov, Thorndike and others are recent landmarks indeed. It has been even more recently that man's language has been considered part of that behavior. Until the pioneering writings of Kantor (1935), Eisenson (1938), and Skinner (1957), the exclusive conception of language was that of the expressive and receptive medium of the mind. Ideas were transmitted from mind to mind via language. Because the mind was considered to operate with a *free will,* its medium was likewise not considered subject to environmental control.

The alternative approach developed most fully by Skinner treats language simply as a form of behavior. This approach proposes that if language is like other behavior, it will be subject to environmental control: control that will enable us to modify disorders of language and control its development.

This naturalistic approach to behavior has been profitably applied to clinical and educational problems under the term *behavior modification.* Although this approach is primarily characterized by its *attitude* that applied psychology should incorporate the methods and questioning spirit of experimental psychology, particularly as they apply to the study of learning, its acceptance is probably due more to the simplicity and effectiveness of its growing stock of *techniques.* It is this same set of techniques that is now being applied to language disorders. The chapters in this text will attest to the effectiveness of the behavior modification approach to language.

BASIC LINGUISTIC TERMS

To maintain a consistent vocabulary, it will be necessary to define some basic linguistic terms as they will be used in the text.

Although they have origins in mentalistic linguistics, they have found a use in behavioral papers and must be given definitions consistent with such a usage. Later, the basic principles of learning that play a role in behavior modification procedures and some basic assumptions of the behavior modification approach will be defined for those who are unfamiliar with them.

Productive and Receptive Language

Language has two aspects in the communication process. It is behavior for the speaker and a stimulus which alters the behavior of the listener. If he is to function appropriately in his linguistic community, the individual must learn to both speak and listen. He must affect the behavior of others in specific ways through his language (productive or expressive language), and in turn he must be affected in specific ways by the language of others (receptive language).

Generative Property of Language

The easiest way to define the term *generative* will be to discuss some of the ways that languages *could* be, but are *not*. Most human interactions would go on unchanged if all utterances were in the form of a large, but fixed set of sentence structures. For example, if the following sentence form were part of the speaker's repertoire,

Article + Noun + Verb + Article + Noun

a large number of *declarative statements* could be made:

The beagle ate the cookie.
A girl won the prize.
The gnome missed the point.

If the speaker's repertoire consisted of a large number of such forms, most utterances could be made without restriction.

Human speakers are not limited to a fixed stock of *sentence frames,* however. We frequently produce *grammatically correct* utterances and respond appropriately to utterances in grammatical forms that we have never before experienced. But, although an unlimited number of unique utterances can be produced and understood by the members of a linguistic community, not all possible utterances will be functional in communication. All appropriate utterances of a speaker will exhibit certain grammatical regularities. This is what is meant by the term *generative:* the production and reception of an unlimited number of utterances which share a limited number of regularities. Stated in formal terms, these regularities are the *rules of grammar.*

Techniques to produce full generative language in individuals who lack it are discussed in Chapters I, II, VI, and VII.

Levels of Analysis

Language can be analyzed into its component parts at two levels: the morpheme-syntax level and the phoneme level. Both levels are important and are not mutually exclusive ways of looking at language.

Morphemes

We typically think of language as being made up of *meaningful* units that we term *words.* The technical unit used by linguists at this level of analysis is the *morpheme,* defined as the smallest indivisible unit of meaning. The category *morpheme* includes simple words that cannot be broken down into smaller units, such as the word *graph.* It also includes meaningful units that cannot stand alone: prefixes (such as *poly*) and suffixes (such as the plural morpheme *s*). Complex words are made up of more than one morpheme:

poly/graph/s

Morphemes that can stand alone (simple words) are termed *free morphemes.* Suffixes and prefixes are termed *bound morphemes.*

Syntax

If the morphemic repertoire is to function effectively in communication, it must show the same *regularities* of sequence and combination as the rest of the linguistic community. These regularities are termed *syntax.*

Phonemes

Language can also be analyzed into units of sound. All utterances are made up of different combinations of a small number of sounds. The smallest indivisible unit of sound is the *phoneme.* Morphemes are made up of one or more phonemes. The morpheme *I* is made up of a single phoneme, as is the morpheme *eye,* whereas the morpheme *by* is made up of two separable sounds. The task of language modification enterprises is frequently to change these repertoires when they are inadequate, nonexistent or deviant.

Language Parameters

A class of language disorders exists in which there is no problem with the phonemic, morphemic or syntactic repertoires, *per se.* The deviance is associated with some characteristic of otherwise normal language, such as fluency, rate or *intelligibility.* The chapter on stuttering by Martin and Ingham and the chapter on cluttering by Simkins demonstrate how behavior modification techniques may be applied to these disorders.

BASIC CONCEPTS IN BEHAVIOR MODIFICATION

The approach demonstrated in the chapters of this book represents an extension of the principles of behavior modification to a kind of behavioral problem that had been previously ignored. It will be in order, therefore, to discuss some of the basic concepts and terms used in the behavior modification approach.

Principles of Learning

As previously stated, the foundation of behavior modification is an acceptance of the methods and attitudes of experimental psychology, especially the study of learning. The science of learning seeks to predict changes in behavior from a knowledge of the environmental events that produce them. It is a short step from this knowledge to behavior modification: if the scientist can learn to control the environmental events that produce behavior change, he can then control the behavior change process itself. Several principles of learning have been worked out, two of which are of special importance to language modification.

Operant Learning

Much behavior change comes about as a result of the consequences of a bit of behavior. The child who gets a handful of cookies as a result of scrambling up on the kitchen counter will be more likely to do so again than before. The child who receives only a sound spanking will be less likely to repeat his action in the future. Because the consequences of an individual's behavior are aspects of his environment, the behavior modifier can gain control over them and use them to establish or eliminate desirable and undesirable behaviors.

PROCEDURES FOR ESTABLISHING DESIRED BEHAVIOR. There are two operant techniques that are used to establish desired behaviors, *positive* and *negative reinforcement.* A positive reinforcer is a response consequence that increases some measure of a response (such as rate, amplitude or precision) above its previous value. Praising a silent preschooler, for example, for his vocalizations will gradually lead to an increase in the frequency of his talking.

A wide range of reinforcers has been found to be effective with children and adults including candy, praise, money, etc. Frequently, convenient objects such as poker chips are used as reinforcers. These can be later exchanged for items such as toys, candy or privileges, and are termed *token reinforcers.* Such reinforcement programs are called *token economies.*

Frequently, reinforcement cannot be effectively used to modify a behavior that rarely or never occurs. If it does not occur, it cannot be reinforced. In such cases, *shaping* or the *method of successive approximations* is used.

At first, responses that are somewhat similar to the target response are reinforced, and then only responses that are successively more similar are reinforced, until the target response itself occurs and can be reinforced. For example, if the target response, *ball* is not in the subject's repertoire, *uh* may be reinforced at first, then *buh,* then *ba,* and finally *ball.* The frequency of desired behaviors may also be increased through negative reinforcement. In this case, the measure of a response is increased when the response terminates or avoids an aversive (although not necessarily *painful*) consequence. Conditioning responses through negative reinforcement is called *escape conditioning* when the response terminates an aversive stimulus and *avoidance conditioning* when the response avoids or postpones an aversive stimulus.

Procedures for Maintaining Desired Behavior. In using positive reinforcement to establish behaviors, it is essential to maximize the frequency of reinforcement, especially in the early stages of acquisition. For this reason, every response is reinforced in most cases, a procedure termed *continuous reinforcement*.

But, the goal of behavior modification is to produce lasting changes in behavior, i.e., behavior changes that will be maintained by the natural consequences of that behavior in the world at large. Unlike the controlled behavior modification setting, however, reinforcement in the natural environment is rarely continuous, but is intermittent. Some responses are reinforced, but most are not.

To protect the new behaviors from an abrupt change in contingencies, the later stages of operant behavior modification frequency consists of thinning out the frequency of reinforcement by placing the individual on a schedule of intermittent reinforcement. Paradoxically, these schedules of reduced reinforcement do not weaken the strength of a firmly acquired behavior, but strengthen them when applied properly.

(i) *Fixed schedules*. In the fixed schedules, reinforcers are delivered after a fixed number of responses (fixed-ratio) or after the first response that occurs after a fixed period of time since the last reinforcers (fixed-interval).

(ii) *Variable schedules*. In the variable-ratio and variable-interval schedules, reinforcement is delivered after a variable number of responses or an interval of variable length. Because these schedules produce the most stable and frequent performance, they are the most often applied schedules in behavior modification.

Stimulus Control. If a behavior occurs more frequently in a given situation than in its absence, such as a child who uses obscene language in the presence of children but not in the presence of adults, the behavior is said to be under *stimulus control*. This is not to say that the stimulus *causes* or *elicits* the behavior, but only that the stimulus is the *occasion* for the occurrence of the behavior. The term stimulus control only implies that there is a reliable relationship between the presence of the stimulus and of the occurrence of the behavior. The controlling stimulus in such instances is termed the *discriminative stimulus*.

Procedures for Eliminating Undesired Behaviors. Consequences can be manipulated in such a way as to eliminate behaviors as well as establish them. The simplest manipulation is simply to withhold positive reinforcement from a response that was previously reinforced. This is termed *extinction.* Aversive consequences can similarly be made contingent on behaviors in the procedure termed *punishment.* These procedures will frequently be useful in language modification, especially when used with positive reinforcement for alternative, desired behaviors. A frequently used alternative to punishment is *time-out from positive reinforcement.* In this procedure, the undesired behavior temporarily eliminates a positive reinforcer, such as turning off a cartoon or being removed from the social situation.

Imitative Learning

Behavior is not changed only as a result of its consequences; much behavior change comes from the observation of the behavior of others. The guest at a formal dinner who is faced for the first time with three forks, will soon be using them in the same manner as the guest who is most easily in view. The preschool teacher who shows a movie of rambunctious children will have a busy afternoon. The same sort of thing is true for a wide variety of situations.

Imitative learning is technically defined as the process through which some measure of a behavior increases above its previous level when the increase can be shown to be produced by observing the same behavior in another individual. The individual whose behavior changed is termed the *observer.* The individual whose behavior is observed is termed the *model,* and the procedure of presenting the model's behavior to the observer is termed *modeling.*

MODELING AND REINFORCEMENT. There is presently considerable debate concerning the origin of limitative learning. Many individuals feel that it is a derived process of learning; that is, that imitative learning is itself learned. It has been suggested that children are frequently reinforced on occasions when they accidentally duplicate the behavior of their parents or others (e.g., saying *hi* like Daddy just did). This, they suggest, could lead to a generalized tendency to imitate.

While this debate need not concern us, it should be pointed

out that modeling and reinforcement are importantly related in language modification. Frequently, children with language problems (especially those termed *autistic* and *mentally retarded*) are deficient in imitation. In these cases, a generalized imitative repertoire can be built by reinforcing the subject for imitating. In other cases, the efficiency of a reinforcement program can be improved by modeling the response that will be reinforced instead of shaping it or waiting for its occurrence.

Prompting

Sometimes it is most convenient to bring about the occurrence of the response that is to be reinforced by instructing the subject to make it by forming an articulation with the therapist's fingers on the subject's lips, giving part of the answer to a question, etc. These techniques are called *prompts* and they find frequent use in the early stages of language modification.

It is usually desirable to discontinue the use of prompts as soon as possible. The most effective way of removing them is to do so gradually. This will produce a minimal disruption of the response. For example, in trying to bring a child to use the therapist's name when asked, the following prompt might be used: "What's my name? Doctor La. . . ." Later, after the response using the prompt is well established, the prompt could be gradually removed; for example, "What's my name? Doctor . . .", "What's my name? Doc . . .", etc. Removing a prompt gradually is termed *fading*.

WITHIN-SUBJECT DESIGNS

There are several scientific strategies which may be used in demonstrating the effects of a controlling variable such as reinforcement or modeling. The one used most often in behavior modification research is the within-subject or the ABAB design. In this design, the target behavior is measured for a period of time, then the controlling variable is introduced. The change in the measure of the response can then be attributed to the variable. To ensure that this interpretation is correct, and the change is not simply due to the passage of time or some related factor, the controlling variable is then removed for a time, and then rein-

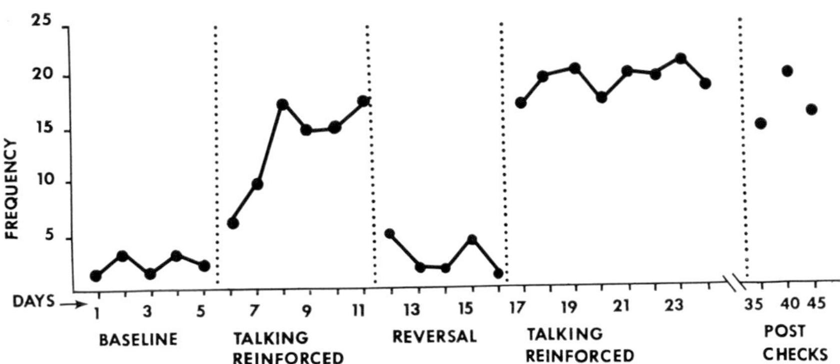

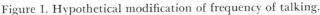

Figure 1. Hypothetical modification of frequency of talking.

troduced. Figure 1 gives an example of a hypothetical graphical presentation of this type of design.

In this study of the effects of social reinforcement (praise, smiles, etc.) on the talking of children, the target behavior is the frequency of vocalizations made to the teacher or other children in a preschool classroom. The frequency of vocalizations is first measured before introducing the controlling variable. This first measurement is termed the *baseline*. The controlling variable is the presentation of social reinforcement when the child talks. This is introduced following the baseline and changes in the target behavior are measured. In Figure 1, it can be seen that there is a decided increase in the talking during the time when the subject is reinforced for doing so. The controlling variable is then removed in the period called *reversal* (or the *second baseline*), and then replaced again in the fourth phase. The measure can be seen to increase, then decrease in these periods. An excellent addition to such a design is a follow-up or *post check* at a later date to check on the permanence of the change. In this experiment, the control of social reinforcement was demonstrated and the behavior was clearly (and rather permanently) modified.

The next most frequently used design is the traditional *between-groups* comparison. In this method, the controlling variable is present in one group, but absent in the *control group,* although all other conditions are identical in the two groups. Differences in the behavior of the subjects in the two groups may be attributed to the controlling variable. Unlike the within-subject design, data is usually considered in terms of groups of subjects rather than individual subjects.

ETIOLOGY

Another aspect of the behavior modification approach that sets it apart is its notions about the origin or etiology of behavior disorders. Since deviant behavior is simply behavior (and not a *symptom* of some inferred underlying *psychic pathology*) it is usually assumed to be produced by deviant experiences, or a deviant environment. Bijou (1963), for example, has suggested that moderate *mental retardation* may be due to inadequate environments during development rather than genetic causes.

One need not necessarily make this kind of assumption regarding etiology, however, to operate within the behavior modification framework. One need not make any assumptions concerning etiologies at all. The behavior modifier is faced with a deviant behavior. He or she knows that the behavior can be changed through specific manipulations of the individual's environment, and that is all he or she needs to know. It is not necessary to know where the behavior came from, just how to change it. The question of etiology is an important question for the construction of a preventive science of deviant behavior, but it need not be answered for the way as to modify it.

CHAPTER HEADINGS

It should be pointed out that the chapter headings of this book were not chosen on the basis of theoretical notions about etiology. There are many problems with categories such as *autism* and *mental retardation*. The language problems of these and other groups may turn out to be quite similar and may in fact turn out to have the same etiology. That information simply is not available. These terms are merely used in this book as a convenient way of dividing the subject matter into sections.

The point of the behavior modification approach should be clear in spite of the use of these categories: regardless of the label given to the individual, determine how the language is deviant through observation, then manipulate the environment in such a individual case.

REFERENCES

Bijou, S. W.: Theory and research in mental (developmental) retardation. *Psychological Record, 13*:95-110, 1963.

Eisenson, J.: *The Psychology of Speech.* New York, Crofts, 1938.

Kantor, J. R.: *An Objective Psychology of Grammar.* Evanston, Principia Press, 1935.

Skinner, B. F.: *Verbal Behavior.* New York, Appleton-Century-Crofts, 1957.

ACKNOWLEDGMENTS

THE editor and authors wish to thank the following copyright owners, authors, and publishers for permission to reprint excerpts from copyrighted materials.

Engelmann, S.: How to construct effective language programs for the poverty child. In F. Williams (Ed.): *Language and Poverty*. Chicago, Markham, 1970, p. 102.

Hart, Betty M.: Investigations of the language of disadvantaged preschool children. Unpublished doctoral dissertation, University of Kansas, 1969, pp. 8-14, 20, 27-28, 68, 74-75, 81, 102, 107-108.

Hartung, J.: A review of procedures to increase verbal imitation skills and functional speech in autistic children. *Journal of Speech and Hearing Disorders, 35*:203-217, 1970.

Holland, Audrey and Matthews, J.: Application of teaching machine concepts to speech pathology and audiology. *ASHA, 5*:474-482, 1963.

From: *Articulatory Acquisition and Behavior,* by Harris Winitz. Copyright © 1969. By permission of Appleton-Century-Crofts, Educational Division, Meredith Corporation.

Labov, W.: The logic of nonstandard English. Paper presented at Twentieth Annual Roundtable Meeting on Linguistics and Language Studies, Georgetown University, March 14, 1969. Reprinted in F. Williams (Ed.): *Language and Poverty*. Chicago, Markham, 1970, pp. 159-161, 171.

Lahey, B. B.: Modification of the frequency of descriptive adjectives in the speech of Head Start children through modeling without reinforcement. *Journal of Applied Behavior Analysis, 4*:19-22, 1971. Copyright 1971 by the Society for the Experimental Analysis of Behavior, Inc.

Langora, J. and Mororek, M.: Some problems of cluttering. *Folia Phoniatrica, 22*:325-336, 1970.

McDonald, E.: *Articulation Testing and Treatment: A Sensory-motor Approach.* Pittsburgh, Stanwix House, 1964, p. 183.

Moore, J.: The effect of certain schedules of reinforcement on the experimental manipulation of fundamental frequency. Unpublished doctoral dissertation, Florida State University, 1968.

Risley, T. R.: Learning and lollipops. In P. Cramer (Ed.): *Readings in Developmental Psychology Today.* Del Mar, CRM Press, 1967. Reprinted from *Psychology Today* Magazine, January, 1968. Copyright Communications/Research/Machines, Inc.

Roll, Joyce: Manipulation of fundamental frequency in functional voice disorders by application of reinforcement principles. Unpublished doctoral dissertation, Florida State University, 1969.

Simkins, L., Kingery, M. and Bradley, P.: Modification of cluttered speech in an emotionally disturbed child. *Journal of Special Education, 4*:81-88, 1970.

From *Voice-Speech-Language* by Richard Luchsinger and Godfrey E. Arnold. Copyright © 1965 by Wadsworth Publishing Company, Inc., Belmont, California 94002. Reprinted by permission of the publisher (Table 12, page 613).

Sloane, H. and MacAulay, B.: *Operant Procedures in Remedial Speech and Language Training.* Boston, Houghton Mifflin, 1968.

Van Riper, C.: *Speech Correction: Principles and Methods* (4th Ed.). Englewood Cliffs, Prentice-Hall, 1963, p. 26.

Weiss, D.: Cluttering. In C. Van Riper (Ed.): *The Foundations of Speech Pathology Series.* Englewood Cliffs, Prentice-Hall, 1964, pp. 7, 34, 36.

CONTENTS

		Page
	Contributors	v
	Preface	vii
	Introduction	ix
	Acknowledgments	xxi
Chapter		
I.	Some Experimental Analyses of Linguistic Development in Institutionalized Retarded Children—*Doug Guess and Donald M. Baer*	3
II.	Establishing Verbal Imitation Skills and Functional Speech in Autistic Children—*Sheila McKenna-Hartung and Jurgen R. Hartung*	61
III.	Stuttering—*Richard Martin and Roger Ingham*	91
IV.	Voice and Articulation—*James L. Fitch*	130
V.	Cluttering—*Lawrence Simkins*	178
VI.	Training Spouses to Improve The Functional Speech of Aphasic Patients—*Robert Goodkin, Leonard Diller and Nandini Shah*	218
VII.	Minority Group Languages—*Benjamin B. Lahey*	270
	Name Index	317
	Subject Index	321

The Modification of Language Behavior

CHAPTER I

SOME EXPERIMENTAL ANALYSES OF LINGUISTIC DEVELOPMENT IN INSTITUTIONALIZED RETARDED CHILDREN[1]

DOUG GUESS AND DONALD M. BAER

LANGUAGE DEVELOPMENT has attracted research effort for many years, for appropriately important reasons. Simply at the descriptive level, it must be recognized as one of the most frequently used response systems in man. At a more analytic level, it is apparent that language is one of the most highly developed systems serving the symbolic capabilities of man, and these symbolic skills underlie a great deal of man's competence. Much of that competence is transmitted across generations primarily by language, frequently without significant loss, and thus contributes to the cumulation of competence in man as a species. Furthermore, the developmental course of language as a behavior system within each human, from infancy to adulthood, is an extreme one: it progresses from virtually no linguistic competence in the infant to a complex usage of perhaps a hundred thousand separate responses (words) in a remarkable variety of chains (sentences), subject to endless variation which nevertheless is usually understood by its well-educated audiences. So important and extreme a course to so grand an outcome would virtually command scientific analysis.

Nevertheless, the bulk of that analysis has been less than experimental. Instead, it has been descriptive of the changing content and structure of language typifying the various stages of development, and has noted some of the gross environmental circumstances correlated with those changes (cf. McCarthy, 1954). In the place of experimental analysis, with its potential for demonstrating cause and effect in language growth, there has occurred instead an occasional use of experimental technique to better display the current characteristics of language as it exists in subjects of a given status (cf. Palermo, 1970, for a concise review), and an abundant flowering of theory (again, Palermo offers an excellent sampling and perspective). Much of this theory has been distinctively linguistic (or mentalistic), in that language development processes were taken as exemplifying unique principles. However, some theory has suggested that language follows the same laws as any other examples of human behavior (Skinner, 1957; Staats and Staats, 1963). The latter approach immediately implies experimental analyses of language development as an environmentally controlled process, perhaps similar to environmentally controlled non-language developments.

Even with such theoretical impetus, abstention from a cause-and-effect oriented experimental analysis would not be difficult to explain. In the realm of human behavior, experimental analysis has never been the predominant research approach, largely because of an unwillingness to do the necessary tampering with the futures of humans which experimental manipulation of their environment suggests. In the case of symbolic language, especially within its developmental stages, reluctance would naturally be extreme, in that no one would wish to deter or distort this remarkable component of future symbolic competence and socialization. As experimental analysis is ordinarily resorted to because of ignorance concerning the underlying processes relevant to a behavioral outcome, experimental manipulation of a child's linguistic environment cannot be guaranteed to do no harm to the language skills already in existence nor to prospective further development.

Nevertheless, there is a case in which experimental analysis could do little harm, might well accomplish considerable good, and also could contribute something to the general understanding of language as a behavioral phenomenon; that case is the language-deficient, institutionalized retardate.

Amongst severely and profoundly retarded children, language development is quite often nil; thus they represent an unusually pure case in which language remains entirely to be developed.

Institutionalization is not often an environmental process which will accomplish this development; too frequently, it seems, it is not even a process which will permit it, let alone accomplish it. Indeed, it is not uncommon to find that institutionalization will be associated with a loss of any previously evident language capabilities. Hence, it would appear that a carefully designed alteration of the institutionalized child's environment, in a manner calculated primarily to accomplish some linguistic development, may, if it succeeds, enrich the child's means of managing his environment, and if it fails, leave him no more impoverished in doing so than he was previously.[2]

Of the institutionalized retardates without language, the most valuable subject for language research is the child who, as best we know, has never had these skills, rather than the child who has previously developed some of them only to lose them in the process of institutional living. To *recover* a previously developed language skill in an institutionalized child is certainly a worthwhile clinical feat; the techniques for doing so are valuable additions to any clinical technology. However, to develop such skills *for the first time* in an institutionalized child is all of that and, as well, represents a challenge to psycholinguistic theory. For such a demonstration will establish that there are environmental conditions under which a given language skill will develop,[3] at least in these children. If these environmental conditions are essentially similar to those conditions used to develop non-language behavior in organisms in general, then a certain presumption has been raised, that *these* language behaviors are not different in origin than any other behaviors, and thus that their principles are not uniquely linquistic principles. This demonstration will not establish that these are the only environmental conditions under which the language skill develops, nor will it establish that these conditions are typical of the conditions under which corresponding language repertoires develop in normal children in more usual environments. Nevertheless, these demonstrations establish at least the feasibility of such an environmental origin. Given a context within which basic argument continues over whether language behavior follows principles of its own, or the same principles governing other behavior systems, a feasibility analysis will have obvious value and relevance for future research aimed *within* what is feasible and what is typical in everyday environments (Baer, 1972).

However, this value, obvious as it may be, can hardly be any greater than the range, breadth, or generality of language behavior which is shown to result from such environmental origins. That is, if only the most primitive rudiments of language can be made to respond to environmental manipulations of the sort which readily generate non-language behaviors, then no worthwhile analysis of language has yet resulted. On the other hand, if every segment, component, or system of language behavior specifiable can be made to develop under these conditions, then an extremely complete *feasibility* account of language as a developmental behavior system is accomplished, one which equates it in status to all other behaviors of organisms in general. To discover whether the former extreme or the latter is the more accurate representation of how language can be made to develop will require a lengthy series of studies. That series might well begin exactly with the most primitive rudiments of language, not merely because starting at the bottom has a certain logical ring to it, but also because the simplest aspects of language are probably the best ones to which to apply new experimental procedures. The implementation of procedures developed to their best with non-language behaviors, but now to be applied to language responses, will not be an obvious exercise; it will instead be full of surprises, and occasionally will require invention. When the behaviors to which these new implementations are being applied are not known to be responsive to them, a double uncertainty results. Consequently, when working with the simplest aspects of language, failure to accomplish an experimental analysis will be most readily analyzed itself, for the causes of that failure and the possible remediation of it, through better implementations of technique which *will* control the target responses. Where the target response is itself complex, the areas within which the *error* may reside are too numerous to allow its easy discovery. Thus, starting at the bottom of the language repertoire may well be good experimental technique, but it cannot contribute much to the analysis of language as a total repertoire until it has progressed well upward into the complexities of that repertoire. This chapter is meant to be a report of one such thrust off rock-bottom.

It must be emphasized that none of the attempts at experimental analysis of language, rock-bottom or higher, are very old. Spradlin (1963), surveying the field in the early 1960's, found it little different than the status of research into language development in general: that is, the focus of research on the language of retarded children cited nonmanipulative, correlative variables such as sex, age, IQ, hypothetical personality states such as anxiety, or diagnostic labels. The majority of these investigations have involved simple correlations between certain indices of language behavior and other variables, or the counting and tabulation of various speech and language skills among etiological or behaviorally similar groups. As pointed out by Spradlin (1963), these types of studies may have some validity in predicting the speech and language behavior of retarded children, but they do not provide a means for the modification of the behaviors. Only more recently have there been attempts to analyze functionally the language behavior of retarded children, and to manipulate these variables responsible for behavioral change (Bricker and Bricker, 1966; Sloan and MacAuley, 1968; and the studies to be cited below).

AN EXPERIMENTAL APPROACH TO THE ACQUISITION OF MORPHOLOGICAL GRAMMAR IN RETARDED CHILDREN

Characteristically, mentally retarded children exhibit varying degrees of delayed linguistic development. This delay offers the excellent opportunity to teach them directly the correct usage of selected grammatical rules, while experimentally manipulating variables theorized to play an important role in acquisition of the learned behavior.

Grammar was chosen as a target of analysis for several reasons. The rudiments of language behavior have been often enough developed by experimental uses of operant conditioning techniques no longer to be at issue as possible outcomes of those techniques. Thus, it is clear that vocal rate, vocal diversity, and specific phonetic characteristics of vocal response can be produced by shaping techniques. Furthermore, it has become apparent that a generalized usage of vocal imitation can be established through the same techniques, such that modeling (suitably backed by reinforcement for occasional correct imitations of models) is sufficient to accomplish the development of new vocal responses throughout a wide range of phonetic content (e.g., Baer, Peterson, and Sherman, 1967). The discrimination of such diverse vocal responses to appropriate social, physical, and relational stimuli has similarly been well extended into useful technique (cf. Lovaas, 1966; Risley and Wolf, 1967), even if with children in whom speech is being recovered rather than established for the first time. That extension, significantly, required no more than appropriate imitation and differential reinforcement. Thus, it may well be wondered whether a more complex level of language—its grammatical organization—will also respond to imitation and differential reinforcement. For, if it will (or, indeed, if it will respond to any other set of environmental procedures) then not only will a more meaningful component of what may be called language behavior have been analyzed in *feasibility* terms, but a wholesale language-expanding skill will have been given to the subject. Grammar is a way of organizing not only a speaker's current language repertoire, but also his future acquisitions. In effect, it may be a behavioral framework within which the speaker can become a self-teaching language acquirer, as well as an already-taught language user. In view of the size of the behavioral repertoires making up language, some such wholesale, self-generating approach is essential to realism, both on theoretical and clinical grounds.

Thus, during the past several years, a concentrated research effort at Kansas Neurological Institute has focused on the experimental analysis of morphological grammar in mentally retarded children functioning in the severely and moderately retarded range. In the area of linguistics, morphology pertains to the forms and grammatical inflections of words as they undergo modification for tense, number, case, person, etc. (Carroll, 1961). Previous studies have observed various forms of morphology in relation to age levels and sex differences in both normal children (Berko, 1961) and educationally subnormal children (Lovell and Brad-

bury, 1967). These investigations, however, made no attempt to provide a functional analysis of the content area.

Morphological grammar was selected specifically for the research described in this chapter because, as a unit of analysis, it was readily amenable to experimental manipulation and, yet, it also represented an area of analysis in which conceptual derivations from learning theory could be systematically explored. The experimental designs and techniques of analysis used in these research studies demonstrated that linguistic development could be approached with the same scientific rigor observed in other areas of investigation. The particular research design varied among the studies, although each design was clearly adequate to show manipulation and control of those variables which were important to the procedures of training.

The basis for training common to these investigations followed procedures of imitation and differential reinforcement, procedures which have evolved from learning theory. Most importantly, however, the research was based on a conceptual approach which has attempted to account for productivity and organization of spoken language.

Some theorists have remained skeptical of the role of imitation in speech and language development (Chomsky, 1957; Lenneberg, 1967), objecting to the fact that spoken language contains many elements which were never taught directly, nor even experienced for later imitation. Needless to say, their objections have been valid, inasmuch as the roles of differential reinforcement and imitative stimulus control in the acquisition of generalized spoken language have not been clearly demonstrated.

Conceptually, the studies pursued in this research were based on the concept of response class (Skinner, 1938; Salzinger, 1967), a term which corresponds closely to the linguists' use of *generative* language (Chomsky, 1957). Each term has been used to describe a significant fact of response development: that there often emerges from the organism more behavior exemplifying the dimensions of his experience than the experience has taught directly to him. The importance of the response-class phenomenon remains partly in the amount of new behavior produced and partly

in the fact that this new behavior can result from a properly unified sequence of instructions. From this conceptual approach, the complexity, diversity, grammatical, and generative characteristics of speech and language can be viewed as response classes—i.e., as highly generalized sets of vocal behaviors which exemplify the same dimensions or rules that characterized their training experiences, whether deliberately or accidentally.

The overall strategy of the present research endeavor was to demonstrate response-class development in mentally retarded children, using different forms of morphology as exemplars for systematic replication of the phenomenon. In the process, several related areas of investigation were pursued to provide a more complete analysis of those variables relevant to the acquisition of morphological grammar in the retarded child. These investigations have been incorporated into the chapter.

STUDIES IN MORPHOLOGICAL GRAMMAR

Productive Acquisition of the Plural Morpheme

As a starting point for the experimental analysis of morphological development, Guess, Sailor, Rutherford, and Baer (1968) used procedures of imitation and differential reinforcement to establish a generative use of the plural morpheme in the speech of a severely retarded girl. The subject, Janet, was a 10-year-old girl who had previously undergone a verbal imitation training program (Sailor, Guess, Rutherford, and Baer, 1968) and had developed a small vocabulary of simple words and phrases. Prior to the imitation training, Janet had been nonverbal. Her retardation was a result of unknown, but presumed psychologic cause.

Procedure

A large number of paired objects which could be pluralized with either the voiced or voiceless allomorphs served as training stimuli. Each object was trained separately, according to a three-stage sequence. In Stage 1, Janet was shown a single object and was asked, "What do you see?" A correct response in the singular form was reinforced with sweets, milk, jello, or mixed fruit. If the subject failed to respond within 20 sec. the experimenter

provided the correct label, withdrew it from sight for 10 sec., and presented it again for the next trial. If the object was labeled incorrectly, the experimenter said "No," and repeated the procedure. A criterion performance in Stage 1 required three consecutive correct responses.

TABLE I.I

SAMPLE DATA SHEET FOR THE TRAINING OF THE PRODUCTIVE PLURAL MORPHEME, ILLUSTRATING THE ORDER IN WHICH ITEMS WERE PRESENTED (SINGLY OR IN PAIRS), AND THE RECORDING AND SCORING OF A PERFORMANCE TO THE CRITERIA OF PLURAL ACQUISITION*

Item: cup (s)

Instructions to observer: star (*) response if correct: cross it (x) if incorrect

Stage 1		Stage 2	
Present:		Present:	
*1. cup	(etc.)	x1. cups	(etc.)
*2. cup		x2. cups	
*3. cup		*3. cups	
4. cup		*4. cups	
5. cup		*5. cups	
6. cup		6. cups	
(etc.)		(etc.)	

Stage 3			
Present:			
*1. cup	(etc.)	(etc.)	(etc.)
*2. cup			
x3. cups			
*4. cup			
*5. cups			
*6. cup			
*7. cups			
*8. cups			
*9. cups			
10. cups			
(etc.)			

* This sample data sheet shows that the subject met the singular criterion of three consecutive correct trials in the first three trials of Stage 1; that she met the plural criterion of three consecutive correct trials on trials 3, 4, and 5 of Stage 2; and that she met the mixed criterion of three singulars and three plurals intermixed without error on trials 4 through 9 of Stage 3. To meet these three criteria required (3 + 5 + 9) = 17 trials; of these 17, 14 were correct, yielding a percentage correct of 82. A plural shift was not recorded for this word, in that the subject did not make a correct plural response on the first trial of Stage 2. For early words, meeting these criteria typically would require many more trials in each stage, and a complete data sheet therefore included more entries of potential trials. These are indicated by (etc.) in this table.

In Stage 2, Janet was presented with two of the same objects and again asked, "What do you see?" Only plural responses were reinforced. Failures to respond or incorrect labels were treated exactly as in Stage 1; again criterion was held at three consecutive correct responses.

A random sequence of single and paired objects was presented in Stage 3. Criterion performance required a sequence including three correct singular responses intermixed with three correct plural responses, without intervening errors.

Criterion for each stage was met before the next stage was begun. Then these stages were repeated for each item presented in each of the experimental conditions. Table I.I displays a sample data sheet illustrating the recording and scoring of data in these stages.

Experimental Conditions

In Condition I, the subject was taught to respond correctly with singulars or plurals when presented with single objects or pairs of objects, respectively. In Condition II, the reinforcement contingencies were *reversed,* such that Janet was required to give a plural response to single objects and a singular response to pairs of objects. Condition III returned to the normal contingencies originally used under Condition I.

Results

The final stimulus control sought in this study was one in which Janet would produce a correct singular label when shown one item, and a correct plural label when presented with two (or more) of them. When Janet had advanced to the point at which her new language acquisitions were automatically organized into these correct singular and plural forms, without direct and specific training in their pluralization, she could then be termed grammatically generative for that specific example of grammar.

Two measures of this generative characteristic were derived from Janet's performance. The first was based on the number of trials required to bring her to the multiple criterion of singular-plural usage for each new word that was trained.[4] This measure was calculated as a percentage of correct response displayed in achieving the criteria required by Stages 1, 2, and 3 throughout training (as explained in the note accompanying Table I). The second evaluation simply measured the probability that on the first presentation of items in pairs (rather than one at a time) she could consistently shift to their plural label without training or correction. This second measure was scored as a successful plural shift if, on the first item of Stage 2 (when first shown the current item as a pair of objects) the subject correctly supplied the plural label. (Refer to the note in Table I.I for an example of this scoring procedure.)

The changes in percentage of correct response over the trials and conditions of the study are shown in Figure I.1. A score of 100 means that no errors were made in achieving the criteria of productive plural usage.

Figure I.1 shows that productive plural usage was achieved by

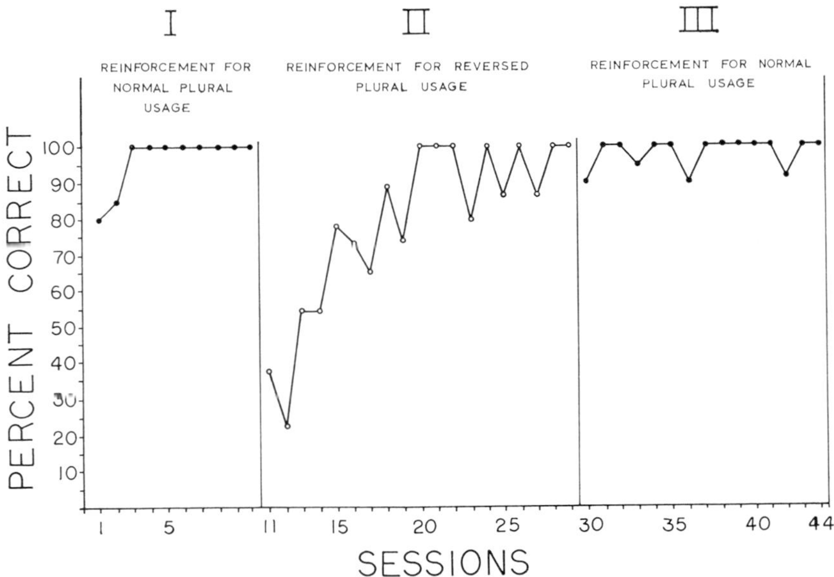

Figure I.1. Percentage of correct responses for three experimental conditions. In Conditions I and III (solid dots) the graph represents percentage of correct responses for those objects trained under standard or normal productive plural usage. (See Table I.I for an example of percentage calculation.) In Condition II (open dots) the graph represents percentage of correct responses on those objects trained under reversed contingencies of reinforcement, and in this case indicates productive plural usage (calculated in the manner identical to Conditions I and II).

the third word of Condition I, and maintained for the remaining seven words of that condition. Upon reversal of the contingencies of reinforcement, Janet's percentage of correct response dropped markedly, but gradually rose as she began to develop a reversed singular-plural usage. Janet almost immediately recovered her mastered singular-plural usage when returned to the normal contingencies of everyday English in Condition III.

In terms of the all-or-none measure of plural shift displayed during the first trial of every Stage 2, Janet showed similar evidence of the development, reversal, and recovery of a productive linguistic class of plurals. Figure I.2 shows the cumulative number of successful shifts over the trials of Conditions I, II, and III.

Further probing analyzed certain error responses occurring during the first experiment, and further displayed the generative nature of Janet's plural usage. It was found that errors were more

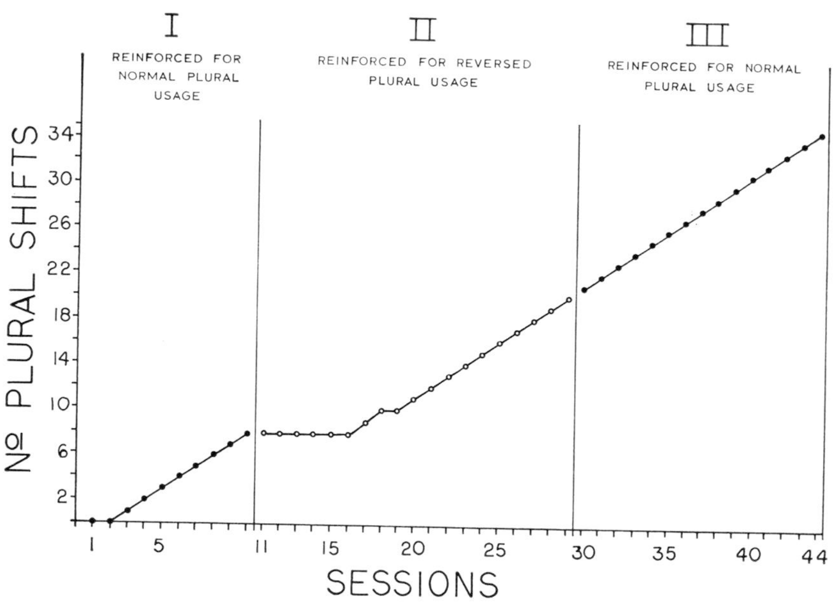

Figure I.2. Cumulative numbers of plural shifts for the three conditions. A plural shift was recorded for Conditions I and III (solid dots) if Janet correctly supplied the plural label on the first item of Stage 2 when first shown a pair of objects. A shift was recorded in Condition II (open dots) if Janet gave a singular response when first presented a pair of objects in Stage 2.

likely to occur in the pluralization of words ending in vowels than of words ending in consonants. Furthermore, several words whose plurals had been learned according to the reversed plural rule, when examined later during reinforcement of normal plural usage, were then found to exemplify the normal rule being reinforced, yet without direct training. Further, five words representing irregular plurals or different plurals than Janet's training had included, were interspersed among the other items presented. To the presentation of two men, Janet's response was "mans," to two children, her response was "childs," and to two leaves, her response was "leafs." When presented with two-item pairs requiring the addition of -es (ordinary orthography) to form the plural, glass*es* and box*es,* Janet simply repeated the singular for these presentations. Finally, Janet correctly provided plural labels to objects presented in trios, thus supporting the basic results in Experiment I: Janet had learned a thoroughly generative morphological rule through imitation and differential reinforcement.

The study just presented provided the background for two other areas of research in the acquisition of morphological grammar, as exemplified by regular plural usage. The first dealt with the relationship of phonological acquisition to the development of correct morphological usage; the second investigated the functional relationship between productive (spoken) speech and receptive (understanding) language.

Productive Acquisitions of Plural Allomorphs

The second experiment in the study by Guess, et al. (1968) indicated that the subject, Janet, had more difficulty (in terms of correct responses) on those items with terminal vowel endings. In conventional speech, pluralization of words ending in voiced consonants (e.g. car) or vowels (e.g. tree) require the voiced sibilant, while pluralization of words ending in voiceless consonant sounds (e.g. cup) require the voiceless sibilant ending. An analysis of Janet's response to the items suggested that, in the course of the training conditions, she had learned to articulate only the voiceless allomorph in the production of plural words. Indeed, four of the first five words trained in the initial condition of the study required a voiceless sibilant ending. Further, tape recordings made during the experiment indicated that Janet was, in fact, pausing and then accentuating the voiceless allomorph on those vowel and consonant ending words which normally required the voiced ending for pluralization. These findings raised the question concerning the relationship of phonological acquisition to the acquisition of correct morphological usage.

A subsequent study by Sailor (1971) sought to determine the extent to which differential reinforcement from an echoic model could control the acquisition of plural allomorphs in previously aplural, mentally retarded subjects. The first Subject, Pam, was a fifteen-year-old girl, diagnosed as severely retarded, with cause resulting from maternal intoxications; the second subject, Willa, was an eight-year-old girl diagnosed as moderately retarded, with unknown but presumed psychologic cause. Neither of the girls emitted plural responses to objects prior to the experiment, as determined by extensive screening tests for plural usage.

Procedure

Both subjects began the experimental procedure with reinforcement training to establish the generative use of plurals, following exactly the three-stage sequence of training used in the study by Guess, et al. (1968). The recording and scoring of a performance to criteria for each item also remained the same. (Refer to Table I.I for a summary of these procedures.) During the initial training session, a Variable Ratio 3 (VR3) schedule of reinforcement was established for correct responses. This schedule was used to accommodate a series of probe items (unreinforced trials), inserted in experimental conditions to measure the extent to which training on one type of plural allomorph generalized to items which normally required a different allomorph.

Subject 1, Pam, received initial training (Condition I) on a series of items whose singular forms have voiced endings, thus calling for the voiced plural allomorph for pluralization (e.g. pens), according to the conventional rule of English morphology. The subject was considered to have acquired generative plural usage when, on ten consecutive objects trained, the voiced plural ending was given on the first presentation of paired objects in

Stage 2 of the training sequence (referred to previously as a plural shift).

Probes in the first condition for Subject 1 consisted of items whose singular form ending was unvoiced, thus calling for the unvoiced plural allomorph (e.g. cups), as dictated by normal English. Probe items were presented in the same manner as items from the training list, except that Stage 3 of the sequence (intermixed singulars and plurals) was omitted. Probe items were alternated with training items once the criterion of ten consecutive correct plural shifts had been obtained in training. Twelve probe items with three presentations of each item were given, for a total of thirty-six probe trials. When all thirty-six probe trials had been administered, the condition was terminated.

In Condition II the reinforcement contingencies were reversed such that Pam was then trained to criterion on items calling for the voiceless plural allomorphs and probed with items which conventionally required the voiced plural allomorphs. Otherwise the procedures were exactly the same as in Condition I.

The procedures for Subject 2, Willa, were the same as for Subject 1, except that Subject 2 was trained on voiceless plural-ending items in Condition I and voiced plural-ending items in Condition II, to counterbalance for possible effects of the initial training list.

Results

Evaluation of the dependent variable was conducted by having sound tapes of the probe responses for each condition, for each subject, rated independently by two speech pathologists for the audible presence of either [-s] or [-z] plural allomorphs. Conditions and items within conditions were scrambled and presented to the raters in random order. Only those responses in which both raters agreed on the allomorphic endings were used to evaluate the results.

Table I.II presents results of Condition I for Subject 1, including the list of probe items used, the raters' judgments of each response, and summary data of the ratings. Results showed that Pam made a plural response to twenty-five of the thirty-six probes, all of which were rated as having the voiced plural allomorph

TABLE I.II

RESULTS OF CONDITION I FOR SUBJECT 1*

Probe Words	*Raters* *A*	*B*	*Agree on Voiceless (vl)*	*Agree on Voiced (v)*	*Dis-agree*
1. Light	v	v		+	
2. Light	v	v		+	
3. Light	v	v		+	
4. Belt	v	v		+	
5. Belt	v	v		+	
6. Belt	v	v		+	
7. Dart	v	v		+	
8. Dart	v	v		+	
9. Dart	v	v		+	
10. Top	—	—		—	
11. Top	v	v		+	
12. Top	v	v		+	
13. Hoop	v	v		+	
14. Hoop	v	v		+	
15. Hoop	v	v		+	
16. Tank	—	—		—	
17. Tank	v	v		+	
18. Tank	—	—		—	
19. Tip	—	—		—	
20. Tip	v	v		+	
21. Tip	—	—		—	
22. Butt	v	v		+	
23. Butt	v	v		+	
24. Butt	v	v		+	
25. Chalk	—	—		—	
26. Chalk	v	v		+	
27. Chalk	—	—		—	
28. Soap	v	v		+	
29. Soap	v	v		+	
30. Soap	v	v		+	
31. Mint	—	—		—	
32. Mint	v	v		+	
33. Mint	v	v		+	
34. Chief	—	—		—	
35. Chief	—	—		—	
36. Chief	—	—		—	

* Subject 1, Pam, was trained on items calling for the voiced allomorph (indicated in this and subsequent Tables by v), and probed for generalization of the voiced ending to items which normally required the voiceless allomorph (indicated in this and subsequent Tables by vl).

Summarizing, the table show thirty-six agreements (+) and no disagreements for 100% rater reliability. Twenty-five of these responses were scored in a direction consistent with the hypothesis. No responses were scored in the unsupportive direction, eleven responses were scored as having no plural ending (—).

TABLE I.III

RESULTS OF CONDITION II FOR SUBJECT 1*

Probe Words	*Raters* A	*Raters* B	*Agree on Voiceless (vl)*	*Agree on Voiced (v)*	*Dis-agree*
1. Tree	vl	vl	+		
2. Tree	vl	vl	+		
3. Tree	vl	vl	+		
4. Bow	vl	vl	+		
5. Bow	vl	vl	+		
6. Bow	vl	vl	+		
7. Flag	vl	vl	+		
8. Flag	vl	vl	+		
9. Flag	vl	vl	+		
10. Can	vl	vl	+		
11. Can	vl	vl	+		
12. Can	vl	vl	+		
13. Car	vl	vl	+		
14. Car	vl	vl	+		
15. Car	vl	vl	+		
16. Ball	vl	vl	+		
17. Ball	vl	vl	+		
18. Ball	vl	vl	+		
19. Horn	vl	vl	+		
20. Horn	vl	vl	+		
21. Horn	vl	vl	+		
22. Deer	vl	vl	+		
23. Deer	vl	vl	+		
24. Deer	vl	vl	+		
25. Comb	vl	vl	+		
26. Comb	vl	vl	+		
27. Comb	vl	vl	+		
28. Bear	vl	vl	+		
29. Bear	vl	vl	+		
30. Bear	vl	vl	+		
31. Record	vl	vl	+		
32. Record	vl	vl	+		
33. Record	vl	vl	+		
34. Penny	vl	vl	+		
35. Penny	vl	vl	+		
36. Penny	vl	vl	+		

* Subject 1 was retrained on a list calling for the voiceless allomorph (vl), and was probed for generalization of the voiceless ending to items calling for the voiced (v) allomorph.

Summarizing, the table shows thirty-six agreements and no disagreements, giving 100% rater reliability. All thirty-six responses were scored in a direction consistent with the hypothesis.

TABLE I.IV

RESULTS OF CONDITION I FOR SUBJECT 2*

Probe Words	Raters		Agree on Voiceless	Agree on Voiced	Dis-
	A	*B*	*(vl)*	*(v)*	*agree*
1. Ball	vl	vl	+		
2. Ball	vl	vl	+		
3. Ball	vl	vl	+		
4. Car	vl	vl	+		
5. Car	vl	vl	+		
6. Car	vl	vl	+		
7. Can	vl	vl	+		
8. Can	vl	lv	+		
9. Can	vl	vl	+		
10. Flag	vl	vl	+		
11. Flag	vl	vl	+		
12. Flag	—	—	—		
13. Bow	—	—	—		
14. Bow	vl	vl	+		
15. Bow	vl	vl	+		
16. Tree	vl	vl	+		
17. Tree	vl	vl	+		
18. Tree	vl	vl	+		
19. Pen	v	vl			+
20. Pen	v	vl			+
21. Pen	vl	vl	+		
22. Card	vl	vl	+		
23. Card	vl	vl	+		
24. Card	vl	vl	+		
25. Key	vl	vl	+		
26. Key	vl	vl	+		
27. Key	vl	vl	+		
28. Man	vl	vl	+		
29. Man	vl	vl	+		
30. Man	vl	vl	+		
31. Spoon	vl	vl	+		
32. Spoon	vl	vl	+		
33. Spoon	vl	vl	+		
34. Gun	vl	vl	+		
35. Gun	vl	vl	+		
36. Gun	vl	vl	+		

* Subject 2, Willa, was trained on items calling for the voiceless (vl) allomorph, and probed for generalization of the voiceless ending to items calling for the voiced (v) allomorph.

Summarizing, the table shows thirty-two agreements and two disagreements for 95% rater reliability. Thirty-two of these responses were scored in a direction consistent with the hypothesis. None were scored in the unsupportive direction. Two responses were scored as having no plural endings.

TABLE I.V

RESULTS OF CONDITION II FOR SUBJECT 2*

Probe Words	*Raters* *A*	*B*	*Agree on Voiceless (vl)*	*Agree on Voiced (v)*	*Dis-agree*
1. Light	v	v		+	
2. Light	v	v		+	
3. Light	v	v		+	
4. Belt	v	v		+	
5. Belt	v	v		+	
6. Belt	v	v		+	
7. Dart	v	v		+	
8. Dart	v	v		+	
9. Dart	v	v		+	
10. Top	v	v		+	
11. Top	v	v		+	
12. Top	v	v		+	
13. Hoop	v	v		+	
14. Hoop	v	v		+	
15. Hoop	v	v		+	
16. Tank	v	v		+	
17. Tank	v	v		+	
18. Tank	v	v		+	
19. Hat	v	v		+	
20. Hat	v	v		+	
21. Hat	v	v		+	
22. Cup	v	v		+	
23. Cup	v	v		+	
24. Cup	v	v		+	
25. Book	v	v		+	
26. Book	v	v		+	
27. Book	v	v		+	
28. Boot	v	v		+	
29. Boot	v	v		+	
30. Boot	v	v		+	
31. Block	v	v		+	
32. Block	v	v		+	
33. Block	v	v		+	
34. Boat	v	v		+	
35. Boat	v	v		+	
36. Boat	v	v		+	

* Subject 2 was retrained on a list calling for the voiced (v) allomorph, and was probed for generalization of the voiced ending to items calling for the voiceless allomorph.

Summarizing, the table shows thirty-six agreements and no disagreements, giving 100% rater reliability. All thirty-six responses were scored in a direction consistent with the hypothesis.

ending, although this ending is inappropriate to the items as indicated by conventional usage.

Pam's responses to the probe trials of Condition II are shown in Table I.III. As observed, the subject made a plural response to all thirty-six items; each response was rated as having a voiceless allomorphic ending, thus showing generalization from phonic training to probe trials as before.

Table I.IV includes the results of Condition I for Subject 2. Willa produced a total of thirty-two plural responses to the thirty-four items judged reliably. All thirty-two responses were rated as having the voiceless plural allomorph ending, again inappropriate to the normal dictates of English morphology.

Results of Condition II are presented in Table I.V. Willa responded to all thirty-six items with a plural response; each response was rated as having the voiced allomorphic ending, thereby clearly showing generalization from the voiceless allomorphic training to the probe trials.

Data from both subjects supported the expectation that allomorphs of the plural class can be taught, using techniques of differential reinforcement and imitation to a retarded child. Further, the child will generalize from training of a specific allomorphic response to a different allomorphic type, regardless of appropriateness by the dictates of common English usage.

Functional Relationship Between Receptive Language and Productive Speech

In the study reported earlier by Guess, et al. (1968), the subject, Janet, showed a very rapid acquisition of productive generative plural usage. This finding raised the question as to whether or not she already had possession of this concept at the receptive or understanding level of language and the reinforcers merely encouraged her to verbalize what she "already knew." Conceivably, then, the plural morpheme, as one rule of grammar, may have been present at the receptive level, even though the child gave no evidence in her productive speech of having acquired this concept. This possibility is in agreement with a common observation in the development of language which indicates that auditory comprehension or reception precedes productive speech. This observation is supported by a review of both theory (Myklebust, 1957) and research (McCarthy, 1954; Fraser, Bellugi, and Brown, 1963).

The relationship between auditory comprehension and expressive speech is especially relevant to the development of grammar. Basically, there is some disagreement as to whether the use of grammar reflects an underlying set of rules which the child develops through maturation (Chomsky, 1959; Lenneberg, 1967), or whether the development of grammar follows primarily an echoic model (Skinner, 1957), in which sequential language stimuli are imitated by the child. In this latter point of view, meaning or understanding is not a necessary component of learning.

The investigations to be reviewed next have explored the functional relationship, or mutual independence, between receptive language and productive speech, again using the plural morpheme as the unit of experimental analysis.

A study by Guess (1969) used the technique of differential reinforcement to establish the receptive identification of singular-plural items in two severely retarded boys. Each subject was trained to an errorless (generative) criterion of correct performance. Unreinforced probe trials measuring the productive use of singulars and plurals were given at the end of the training sequence for each object to measure for possible generalization from receptive training to productive speech.

Subject 1, Bob, was a thirteen-year-old male diagnosed as Down's Syndrome. The second subject, Ken, also had a diagnosis of Down's Syndrome, and was fourteen years old. Prior evaluations of the subjects indicated that neither had acquired the plural rule at the receptive or productive levels, yet each was capable of producing both the voiced and voiceless phonemes in the final position of words, necessary, of course, for the articulation of plural words.

Procedure

In Conditions I and II of the study (discussed later) the subject was trained to point to single or paired objects in response to singular or plural labels presented by the experimenter. In the process he was to be probed repeatedly to determine whether this receptive training generalized to his ability to label productively singular and plural items. Because the probing technique was interspersed repeatedly between series of training trials and involved unreinforced responding, the subject had to be adapted to not receiving a reinforcer for every correct response. Accordingly, pretraining sessions were held in which the subject was required to point to either a big or small ball, labeled in random order by the experimenter. During these sessions the subject was trained to respond on a VR3 schedule of reinforcement which was used throughout the remaining conditions of the study. Chips were used as reinforcers for correct responses and were redeemed at the end of each session for a variety of sweets and/or toys.

CONDITION I. RECEPTIVE TRAINING. Receptive training again used the three-stage sequence followed in the studies previously discussed (Guess et al., 1968; Sailor, 1971). The only deviation from the previous procedure was that now the subject was required to point to objects presented singly or in pairs, in response to the appropriate singular or plural label provided by the experimenter. Training items were placed on the table in front of the subject (i.e., one object on one side of the table and a pair of the same objects on the other side). The positions of the objects, single or paired, were changed frequently to avoid a position bias. In Stage 1, the subject was reinforced for pointing to the single item until criterion of three consecutive correct responses; Stage 2 required the subject to point to pairs of items in response to a plural label for three consecutive correct trials; Stage 3 intermixed singular and plural trials until the criterion of three consecutive plural responses and three consecutive singular responses was reached. A pool of thirty separate objects (each represented in trios) was available for the study.

A probe for productive plural acquisition was given at the end of the training sequence (where the three-stage criterion was met) for each object trained. For this probe, the subject was presented the objects which had just been trained plus the objects to be used next in the training series. The subject was shown first the single item just used in the receptive training task and asked "What do you see?" He was then shown a pair of those objects and asked the same question. Next, he was presented with the object (s) to be used in the subsequent training series in an identical manner. Accordingly, the subject was required to give four productive responses during each probe: he was never reinforced for these responses and was corrected only if he mislabeled the single item (this occurred rarely since familiar items were used in the study).

CONDITION II. PRODUCTIVE TRAINING. The next phase consisted of productive plural training.[5] Now instead of pointing to the item, or pair of items, the subject was required to respond productively with their singular or plural labels. The subject was shown either one or a pair of objects and asked, "What do you see?" Criterion of performance was again measured by the three-step sequence of training. There were no probes of any sort.

CONDITION III. REVERSED RECEPTIVE TRAINING. This condition consisted of reversed receptive plural training wherein reinforcers were delivered for pointing to a single item when given its plural label and for pointing to the pair of items when presented with their singular label. Productive plural probes again were used, exactly as in Condition I.

Results

A summary of results for Subject 1, Bob, is found in Figure I.3 graphed as percent correct responses for the training and probe trials across the three experimental conditions. Receptive plural training trials in Condition I, productive plural training trials in Condition II, and reversed receptive plural training trials in Condition III are all represented by line graphs. In order to condense the figure, each point represents the average percent correct for three separate objects trained in succession. The percentages for each object were calculated by dividing the total number of trials by the total number of responses needed to meet the criteria of training Stages 1, 2, and 3 (refer to Table I.I).

Performance on the productive probes of Condition I and III are portrayed by a series of bars superimposed over the line graphs of receptive training. The productive probes are grouped separately for singular responses (open bar) and plural responses (mottled bar). Each open bar represents percent correct responses

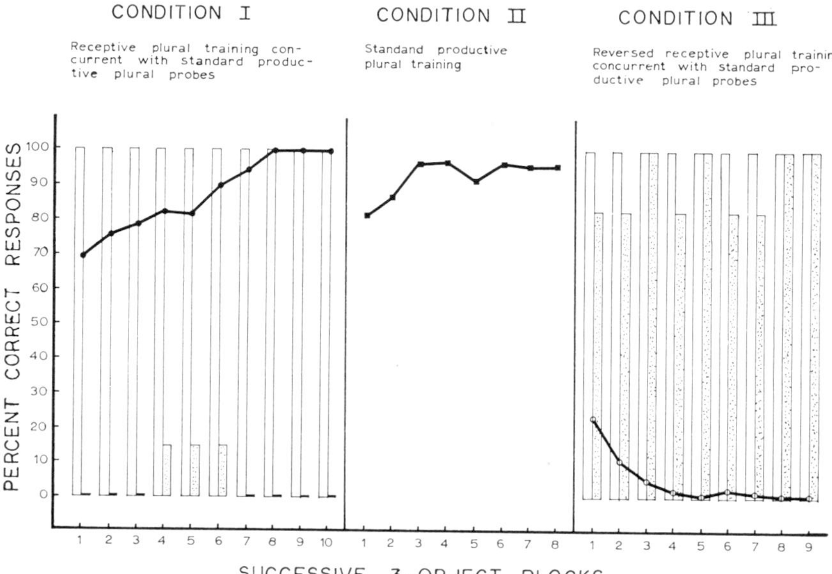

Figure I.3. (Subject 1, Bob.) Percent correct responses for training conditions and their associated probes. The graphs represent performance on the three training conditions. Each point depicts average percent correct for three successive object training series. Productive verbal probes are shown as bars. Each open bar represents percent correct responses for six singular probes; each mottled bar denotes percent correct for six plural probes.

for six singular probes (i.e., probes before and after training on three separate items). The mottled bars similarly depict percent correct responses for paired objects.

Results of Figure I.3 show that Bob acquired slowly the receptive discrimination between single and paired objects across the thirty training items used in Condition I. Errorless performance was manifest on the final three object blocks of this condition, indicating generative acquisition of receptive plural usage. However, as noted in the probe trials (bar graphs) there was negligible generalization from training to the productive labeling of single and plural items; instead, Bob continued to provide singular labels to items presented both singly and in pairs.

Productive plural usage emerged rapidly in Condition II, as indicated in the line graph of Figure I.3. And now, after having been trained in the productive use of singulars and plurals, the third condition was implemented to test again the original findings of Condition I: that generalization failed to occur from receptive training to productive speech.

Condition III (Figure I.3) depicts performance under the reversed singular-plural contingencies, and shows a rapid decrease in percent correct responses, indicating that Bob quickly learned the reversed receptive plural contingencies of this training condition. (In viewing Condition III the reader should keep in mind that percent correct responses, as depicted on the ordinate, refer to the normal or standard use of plurals; thus successful reversed singular-plural training is reflected in a low percentage of correct responses.)

Productive probes were again administered concurrent with the reversed receptive training of Condition III. They were presented in a manner identical to Condition I. Results show errorless performance with all the singulars and a high percentage of correct plurals (never dropping below 83%). Thus, while the subject was trained to point to a single item when given a plural label and point to a pair of items when provided with a singular label, he nevertheless gave appropriate and correct singular and plural labels in the productive probe trials.

Results for Subject 2, Ken, are presented in Figure I.4, again showing training and probe trials in three experimental conditions. His performance in each condition was almost identical to that of Subject 1. There was no generalization from receptive training to productive probes in Condition I; he rapidly acquired productive singular-plural usage in Condition II; and he continued to label correctly singular and plural items in the probe trials of Condition III even though his training had produced a reversed singular-plural usage at the receptive level.

Harrelson (1969) used the same research design as the study just reviewed, except he trained plural usage among retarded subjects at the productive level and probed for generalization to receptive language. His results supported those of Guess (1968), again indicating the functional independence possible between the two language repertories: training productive plural usage to errorless performance did not increase receptive discrimination between singular and paired items.

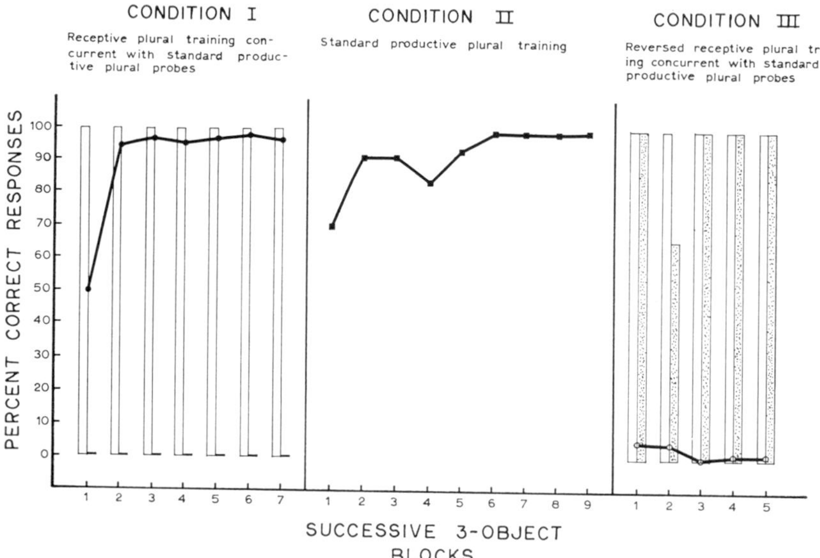

Figure I.4. (Subject 2, Ken.) Percent correct responses on the training and probe conditions. Refer to Fig. I.3 for an explanation of the graphs.

However, neither the Guess (1968) nor the Harrelson (1969) study was competent to demonstrate that training one language repertoire (either productive or receptive) would not facilitate *acquisition* of the other repertoire, even though there was no direct generalization from one to the other. Consequently, a third study was conducted in which both receptive and productive training were programmed concurrently, using two different classes of plurals as concurrent baselines for this training (Guess and Baer, 1972). These two classes,[6] defined by the plural endings (voiceless) [-s] and [-es] (extra syllable and voiced), provided a useful experimental situation: one in which the topography of the response remained constant—i.e., it discriminated singular and plural objects. The major question was whether a plural rule would generalize between the two language repertories (receptive and productive) if *both* repertoires were being maintained and extended simultaneously, a variable which had not been explored in the previous research on plural morphemes.

Method

Four subjects were selected for the study who, according to results of an extensive screening test, did not display already generalized plural usage at either the receptive or productive level in either of the two classes of plurals used. All subjects, however, were able to label objects and articulate the [s] and [es] sounds necessary for plurals. The subjects were all measured to be functioning in the severely retarded range. Subject 1, David (CA 11), was considered retarded, but of unknown cause; Subject 2, Dan (CA 21), Subject 3, Kevin (CA 20), and Subject 4, Gary (CA 13), were diagnosed as Down's Syndrome.

The training materials used in the study were seventy-four trios of identical items, the labels of which are pluralized with either (voiceless) -s or (extra syllable and voiced) -es endings. Forty sets of items required (voiceless) -s endings in the formation of plurals; thirty-four sets required (extra syllable and voiced) -es endings.

Training and Probe Baselines. The basic experimental procedures consisted of concurrent training of both productive speech (labeling) and receptive comprehension (pointing), as separate training baselines representing the basic modalities of language. Training in one baseline (modality) was restricted to objects requiring -s endings for pluralization (e.g., hat/hats, cup/cups); training in the other baseline (modality) was restricted to objects requiring -es endings for pluralization (e.g., bus/buses, horse/horses).

Possible generalization of either type of training to the other modality (within the same plural-ending baseline) was measured by probes interspersed among training trials within each training baseline. These probes were presented in the response modality opposite to the one being trained in that baseline. Thus, probes of the productive (labeling) baseline were presented as receptive (pointing) trials; probes of the receptive (pointing) baseline were presented as productive (labeling) trials. Items used for probes were always pluralized with the same ending (-s or -es) characterizing the training baseline in which they were inserted.

TABLE I.VI

ASSIGNMENT OF -S AND -ES PLURAL ENDINGS TO THE TRAINING BASELINES AND PROBES, AND INITIAL SEQUENCE OF TRAINING PROCEDURES, ACROSS SUBJECTS

Subject	*Initial Sequence*	*Plural Ending*	*Training Baselines*	*Probe*
S1, David	1st object	-s	productive	receptive
	2nd object	-es	receptive	productive
S2, Dan	1st object	-es	productive	receptive
	2nd object	-s	receptive	productive
S3, Kevin	1st object	-es	receptive	productive
	2nd object	-s	productive	receptive
S4, Gary	1st object	-s	receptive	productive
	2nd object	-es	productive	receptive

Two subjects were trained to use -s-ending plurals productively and respond to -es-ending plurals receptively. For one of these subjects, the first item of each session was taught productively, and the second receptively (alternating thereafter); for the other subject, the reverse order was used. Two other subjects were trained to use -es-ending plurals productively and respond to -s-ending plurals receptively. For one of these subjects, the first item of each session was taught productively, and the second receptively (alternating thereafter); for the other subject, the reverse order was used. This counter-balancing of plural endings, modalities of training and probes, and sequence of trainings across subjects is shown in Table I.VI.

Procedures

Plastic tokens were used as reinforcers for correct responses. The tokens were redeemed for a variety of personal items, toys, games, and privileges (e.g., trip to the local candy store).

The experimental design required that the probes be interspersed within a sequence of training trials. Thus, it was necessary to adapt the subject to nonreinforcement of some correct responses. A simple size discrimination task (point to a big or little ball) was used as a preliminary problem in which to establish an intermittent reinforcement schedule, specifically, variable ratio two. This schedule was used to accommodate probe trials in all further training conditions.

Training. The procedures for receptive plural training were identical for items requiring either -s or -es pluralization. Training involved pointing to either the single or paired item upon request of the experimenter who labeled the item (s) in singular or plural form. The same three-stage sequence of training described in the previous studies (Guess, et al., 1968; Sailor, 1971; Guess, 1969) was used to measure criterion performance for each item trained.

The procedures followed for productive training were identical for items requiring either -s or -es pluralization. Subjects were reinforced for providing the correct singular response when shown a single item and for giving a plural label response to paired items. Again, the three-stage sequence of training was followed to determine criterion performance for each item.

Probes. Probes were administered to determine the extent to which training at the productive level with a given plural ending generalized to receptive comprehension (pointing) with that ending; and, conversely, to determine the extent to which training at the receptive level with a given plural ending generalized to productive response (labeling) with that ending.

Receptive probes were administered in a manner identical to receptive training trials, but without any reinforcement of correct responses, correction of incorrect responses, or repetition after no response. Similarly, productive probes were presented exactly as for the productive training trials, but again without reinforcement, correction, or repetition.

Eight probes were inserted within the training of each item, following Stage 3 (intermixed singulars and plurals) of the training sequence. Four probes, two single-object presentations and two paired-item presentations, were given using the item (s) just trained; and then four more probes, again two single-object and two paired-item presentations, were presented using the item (s) to be taught next in the training sequence. (Almost without exception, all of the subjects already knew the name of each "new" item presented. Thus, incorrect response to these "new" probes almost invariably represented a singular-vs.-plural error, rather than a failure to respond.)

An example of a typical sequence of training and probe trials is shown in Table I.VII.

TABLE I.VII

AN EXAMPLE OF THE SEQUENCE OF TRAINING AND PROBE PROCEDURE FOR THE TRAINING OF TWO SUCCESSIVE OBJECTS PER BASELINE*

	Training Sequence for "Cup" and "Axe"				*Next Training Sequence for "Hat" and "Bus"*				*Etc.*
Plural Ending	*Objects Being Trained*	*(Objects to Be Trained Next)*	*Productive Training (Label)*	*Receptive Training (Point)*	*Objects Being Trained*	*(Objects to Be Trained Next)*	*Productive Training (Label)*	*Receptive Training (Point)*	*Etc.*
/s/	cup	(hat)	Stage 1: cup Stage 2: cups Stage 3: cup/cups VR 2 schedule, *receptive probes:* cup/cups, hat/hats		hat	(truck)	Stage 1: hat Stage 2: hats Stage 3: hat/hats, VR 2 schedule, *receptive probes:* hat/hats, truck/trucks		etc.
/es/	axe	(bus)		Stage 1: axe Stage 2: axes Stage 3: axe/axes, VR 2 schedule, *productive probes:* axe/axes, bus/buses	bus	(fox)		Stage 1: bus Stage 2: buses Stage 3: bus/buses VR 2 schedule, *productive probes:* bus/buses, fox/foxes	etc.

* This example sequence of training and probe procedures corresponds to the assignment of plural endings for Subject 1 (See Table I.VI).

Results

The results of training and nonreinforced probing in the four subjects are presented in Figure I.5, graphed as the percentage of correct responses in the trials of each consecutive object. Responses to training trials, both receptive and productive, are depicted as bar graphs; responses to nonreinforced probe trials are presented as line graphs superimposed on the bar graphs, corresponding point-for-point with the objects used in that training condition. It will be recalled that probe trials included the objects currently being trained plus the set of objects which followed in the training sequence.

In general, Figure I.5 shows that the concurrent training of productive and receptive plurals (with different endings) was successful. Each subject's training baselines (bar graphs) rose promptly from the 50% levels that might be expected initially, toward roughly 90% levels of correct response.

However, Figure I.5 also shows that generalization from this training to its unreinforced (opposite modality) probes within the same plural ending (line graphs) was extremely variable, both within and across subjects. In fact, these results indicated strong generalization from training to probe trials only in the case of Gary (Subject 4). As receptive training with objects requiring -s plural endings progressed with Gary, his percentage of correct labels increased to a high level in the productive probe trials; similarly, as he learned to label paired objects correctly with the -es plural form, he also began to point correctly to single or paired objects in response to singular or plural labels in the receptive probe trials. Subject 1, David, showed some generalization from productive training using -s plurals to their receptive probe trials; however, his receptive training (-s plurals) did not generalize to correct productive labels in the probes. Subject 2, Dan, showed partial generalization from productive training (-es plurals) to their productive probes. However, in both training conditions, the probe trials were highly variable and well below the level of accuracy maintained in the training conditions. Kevin, Subject 3, showed the least amount of generalization from training conditions to their corresponding nonreinforced probe trials. Correct

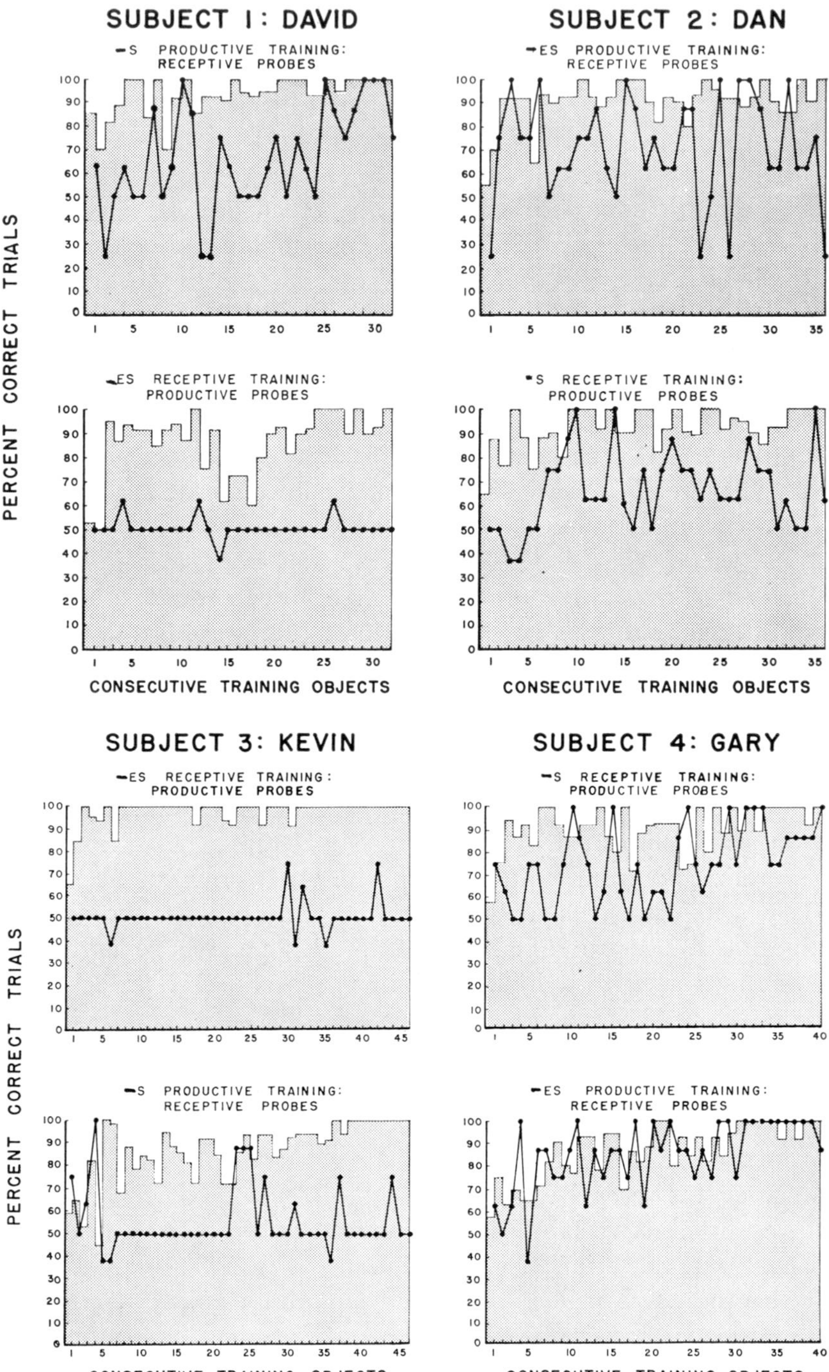

Figure I.5. Percent correct trials for two training conditions and their associated probes in four subjects. Bar graphs depict reinforced training trials in each of two response modalities. Each corresponding point on the line graphs represents percent correct responses for eight probe trials; two singulars and two plurals for the trained object; two singulars and two plurals for the object appearing next in the training sequence.

responding in the receptive -es plural training condition was very high across objects, yet productive probes of that baseline varied little from the 50% level of correctness. Similarly, productive training (-s plurals) showed a steady acquisition across objects, yet its receptive probes remained at chance (50%) level of pointing.

Thus, despite the fact that the subjects had learned near-perfect generative pluralization rules *concurrently* in both receptive and productive modalities, and were being reinforced for maintaining these rule-bound behaviors, nevertheless, as a group they showed relatively little tendency to generalize these rules across modalities, even though the rules were separated by no more than the use of -s or -es endings for correct pluralizations.

A second part of this study (Experiment II) was conducted to analyze the patterns of generalization found in Experiment I by

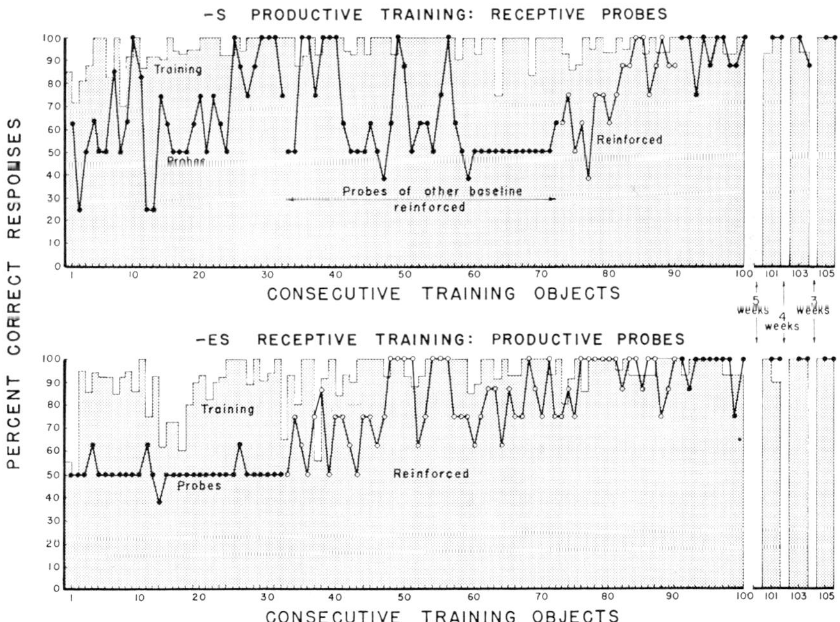

Figure I.6. (Subject 1, David.) Percent correct trials for two training conditions and their associated probes. Reinforced probe trials are indicated by open dots. (Previous data from Figure I.5 are included for comparison.)

using a procedure to produce or solidify generalization between the two language repertories where it was absent or weak, and to reduce generalization where it was strong. The procedure used was an appropriate contingency of reinforcement in each case. As recalled in Figure I.5, Subjects 1, 2, and 3, showed an absence of generalization or only weak generalization from receptive training to productive (labeling) probes in one class of plural endings, with the same pattern observed from productive training to receptive (pointing) probes in the other class of plural endings. Thus, for each of these subjects, probe trials, both receptive and productive, were temporarily reinforced, either separately or concurrently. The data resulting from these procedures are summarized in Figures I.6, I.7, and I.8, for Subject 1 (David), Subject 2 (Dan), and Subject 3 (Kevin), respectively.

Results of the reinforcement contingency in probe trials pro-

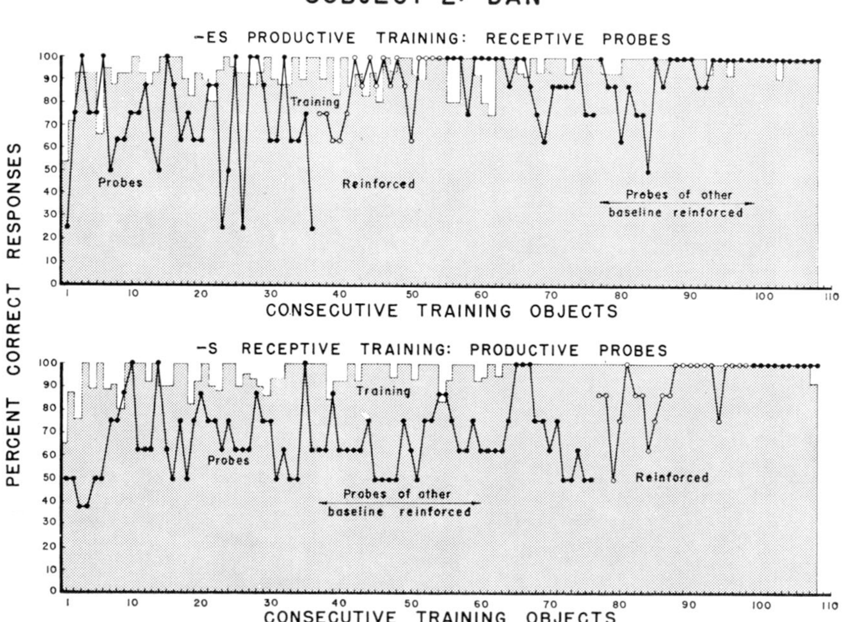

Figure I.7. (Subject 2, Dan.) Percent correct trials for two training conditions and their associated probes. Reinforced probes are depicted by open dots. (Data from Figure I.5 included.)

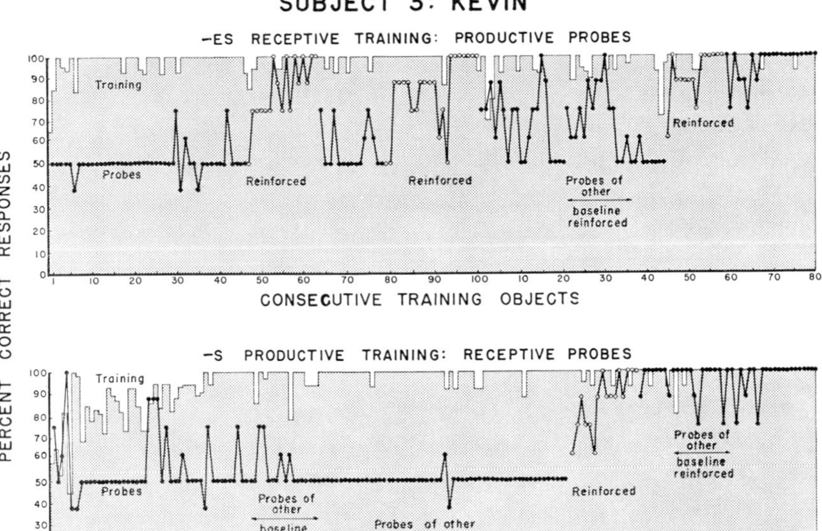

Figure I.8. (Subject 3, Kevin.) Percent correct trials for two training conditions and their associated probes. Reinforced probe trials are indicated by open dots. (Data from Figure I.5 included.)

duced eventually a durable generalization between the two repertoires in each subject, although in the case of David[7] (Subject 1) a lengthy exposure to reinforced productive probe trials was necessary and for Kevin (Subject 3) repeated sequences of reinforced probe trials were required before strong generalization occurred.

For the one subject, Gary (Subject 4), who showed initial generalization, incorrect generalization was briefly reinforced. Labeling single objects in plural form and pairs of objects in the singular were reinforced in probe trials of the receptive training baseline; pointing to single items when provided with a plural label and pointing to paired objects when presented with a singular label were reinforced in probe trials of the productive training baseline. Gary proved responsive to the reinforcement only so long as it was continued; when reinforcement of incorrect generalization ceased, correct generalization re-emerged. Gary's data reflecting performance under the reversed contingencies of Experiment II are summarized in Figure I.9.

In summary, the findings of Experiment I indicate that generalization between the language modalities (productive and receptive) is unlikely in language deficient retarded children even when both are trained concurrently, at least with the procedures and area of morphological grammar used in this study. However, further results of Experiment II demonstrated that appropriate contingencies of reinforcement were effective in establishing durable generalization between the two language repertories when it was initially absent, and reversed contingencies of reinforcement were effective in decreasing generalization between the two repertoires when generalization was initially present.

These results contrast somewhat with related research which

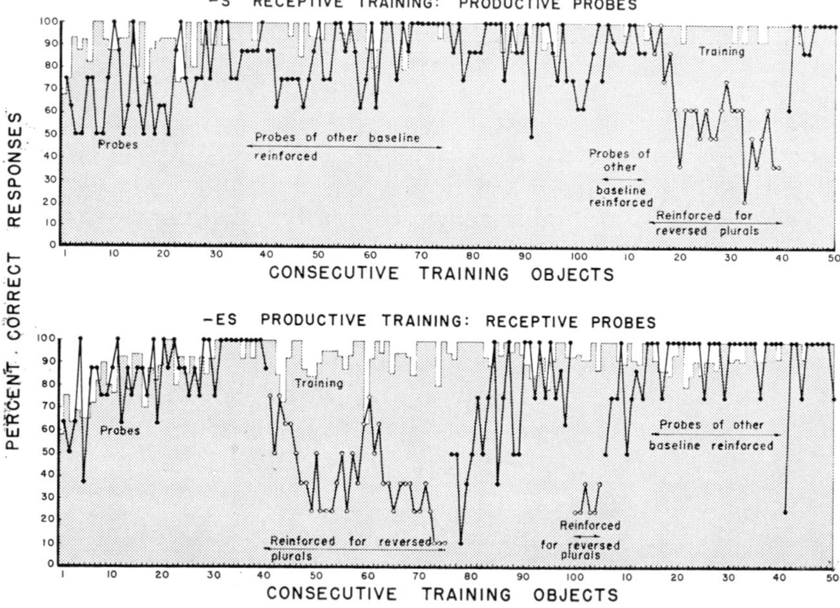

Figure I.9. (Subject 4, Gary.) Percent correct trials for two training conditions and their associated probes. Reinforced probe trials for reversed (incorrect) plural usage are shown by open dots. (Data from Figure I.5 included.)

has indicated that generalization between production and reception can occur in concept development tasks among retarded children (Hamilton, 1966; Dickerson, Girardeau, and Spradlin, 1964), and in the improvement of articulation among normal children (Winitz and Preisler, 1965; Mann and Baer, 1971). Thus, the variety of relationships that may hold between receptive language and productive speech remain unclear: some conditions under which a functional relationship can exist have been indicated; and some other conditions allowing independence have been shown; but the dimensions and parameters connecting these conditions need further exploration.

FURTHER STUDIES IN MORPHOLOGICAL GRAMMAR

Thus far, all the studies reviewed have used the plural morpheme as the unit of experimental analysis. The first showed acquisition of a generative response class as a function of direct training using procedures of imitation and differential reinforcement (Guess, et al., 1968); second, a study by Sailor (1971) demonstrated that allomorphic usage within the class of plurals is susceptible to generalized training effects within a context of echoic reinforcement; and, third, a series of investigations by Guess (1969). Harrelson (1969), and Guess and Baer (1972), demonstrated that retarded children might not *automatically* generalize between the receptive and productive repertoires, as exemplified by the training of generative plural usage.

Additional studies conducted at the Kansas Neurological Institute have used the response class concept to analyze generative speech and language acquisition in other areas of morphological grammar, thus extending the experimental analysis of linguistic development in retarded children, and providing systematic replications of the techniques and procedures which have been used in these training programs.

Acquisition of Productive Noun Suffixes

An unpublished study by Baer and Guess (1971) used procedures of differential reinforcement and imitation to teach mental retardates the usage of productive noun suffixes when labeling stimuli exemplifying the verb form of an action or activity. The noun suffix is a bound morpheme which may be added to many verbs to convert them to nouns, specifically, to nouns meaning one who engages in or displays the action denoted by the verb. This suffix may take several forms: one who works is a work*er,* a flute-player is a flut*ist,* etc. In the present investigation, the -er morpheme was the prime subject of study; the -ist morpheme was used (gramatically, misused) to display experimental control of the imitation-and-reinforcement-based teaching process.

Four children were selected who had a modest vocabulary, but demonstrated no productive usage of noun suffixes, as determined by a series of screening tests. All subjects were diagnosed as severely retarded. Subject 1, Mary (CA 16), Subject 2, Tom (CA 16), and Subject 3, Gene (CA 13) all resided in a state residential facility for the retarded. Subject 4, David (CA 11) lived in the community and attended a day care center for the retarded.

Procedure

Pictures showing persons engaged in various actions and activities were used as training stimuli. The pictures, numbering fifty-seven, were taken from magazines and mounted on 8½″ x 11″ pieces of cardboard. Plastic chips, redeemable for a variety of sweets and toys, were dispensed for correct responses on a continuous schedule of reinforcement.

Training Conditions. In Condition I, each training picture was shown to the subject while the experimenter simultaneously described the ongoing action (e.g., "This man writes."). The experimenter next provided the stimulus phrase, "He is a ....?", and reinforced the subject for producing the verb with the correct suffix (e.g., *writer*). If the subject gave an incorrect response, the experimenter said "No," provided the correct label, and again presented the picture and stimulus phrase after a ten-second delay. If no response was given within ten seconds on any trial, the training procedures were repeated, as if for a new trial. Criterion for each word trained was five correct consecutive responses; the next picture was then introduced, and similar training procedures were applied to it. Training continued in this way until it appeared that the subject would reliably give the correct noun on the first five trials of each new verb presented.

In Condition II the subject was reinforced for producing the verb with a different suffix ending, specifically the -ist suffix, although these verbs conventionally take the -er suffix. For example, in response to the stimulus phrase, "This boy swims. He is a . . . .?", subjects were reinforced for saying "swimmist" rather than "swimmer." The training procedures, trials to criterion, and schedule of reinforcement remained the same as in Condition I. Training under this condition continued until experimental control was apparent, i.e., the subject gave the correct noun on the first six trials of each new verb presented (one trial more than criterion).

In Condition III subjects were again trained to give each verb the correct -er suffix, exactly as in Condition I. As before, this training continued until correct nouns were being given reliably on the first five trials of each new verb presented.

Results

Performance of a subject could be considered as generative when each new verb was converted into its correct noun suffix without any error, that is, when no training trials were required to achieve criterion of five consecutive correct responses. Trials to criterion, across the three experimental conditions, are shown in Figure I.10 for the four subjects.

In general, this figure shows that in each experimental condition, a decreasing number of trials was required to reach each successive criterion. In particular, it is apparent that training during Conditions I and III was finally sufficient to produce a generative outcome, in which each successive verb presented was immediately converted into a conventionally correct noun suffix without error, prompting, or differential reinforcement. Training during Condition II was also sufficient to approach this kind of outcome very closely (albeit with a conventionally incorrect suffix), and was pursued no further.

A more sensitive but less stable measure of a generative performance was the correct production of the noun suffix as the *first* response to each new verb presented. Often enough, a subject would give correct responses to the first, or first few, presentations of a new verb, but would not give five successive correct responses

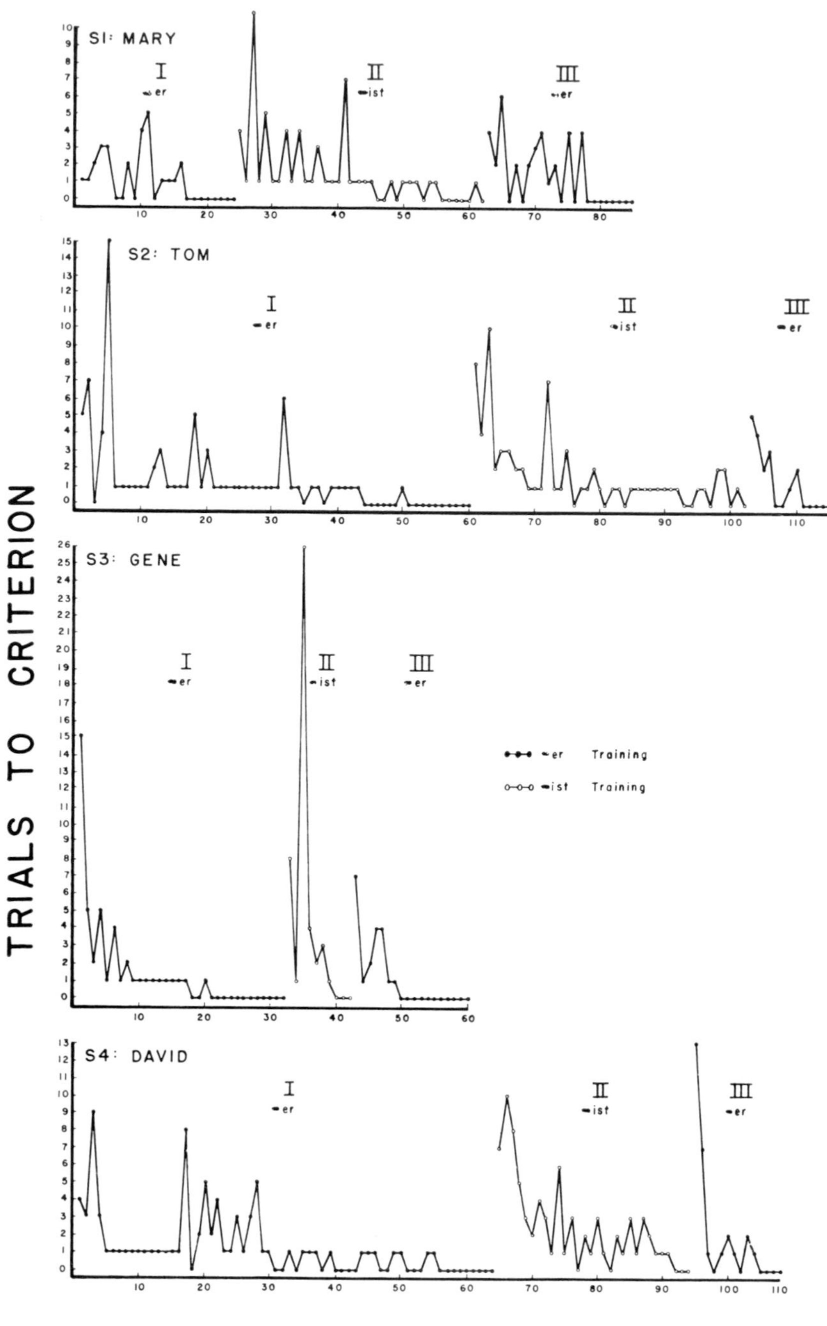

Figure I.10. Trials to criterion for the training of verbs in three experimental conditions for Subjects 1, 2, 3, and 4.

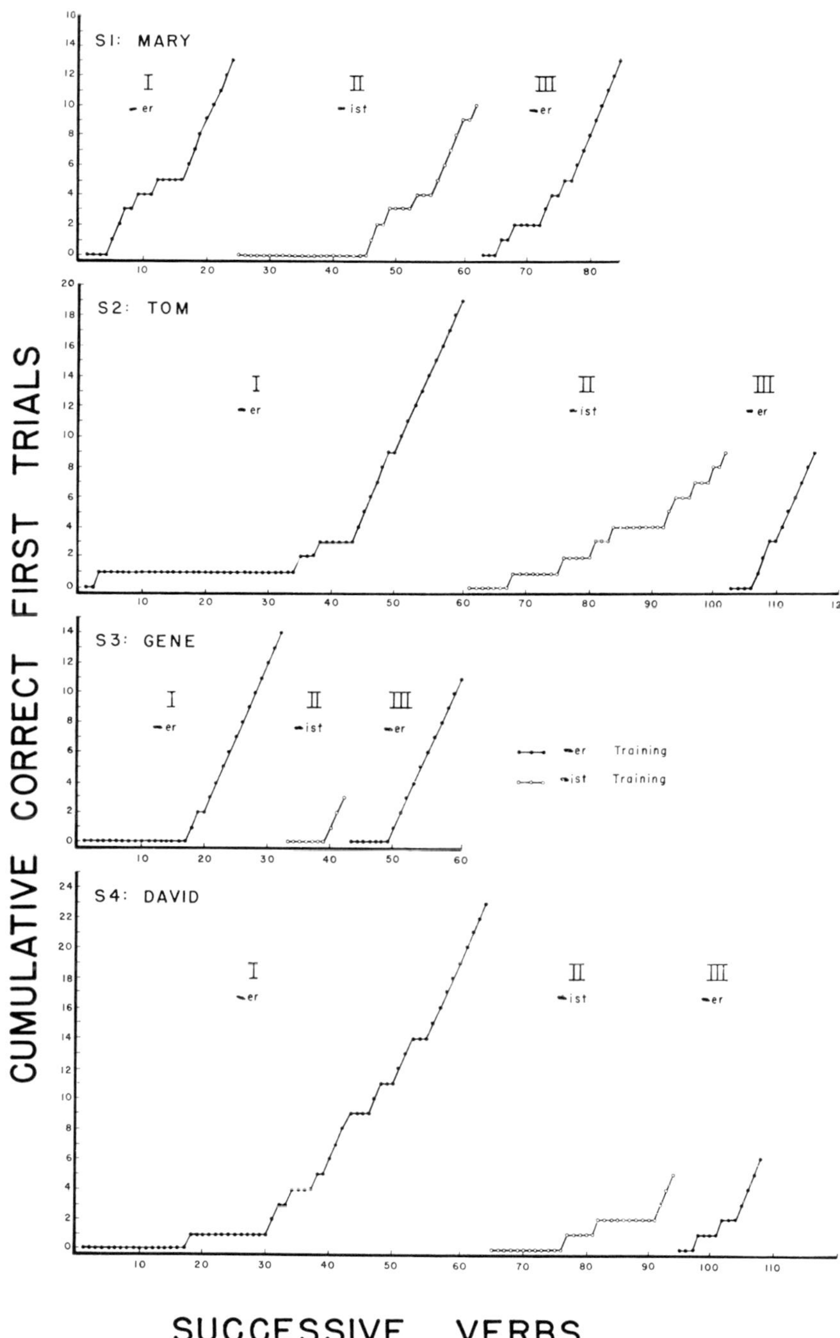

Figure I.11. Cumulative correct first trials for the training of verbs in three experimental conditions for Subjects 1, 2, 3, and 4.

so as to yield a zero trials-to-criterion score. Correctness on the first trials suggests that the subject is generative; subsequent error may suggest that he is not stably generative, or simply that his attending behaviors are not under thorough experimental control. The cumulative number of correct first responses to each verb presented, across the three experimental conditions are shown in Figure I.11, for the four subjects.

In general, this figure displays the same effects seen in the trial-to-criterion data of Figure I.10: probability of a correct first trial increased steadily as training progressed. In Conditions I and III this probability rose to an apparently stable level of 100%. Change in Condition II was similar, but was not pressed to a similar stability.

Receptive Training of Adjectival Inflections

This study (Baer and Guess, 1971) was designed to extend further the experimental analysis of language development in mental retardates to the case of adjectival inflections which, again, can be defined as a generalized response class. In morphological grammar, many adjectives can indicate relative degree of quantity or quality simply by standardized comparative and superlative suffixes: the comparative suffix, -er (e.g., slow*er*), expresses a quantitative degree of difference between a pair of referents, and -est (e.g., slow*est*), indicates the maximum quantitative degree holding between three or more referents. These suffixes can be correctly generalized to a very large number of adjectives; thus, those adjectives potentially constitute a response class conditionable by teaching correct suffix usage with a relatively small number of representatives. The present investigation explored that possibility at the receptive or *understanding* level of language.

Method

Three severely retarded subjects, all residents of a state facility for the mentally retarded, were selected as subjects. An extensive screening test indicated that none of the subjects possessed already the grammatical rule regulating use of comparatives and superlatives. Subject 1, Jim, was 13 years old and diagnosed as Down's Syndrome. Subject 2, Gene, was 12 years of age with cause of retardation due to metabolic disorder. Subject 3, Barb, was 7½ years old, with retardation due to unknown cause.

The training materials used in the study consisted of nineteen sets of pictures. Each set contained four cards (5″ x 8″), each card of a set displaying a quantitatively different picture of the same basic stimulus. For example, the first set consisted of four cards each displaying a circle; the four cards differed clearly and regularly in size. Thus each set of cards could be used to exemplify opposites (*big* and *small*), comparatives (*big, bigger* and *small, smaller*), and superlatives (*big, bigger, biggest* and *small, smaller, smallest*). Table I.VIII describes the nineteen sets of stimulus cards and lists the adjectives exemplified by each set.

TABLE I.VIII

THE NINETEEN SETS OF FOUR STIMULUS CARDS USED TO EXEMPLIFY ADJECTIVES

Set Number	*Descriptions of the 4 Cards in the Set*	*Adjectives*
1	Circles differing in diameter (0.5, 1, 2, 4 in.)	small-big
2	Faces differing in degree of up- or down-curved mouth (0.25 or 0.5 in. deep)	happy-sad
3	Flowers differing in size, esp. height (2, 4, 6, 8 in.)	tiny-huge
4	Squares differing in shading (clear, lined, cross-hatched, black)	light-dark
5	Beetles differing in width (0.25, 0.5, 1, 2 in.)	skinny-fat
6	Triangles differing at apex (60° angle or half-circle of 0.125, 0.25, or 0.5 in. radius)	sharp-blunt
7	Glasses differing in fullness (2%, 10%, 70%, 100%)	empty-full
8	Rings differing in tightness around rod (tight or 33%, 67%, 100% larger in diameter)	tight-loose
9	Rectangles differing in length (0.125 by 0.5 in. by 1.25 by 2.5 by 4 in.)	short-long
10	Striped poles differing in width (0.125, 0.25, 0.75, 1 in.)	narrow-wide
11	Houses differing in height (0.75, 1.5, 4.5, 6.5 in.)	little-tall
12	Birds differing in distance from point (1, 2, 4, 6 in.)	near-far
13	Angles (10°, 45°, 120°, 150°)	acute-obtuse
14	Diamonds differing in one axis (3 by 0.5 by 1, by 2, by 3 in.)	thin-thick
15	Squares differing in density of dots (1, 4, 20, 40 dots/ sq. in.)	sparse-dense
16	Running men differing in perspective "distance" from viewer (12°, 9°, 6°, 3° retinal angle)	slow-fast
17	Grids differing in lines per inch (1, 2, 8, 16 lines/inch)	coarse-fine
18	Sine waves differing in amplitude (0.25, 0.5, 1, 2 in. crest-to-trough)	steady-shaky
19	U's differing in depth (0.25, 0.75, 1.5, 3 in. deep)	shallow-deep

Experimental Design

Control and evaluation of the training procedures were accomplished by a multiple baseline technique which incorporated probes of the subject's ability to transpose from trained combinations of stimuli to untrained combinations. The multiple baseline design was built on two baselines of such probes: a Comparative and a Superlative baseline. First, however, there was a preliminary teaching of opposites (e.g., *big* and *small*). Next, training established the receptive identification of comparatives, exemplified by successive pairs of stimuli showing a quantitative difference (e.g., *big, bigger* and *small, smaller*). This training, called the Comparative Phase, was probed repeatedly for generalization to novel combinations of stimuli: response to these probes constituted the Comparative baseline of the design. Periodically during Comparative Phase training and probing, the subject was probed further for correct response to the superlative. Data from these probes comprised the Superlative baseline of the design. After training in comparatives had produced a satisfactory level of correct response on comparative probes, training was shifted to the development of superlatives and discontinued for the still ongoing comparative presentations. This was called the Superlative Phase. Ongoing probes continued to measure response to untrained comparatives and superlatives.

Procedure

OVERVIEW. Three sequential training conditions were used within each set of stimuli. (1) Using two cards of the set, training established the receptive identification of two opposite adjectives (e.g., *big* and *small*); (2) Using three cards from the set, one of these opposites (e.g., *big*) underwent comparative training *(big, bigger)* if this was the Comparative Phase of the multiple baseline design, or superlative training *(big, biggest)* if this was the Superlative Phase of the design; (3) Again with three cards (but including one not previously used) the other opposite *(small)* underwent comparative training *(small, smaller)* if this was the Comparative Phase of the design, or superlative training *(small, smallest)* if this was the Superlative Phase.

As many as three types of probes were interspersed within these training conditions, to display any effects of training on as yet untrained responses of stimulus combinations. In the Comparative Phase of the design, (1) Superlative probes, always involving the three stimuli used so far, were applied after the first comparative had been trained, to see if that training had evoked any pre-existing discrimination of the superlative; (2) late in the Comparative Phase, transpositional superlative probes, involving stimulus trios not used so far, were added to the nontranspositional superlative probes previously used, to see if any combination of stimuli, familiar or novel, would evoke correct superlative discrimination, and to provide a baseline for the upcoming Superlative Phase; (3) transpositional comparative probes, always involving stimulus pairs not used so far, were applied during the Comparative Phase after the second comparative of each set had been trained, to see if the comparative training (now complete for that stimulus set) had established any generalized skill in identifying comparative relationships.

In the Superlative Phase of the design, nontranspositional superlative probes, supplemented by transpositional superlative probes, were applied after the first superlative of each set had been trained, and again after the second superlative of each set had been trained (to display the generalized effects of superlative training); and transpositional comparative probes were applied after the second superlative of each set had been trained (to display any maintenance of the previously trained comparative skills with new stimuli, now that such training had stopped).

A detailed account of the reinforcement technique, of each type of training condition, and of each type of probe, follows. The overall plan of training and probes is exemplified in Tables I.IX and I.X, for the first stimulus set used in each phase.

Reinforcement. Subjects were reinforced for correct responses on a VR3 schedule with plastic chips, which they redeemed at the end of the session for a variety of sweets, toys, games, etc. The VR3 schedule was established gradually with the first set of opposites taught to the subject; thereafter, it was put quickly into effect for each training condition that followed.

Training the Opposites. The subject was trained to point

correctly to one of the two pictures labeled by the experimenter as opposites (e.g., *big* and *small,* as exemplified in Table I.IX. The two pictures (stimulus cards) were placed in front of the subject; the experimenter then said, "Point to. . . ." If an incorrect response was given, the experimenter said "No," provided the correct label, removed the cards, and presented them again after a 10-sec. time-out. The positions of the training cards were changed unsystematically, to control for position biases. The order of requesting the two opposites (e.g., *big* or *small*) was random. Criterion for successful performances in this condition, as well as all subsequent training conditions, was ten consecutive correct responses.

TRAINING THE TWO COMPARATIVES. In the Comparative Phase

TABLE I.IX

EXAMPLES OF THE SEQUENCE OF TRAINING AND PROBE CONDITIONS USED DURING THE COMPARATIVE PHASE

Train (Reinforced)	*Request ("Point to —")*	*Stimuli Presented: * Correct Response: (*)* ·	•	●	⬤	*No. of Trials*	*Probe (Unreinforced)*
	small		(*)	*		to	
Opposites	big		*	(*)		criterion	
First	small	*	(*)	*		to	
Comparative	smaller	(*)	*	*		criterion	
	smallest	(*)	*	*		4	Superlative[a]
Second	big		*	(*)	*	to	
Comparative	bigger		*	*	(*)	criterion	
	biggest		*	*	(*)	4	Superlative[a]
	smaller	(*)			*	1	
	bigger	*			(*)	1	
	smaller		(*)	*		1	
	bigger		*	(*)		1	Transpositional
	smaller		(*)		*	1	Comparative
	bigger		*		(*)	1	
	smaller			(*)	*	1	
	bigger			*	(*)		

[a] These superlative probes were modified, three stimulus sets before the Comparative Phase ended, to include transpositional superlatives as well. Table I.X describes the modified transportational superlative probes.

TABLE I.X

EXAMPLE OF THE SEQUENCE OF TRAINING AND PROBE CONDITIONS USED DURING THE SUPERLATIVE PHASE

Train (Reinforced)	*Request ("Point to —")*					*No. of Trials*	*Probe (Unreinforced)*
	shallow		(*)	*		to	
Opposites	deep		*	(*)		criterion	
First	shallow	*	*	(*)		to	
Superlative	shallowest	(*)	*	*		criterion	
	shallowest	(*)		*	*	2	
	shallowest	(*)	*		*	2	Transpositional
	shallowest		(*)	*	*	2	Superlative
	shallowest[a]	(*)	*	*		2	
Second	deep		(*)	*	*	to	
Superlative	deepest		*	*	(*)	criterion	
	deepest	*	*		(*)	2	Transpositional
	deepest	*		*	(*)	2	Superlative
	deepest	*	*	(*)		2	
	deepest[a]		*	*	(*)	2	
	shallower	(*)			*	1	
	deeper	*			(*)	1	
	shallower		(*)	*		1	
	deeper		*	(*)		1	Transpositional
	shallower		(*)		*	1	Comparative
	deeper		*		(*)	1	
	shallower			(*)	*	1	
	deeper			*	(*)	1	

[a] These probes were not transpositional; they were identical to the training stimuli of the Superlative Phase and analogous in form to the Superlative probes of the Comparative Phase (Table I.II).

of the design, after training of the opposites, the subject was taught to identify the comparative of one of the opposites. Three stimulus cards were shown to the subject; they included those originally trained as opposites (e.g., *big* and *small*) plus a new stimulus card which, quantitatively, represented the comparative of one of the opposites (e.g., *smaller*) as exemplified in Table I.IX. The subject was reinforced for pointing to the picture previously taught as one of the opposites when requested (e.g., *small*), and to the new stimulus card when the experimenter asked for its comparative (e.g., *smaller*). These requests were made in random order. No requests were made for the remaining stimulus cards, originally trained as the second opposite (e.g., *big*). This card remained in the three-card series as a neutral stimulus, both to reduce the probability of chance correct responses and perhaps to facilitate the discrimination between the first opposite and its comparative. As before, the positions of the cards were changed unsystematically; and the subject was required to meet a criterion of ten successive correct responses.

Procedures for training the second comparative were identical to those used for the first comparative. However, the subject was now shown the two cards originally taught as opposites, plus the stimulus card depicting the comparative for the second opposite (e.g., *bigger*). The first opposite *(small)* was presented as the third stimulus card but was not requested by the experimenter.

TRAINING THE TWO SUPERLATIVES. Training of each first superlative in the Superlative Phase of the design was always preceded by the establishment of two opposites (e.g., the *shallow* and *deep* of Table I.X) just as was training of comparatives in the prior phase. The subject was then shown the two stimulus cards originally trained as opposites, plus an additional card which represented the superlative of one of the opposites (as shown in the example of Table I.X). This logically converted the stimulus trained previously as the other opposite to the anchor item of the superlative series to be trained. For example, *deep* now became *shallow, shallow* implicitly became *shallower,* and the additional third stimulus represented the explicitly trained superlative, *shallowest* (see Table I.X, first Superlative). On the first trial only, the experimenter therefore re-labeled the *deep* card as *shallow* ("This is shallow") and then began a random series of requests to point to either *shallow* or *shallowest.* The middle card (originally trained as *shallow* and now implicitly *shallower)* remained in the training series but was not requested by the experimenter. Again, the positions of the cards were changed unsystematically during the training trials; and the subject was required to meet a criterion of ten consecutive correct responses. The second superlative was trained by the same procedures. As indicated in the example of Table I.X, the combination of stimulus cards was changed for this training (the *shallowest* card was removed, the card originally trained as *shallow* now became *deep,* and the newly added stimulus was labeled *deepest*).

General Probe Conditions

One or another of the three types of probes described in this section was given to the subject interspersed within the training trials, following that point at which the subject had reached criterion in the particular training condition to be probed. The subject was then being reinforced on a VR3 schedule, thus allowing insertion of the probes within the established level of reinforcer density. Responses to all probes, correct or not, were never reinforced.

TRANSPOSITIONAL COMPARATIVE PROBES. These probes measured the extent to which the subject applied the comparative rule to stimulus combinations which had not been taught directly in the comparative training conditions. The subject was requested to point to one of two opposite stimuli, now labeled as a comparative. In the example of Table I.IX, the subject was asked to point to either the *smaller* or *bigger* pattern. Eight transpositional comparative probes were given for each stimuli series, covering pairs of stimulus cards not trained directly as comparatives in the preceding conditions. Table I.IX lists the eight combinations of paired stimuli used for these probes.

SUPERLATIVE PROBES. Nontranspositional superlative probes were taken (as a second baseline) during the early comparative training conditions. The subject was presented with the same three stimulus cards used in training. He was then requested to point to the stimulus card which, quantitatively, would be the superlative. For example, the subject was shown the three stimulus cards originally labeled as *big, small,* and *smaller* in the first comparative training condition. He was then asked to point to the *smallest* of the three patterns. For the second comparative training condition, the subject was asked to point to the *biggest* of the three patterns. The nontranspositional superlative probes were presented four times following training of the first comparative, and four times again following training of the second comparative.

TRANSPOSITIONAL SUPERLATIVE PROBES. The transpositional

superlative probes were administered in a manner identical to the nontranspositional superlative probes. The only difference between them was in the trios of stimulus cards shown to the subject. Whereas the nontranspositional superlative probes used the same three stimulus cards presented in the training condition, the transpositional superlative probes included every other possible trio of stimuli contained in each four-card series (as exemplified in Table I.X). Each of the three possible transpositional superlative probes was presented twice, and the nontranspositional superlative probes now were presented twice. Transpositional superlative probes were introduced to each subject three stimulus sets prior to the beginning of superlative training.

Results

Training. The number of trials required by each subject to reach criterion performance during the training of successive sets

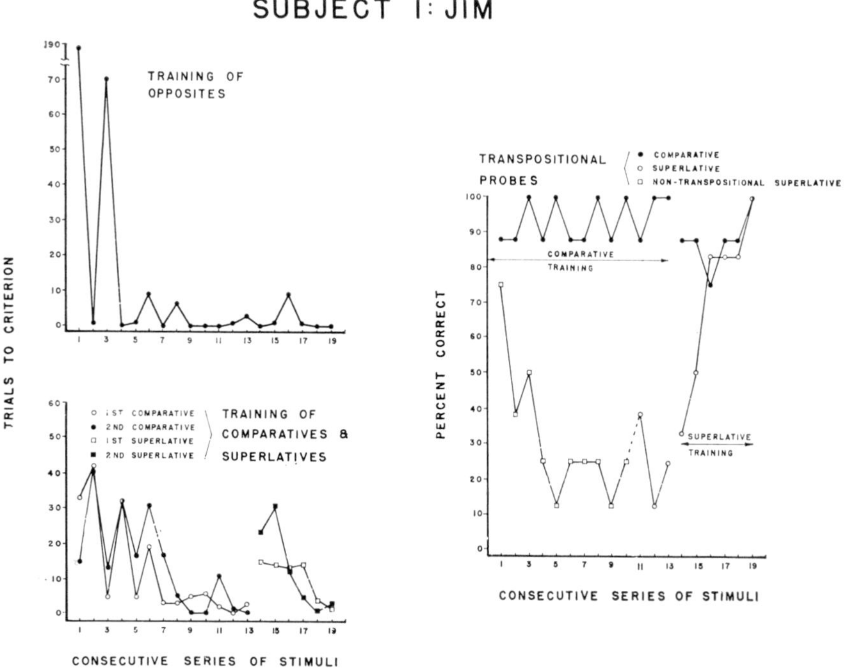

Figure I.12. Trials to criterion for the training of opposites, comparatives, and superlatives, and percentage of correct response to comparative and superlative probes for Subject 1, Jim.

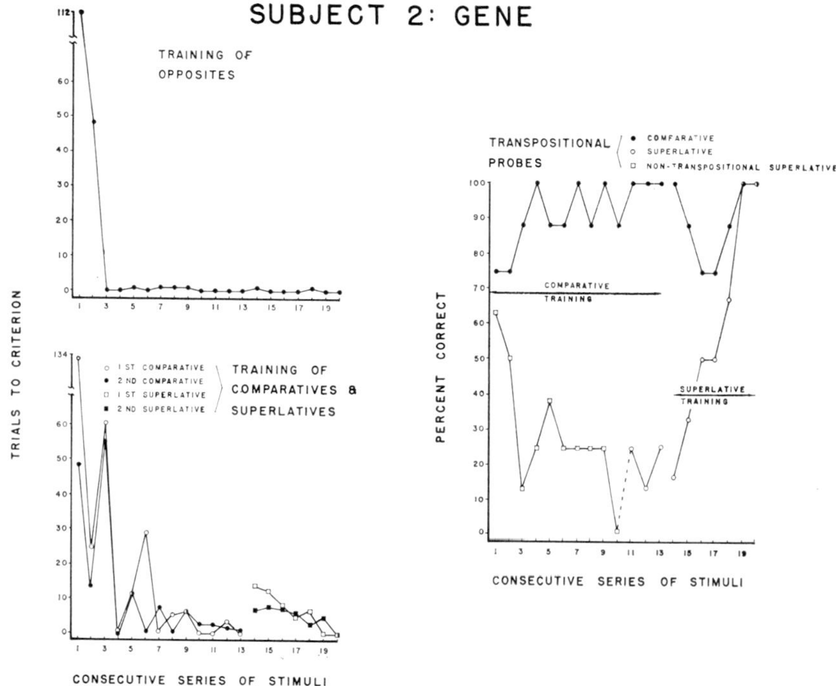

Figure I.13. Trials to criterion for the training of opposites, comparatives, and superlatives, and percentage of correct response to comparative and superlative probes for Subject 2, Gene.

of opposites, first and second comparatives, and first and second superlatives, is shown in Figures I.12, I.13, and I.14, each figure displaying the results for a single subject. In general, fewer and fewer trials were required to reach each criterion, the minimum number being achieved repeatedly by the end of training.[8] However, Subject 3, Barb, required little or no training in opposites; and Subject 1, Jim, was not quite at the minimum level of trials required for learning new superlatives by the end of training.

Probes

The percentage of comparative and superlative probe trials responded to correctly is shown in Figures I.12, I.13, and I.14, each figure displaying the results for a single subject. It will be recalled that the comparative probes were always transpositional; the superlative probes were nontranspositional during most of the

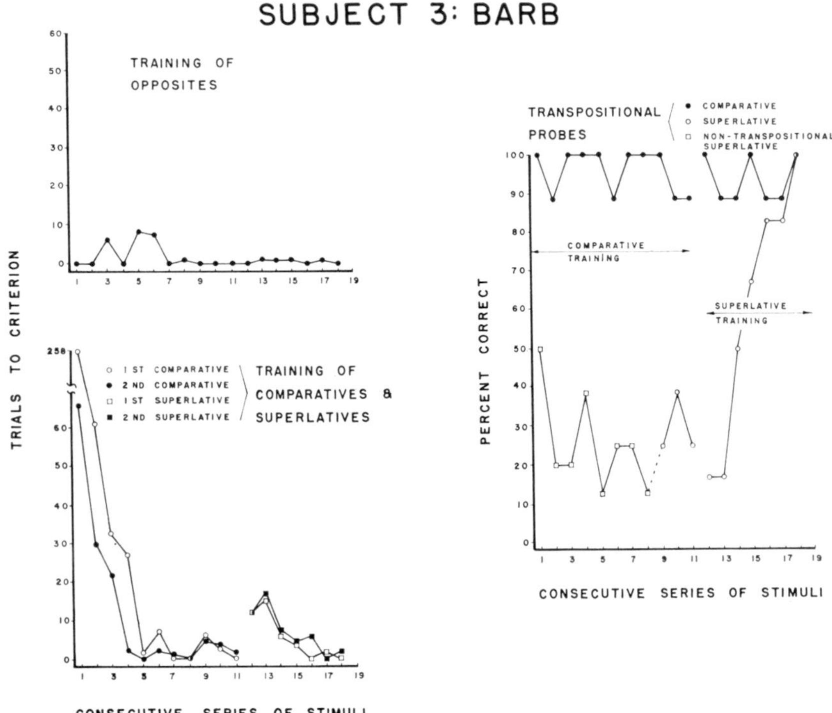

Figure I.14. Trials to criterion for the training of opposites, comparatives, and superlatives, and percentage of correct response to comparative and superlative probes, for Subject 3, Barb.

comparative training condition, but became transpositional three stimulus sets before superlative training began. In general, the three subjects responded accurately to the comparative probes from the outset, generally scoring 87.5% or 100% correct (i.e., seven or eight correct of eight trials). However, Subject 2, Gene, showed some evidence of a more gradually acquired generalization, his initial points being 75% correct and his subsequent scores then showing the usual 87.5% to 100% level.

When comparative training gave way to superlative training, response to comparative probes remained relatively accurate, although Subjects 1 and 2 declined briefly to the 75% level (Subject 1 for only one stimulus set, Subject 2 for two stimulus sets). And, as superlative training progressed, accuracy of response to the transpositional superlative probes steadily increased to the 100% level in all three subjects. During comparative training, the superlative probes had shown only chance (33%) or lower accuracy levels, except for relatively high scores on the first (or first few) stimulus sets shown uniformly by the three subjects.

SUMMARY AND DISCUSSION

In the studies reviewed, severely and moderately retarded children were taught grammatical rules of English morphology using procedures of imitation and differential reinforcement, in the case of plurals (Guess, et al., 1968), noun suffixes (Baer and Guess, 1971), and adjectival inflections (Baer and Guess, 1971). Another excellent study by Shumaker and Sherman (1971) applied the same procedures to train generative usage of verb inflections in severely and moderately retarded children. Taken as a group, these investigations provide a modest step in the experimental analysis of linguistic development in retarded children. In each study, the concept of response class was utilized to demonstrate the generative nature of speech and language skills resulting from the imitation-and-reinforcement-based procedures of training; namely, that teaching a small number of exemplars in a class of linguistic behavior generalizes to other members of that class which were not taught directly. This consistent finding is conceptually important to the contribution of learning theory to the study of linguistic development, and also of practical importance to training programs designed to enhance the speech and language repertoires of mentally retarded children. Studies currently in progress at the Kansas Neurological Institute are attempting to extend the experimental analysis of linguistic development in retarded children to the area of syntax, again using the response class concept to describe the productivity of syntactical usage aimed at in the training programs.

In the introduction to this review, it was argued that experimental analyses of aspects of language behavior above the rudimentary level were essential to establishing the relevance of behavior theory to the phenomenon of language development. Naturally, it may be asked whether this review, and the future lines of research sketched, have indeed advanced that relevance.

Surely, it remains still to be seen. More and more complex aspects of language usage exemplified by normal speakers have been brought under analysis primarily through differential reinforcement and imitation techniques. If sentence usage eventually succumbs to the same approach, will we say that *language* is now understood, at least at the level of a feasibility analysis? The answer must depend on a proportion: what proportion of the language behavior of a normal speaker can be accounted for by these components, aspects, mechanisms, or structures? Put differently, the question might be: if a language deficient retardate were subjected successfully to each of these programs, would his net integrated result be a respectable proportion of the language behavior we note in normal speakers? For psycholinguistic theory, a *respectable* proportion will not be enough—the goal of such theory is apparently to account for all possible sentences generated by any speakers anywhere, any lesser explanation remaining only a special case. For behavior modification, the larger the proportion, the greater its significance—total language capability is of much less significance than *effective* language capability. The proportion remains unassessed, of course. But the point of these researches is that they may produce the building blocks of an eventual (and somewhat heroic) program which could allow a preliminary assessment of that proportion. Indeed, it may well be the case that such an assessment is impossible without these components. That is the logic underlying their pursuit.

As a final point of discussion, we emphasize that many of the children serving as subjects in the research described had obvious neurological damage in addition to their intellectual impairments. Some subjects had diagnosed genetic aberrations; most were mentally retarded as a result of unknown factors. Thus it remains even more a matter of conjecture whether the results from these studies represent the same variables of learning which govern speech and language acquisition in normal children, or, for that matter, in other groups of deviant children. Nevertheless, data derived from these investigations were observable, reliable, and predictable—predictable from principles of learning theory.

REFERENCES

Baer, Donald M.: The control of developmental process: Why wait? In J. R. Nesselroade and H. W. Reese (Eds.): *Life-Span Developmental Psychology: Methodological Issues.* New York, Academic Press, 1972.

Baer, D. M. and Guess, D.: Receptive training of adjectival inflections in mental retardates. *Journal of Applied Behavior Analysis, 4*:129-139, 1971.

Baer, D. M., Peterson, R. F., and Sherman, J. A.: The development of imitation by reinforcing similarity to a model. *Journal of the Experimental Analysis of Behavior, 10*:405-416, 1967.

Berko, Jean: The child's learning of English morphology. In S. Saporta (Ed.): *Psycholinguistics.* New York, Holt, Rinehart, and Winston, pp. 359-375, 1961.

Bricker, W. A. and Bricker, Diane D.: The use of programmed language training as a means for differential diagnosis and educational remediation among severely retarded children. *Peabody Papers in Human Development, 4,* Nashville, George Peabody College for Teachers, 1966.

Carroll, J. B.: Language development in children. In S. Saporta (Ed.): *Psycholinguistics.* New York, Holt, Rinehart, and Winston, pp. 331-345, 1961.

Chomksy, N.: *Syntactic Structures.* Hague, Mouton, 1957.

Chomsky, N.: The general properties of language. In C. Millikan and F. Farley (Eds.): *Brain Mechanisms Underlying Speech and Language.* New York, Grune and Stratton, 1959.

Dickerson, D. J., Girardeau, F. L., and Spradlin, J. F.: Verbal pre-training and discrimination learning by retardates. *American Journal of Mental Deficiency, 68*:476-484, 1964.

Fraser, C., Bellugi, Ursula, and Brown, R.: Control of grammar in imitation, comprehension, and production. *Journal of Verbal Learning and Verbal Behavior, 2*:121-135, 1963.

Gleason, H. A.: *An Introduction to Descriptive Linguistics.* New York, Holt, Rinehart, and Winston, 1965.

Guess, D.: A functional analysis of receptive language and productive speech: Acquisition of the plural morpheme. *Journal of Applied Behavior Analysis, 2*:55-64, 1969.

Guess, D., Sailor, W., Rutherford, G., and Baer, D. M.: An experimental analysis of linguistic development: The productive use of the plural morpheme. *Journal of Applied Behavior Analysis, 1*:297-306, 1968.

Guess, D. and Baer, D. M.: An analysis of individual differences in generalization between receptive and productive language in retarded children. In press, *Journal of Applied Behavior Analysis,* 1972.

Hamilton, J.: Learning of a generalized response class in mentally retarded individuals. *American Journal of Mental Deficiency, 71*:100-108, 1966.

Harrelson, A.: *Effects of Productive Speech Training on Receptive Language.* Master's thesis, University of Kansas, 1969.

Lenneberg, E. H.: *Biological Foundations of Language.* New York, John Wiley and Sons, Inc., 1967.

Lovaas, O. I.: A program for the establishment of speech in psychotic children. In Wing, J. K. (Ed.) : *Early Childhood Autism.* London, Pergamon, 1966, pp. 115-144.

Lovell, K. and Bradbury, B.: The learning of English morphology in educationally subnormal special school children. *American Journal of Mental Deficiency, 71*:609-615, 1967.

Mann, R. and Baer, D. M.: The effects of receptive language training on articulation. *Journal of Applied Behavior Analysis, 4*:291-298, 1971.

McCarthy, Dorthea: Language development in children. In L. Carmichael (Ed.): *Manual of Child Psychology* (2nd ed.). New York, John Wiley and Sons, 1954, pp. 492-630.

Myklebust, H. R.: *Auditory Disorders in Children.* New York, Grune and Stratton, 1957.

Palermo, D.: Language acquisition. In H. W. Reese and L. P. Lipsitt (Eds.) : *Experimental Child Psychology.* New York, Academic Press, 1970, pp. 425-477.

Risley, T. R. and Wolf, M. M.: Establishing functional speech in echolalic children. *Behavior Research and Therapy, 2*:43-47, 1967.

Sailor, W.: Reinforcement and generalization of productive plural allomorphs in two retarded children. *Journal of Applied Behavior Analysis, 4*:305-310, 1971.

Sailor, W., Guess, D., Rutherford, G., and Baer, D. M.: Control of tantrum behavior by operant techniques during experimental verbal training. *Journal of Applied Behavior Analysis, 1*:237-243, 1968.

Salzinger, K.: The problem of response class in verbal behavior. In K. Salzinger and S. Salzinger (Eds.) : *Research in Verbal Behavior and Some Neurophysiological Implications.* New York, Academic Press, 1967, pp. 35-54.

Schumaker, Jean and Sherman, J. A.: Training generative verb usage by imitation and reinforcement procedures. *Journal of Applied Behavior Analysis, 3*:273-287, 1970.

Sidman, M.: *Tactics of Scientific Research.* New York, Basic Books, 1960.

Skinner, B. F.: *The Behavior of Organisms: An Experimental Analysis.* New York, Appleton-Century-Crofts, 1938.

Skinner, B. F.: *Verbal Behavior.* New York, Appleton-Century-Crofts, 1957.

Sloane, H. N. and MacAuley, Barbara D.: *Operant Procedures in Remedial Speech and Language Training.* Boston, Houghton Mifflin Co., 1968.

Spradlin, J. E.: Language and communication of mental defectives. In N. R. Ellis (Ed.) : *Handbook of Mental Deficiency.* New York, McGraw-Hill, 1963, pp. 512-555.

Staats, A. W. and Staats, C. K.: *Complex Human Behavior: A Systematic Extension of Learning Principles.* New York, Holt, Rinehart, and Winston, 1963.

Winitz, H. and Preisler, Linda: Discrimination pretraining and sound learning. *Perceptual Motor Skills, 20*:905-916, 1965.

FOOTNOTES

1. The studies reviewed in this chapter were funded in part by two grants from the State of Kansas, *Studies in the Morphological Language Development of Mentally Retarded Children* (1969-1970), and *Studies in Generative Grammar and Related Language Problems Among Retarded Children* (1970-1971); and in part by a program project grant to the Bureau of Child Research, University of Kansas, by the National Institute of Child Health and Human Development (HD00870). The authors are grateful to Mrs. Muriel Saunders, Mrs. Erminda Garcia, Miss Linda Weir, and Miss Deborah Connole, for their assistance in carrying out the procedures and gathering the data of the experiments described in this chapter. Thanks for helpful editing are also due to German' Casas-Ruiz, and Dr. Wayne Sailor.

2. Indeed, the usual operant conditioning program of language development in such cases, even should it fail, would be expected to leave the child better off than before. The child will have collected a very considerable number of reinforcers, he will have experienced close face-to-face contact on a typically daily basis with an even-tempered, pleasant adult, and very likely he will have developed some general attentional responses. He is quite likely to react to his daily session as play rather than work, and usually will greet the experimenter-teacher in the ward with smiles, giggles, and an immediate start for the experimental room.

3. It is sometimes argued that the *development* of a behavior may be a different process than the *recovery* of a previously developed behavior. If so, it is formally possible that environmental procedures capable of recovering a previously existent but currently absent language skill will have no relevance to the conditions under which the skill first emerged, and consequently do not provide a *developmental* analysis. The argument is a direct descendant of earlier disputes about a distinction between *learning* and *performance*. Some reasons for analyzing *recovery* as well as *first acquisitions* despite this formal possibility are offered by Sidman (1960, p. 100) and, less directly, by Baer (1972). However, while the merits of the dispute are being considered, there remains the challenging possibility of obviating the issue by analyzing *first acquisitions* as thoroughly as possible, to see what will prove possible. The institutionalized retardate with no prior history of a given language skill, or, preferably, of any language skill, offers exactly such a possibility.

4. Measures of inter-observer reliability were calculated for responses trained in each condition of this study, as well as all conditions of subsequent investigations included in this chapter. For purposes of saving space, the procedures for taking reliability and the results of these measures are not included as data, except for one study (Sailor, 1971) in which inter-observer agreement was directly related to the procedure of scoring. However, in all the studies reviewed, agreement between the experimenter and independent observer met more than adequately the reliability requirements generally accepted for speech and language research—i.e., above 85%.

5. It should be noted that Conditions II and III of the study were alternate procedures based on the findings of Condition I. If, in fact, generalization from receptive training to productive speech had occurred in Condition I, the contingencies of reinforcement for receptive training would have been reversed in Condition II, to see if the subjects' productive usage also reversed. Condition III would have then re-reversed the reinforcement contingencies and, again, probed for changes in productive usage.

6. Both the -s and -es plural endings follow the notations of ordinary orthography. Linguistically, they are categorized (Gleason, 1965) under the plural morpheme $\{Z_1\}$, [-s∼-z∼-iz]; the voiceless -s is noted in linguistic terms as [-s], and follows stems ending in [p t k f ⊖]; the -es ending, extra syllable plus voice, is noted as [-iz], and is added to stems that end in [s z ŝ ẑ ĉ ĵ]. The remaining voiced plural allomorph [-z] was not evoked in the training procedures of the study.

7. The durability of effects from reinforced probes could not be examined as thoroughly as desired, because David was assigned to a different program within the institution which did not allow for the scheduling of regular experimental sessions at the necessary times. However, he was spotchecked at five, eight, and twelve weeks following the last experimental session (object 100), and his pattern of correct generalization in the unreinforced probes was still near-perfect at those times.

8. The minimum number of trials to reach criterion during comparative and superlative training was 0, if the first ten trials were correct, as they might well be in a generative subject. During the training of opposites, the minimum number was either zero or one: zero if the subject by chance pointed correctly on the first trial, one if he made an error on that trial. In either case, the trial had enough cue function to allow a generative subject to be correct on all further trials. Nevertheless, in the latter case the subject was scored as making an error (even though he could not be expected to know the opposite labels exemplified by the first presentation of a new stimulus set).

CHAPTER II

ESTABLISHING VERBAL IMITATION SKILLS AND FUNCTIONAL SPEECH IN AUTISTIC CHILDREN[1]

SHEILA MCKENNA-HARTUNG AND JURGEN R. HARTUNG

THE OBJECTIVES of this chapter are threefold. First, an attempt is made to demonstrate the importance of establishing verbal behavior in nonspeaking autistic children. Second, some of the theoretical foundations underlying verbal conditioning are discussed. And finally, the procedures and related theoretical implications are reviewed in some detail.

We also hope to compensate for the lack of direction and guidance given to the reader in previous verbal conditioning reports. Instead of reviewing many different methods completely, the important stages and trends of the verbal conditioning process are presented in a step-by-step fashion, incorporating the ideas and work of many contributors. The chapter thus outlines a procedure by which speech may be established. What follows is a convenient, nonexhaustive list of suggestions, and some theoretical foundations, which have been useful to us and which may prove useful to others. It is important to keep in mind that the following procedures must be adapted to fit the needs of the individual child. A cookbook approach does not do justice to the child's level of functioning, nor does it recognize the sensitivity of operant work to individual variation.

INFANTILE AUTISM

Leo Kanner coined the diagnostic phrase *early infantile autism* in 1944 (Kanner, 1944) to apply to that baffling, bizarre syndrome which he had described one year earlier in an article appearing in

The Nervous Child (Kanner, 1943). These children were aloof and withdrawn, seemingly in a dreamworld—hence, *autistic*. They seem to have been unusual from birth on; thus the onset was *early*.

Rimland (1964) gives an excellent summary of the symptomatology of this group of children. They are apathetic and unresponsive. Headbanging is common, as is rhythmic rocking or twirling. They become very attached to particular toys or objects, and become easily upset if the environment is changed in any way. The child may sit and stare for hours into space. These children tend to be so unresponsive, in fact, that the parents generally suspect that they are deaf, causing them to seek professional help. Unlike a child with a true hearing loss, however, an autistic child will sometimes react to a certain sound, or repeat tunes or things others have said.

Nor are these children mentally retarded. Indeed, their development is sometimes precocious up until the second year of life. Often, the child begins talking early and then suddenly, around his second birthday, stops speaking altogether or retains a few words which he repeats endlessly (Rimland, 1964; Turner, 1970).

There is some recent evidence (Lovaas, Schreibman, Koegel, and Rehm, 1971) on the nature of autism from Ivar Lovaas, who was one of the pioneers in using operant techniques to train autistic children in verbal and social skills (Lovaas, Berberich, Perloff, and Schaeffer, 1966; Lovaas, 1968). He suspected that the autistic child's classic lack of responsivity may result from an attentional deficit. Specifically, Lovaas hypothesized that these children cannot attend to a complex stimulus, but react to such a stimulus with *over-selectivity* (attending to only one aspect). Thus, after a great many trials, the child may come to reliably respond with "mm" when presented with the therapist saying "mm" while he is watching her face. If, however, she turns her head away and says "mm," there is no response. It is as if the child never heard the auditory cue, and had become conditioned to respond to the visual cue alone.

To check this out, Lovaas and his co-workers devised a threefold stimulus (auditory, visual, and tactile) and taught normal, retarded, and autistic children to respond to the discriminatory stimulus (S^D) with a bar-press. They then tested each group on responsiveness to each of the three stimuli presented separately. They found that the normal children responded to all three, the retarded to two, and the autistic to only one of the three parts of the S^D.

If this finding is borne out with other autistic children, it has definite implications for any training program. As Lovaas points out, most learning is based on the contiguous or near-contiguous presentation of two stimuli. If the autistic child cannot attend to both stimuli at once, perhaps each stimulus needs to be presented separately in order for both to be learned. One way we could envision doing this in a verbal learning paradigm would be to present the visual and auditory stimuli in relays: e.g., hold up a picture and turn the child's face toward it; cover the child's eyes and say "What is this?"; uncover his eyes, turn his face toward picture; cover his eyes, and say "This is a ball." This technique would, of course, have to be tried out before one could assess its value in comparison to the more *traditional* methods to be covered in this chapter.

THE VITAL ROLE OF SPEECH FOR RECOVERY

Experience with autistic children has disclosed that about half of all autistic children use speech, while the others are mute. For example, from a sample of twenty-four autistic children, Rimland (1964) found ten who did not speak. These nonspeaking children can be extremely poor prognostic risks. From follow-up studies, Kanner and Eisenberg (1955) found that the presence or absence of speech by age five has important prognostic implications. Almost without exception, those children who had not developed speech by the age of five failed to improve their level of socialization in later years. From a study of the autistic child in adolescence, Eisenberg (1956) showed the significant relationship of speech to recovery. He reported that of thirty-two children who had useful speech by the age of five, sixteen obtained *fair* to *good* social adjustment, while only one out of thirty-one from the nonspeaking group reached the *fair* level. Early speech, then, seems to be an important factor. At the present state of our knowledge and experience, it is almost impossible to determine how useful speech must be before a child can make some degree of social adjustment. It is also unclear as to how socialized the child must be in order for speech to develop. Although speech sometimes can be developed via special procedures, this does not necessarily insure good social adjustment. What we do know is that the child who fails to use speech before the age of five is often the one who makes the worst social adjustment and suffers the most in later years (Eisenberg, 1956).

SPEECH PATTERNS IN AUTISM

Those autistic children who do speak tend to have a highly characteristic form of speech. The main feature of their speech is that it is not generally used as a means of communication, but rather as a response to certain stimuli. Thus, they may name objects, but they will rarely ask or answer questions. The word *yes* is almost never used, affirmation being indicated by simply repeating the question. Pronouns tend to be absent, and when they are used they are often reversed, e.g., *you* rather than *I* (Rimland, 1964). Cunningham (1966) feels that this pronoun reversal is purely a linguistic confusion and not a matter of identity. In the five years that he studied Jimmy, an autistic boy, the child often said *me* rather than *you* and vice-versa, but never once referred to the investigator as *Jimmy* or to himself as *Cunny*.

At age 6½, when Jimmy was first studied, his speech was classified at the twenty-four to thirty month level, and it did not change appreciably in the next five years (Cunningham, 1966). The child exhibited all the speech characteristics of autism mentioned above (pronominal reversal, affirmation by repetition, lack of questions). In addition, Cunningham found that:

1. Articulation was variable—sometimes very good, sometimes very poor;

2. More incomplete sentences were used than the normal twenty-four to thirty-month-olds—words would simply be omitted seeming to indicate a poor grasp of the rules of syntax;

3. More *egocentric* and *emotionally toned* remarks were made by Jimmy then the normals—he tended to make demands and requests rather than give information;

4. There was more immediate repetition of his own or E's remarks than the normals;

5. Variety of words, length of sentences, and frequencies of various parts of speech (nouns, verbs, adjectives, articles, adverbs, prepositions, conjunctions, and interjections) were no different from the average twenty-four to thirty-month-old.

Ferster (1961) has described the speech of autistic children as characterized by mands rather than tacts. Similar to Cunningham's *egocentric* and *emotionally toned* phrases, the mand is a simple verbal response like "Candy" or "Let me out." People tend to reinforce mands by responding to them in order to end the aversive effect of continuous manding. The mand benefits only the speaker, and is usually relevant to his current state of deprivation. On the other hand the tact, which benefits the listener and has nothing to do with the internal pressures of the speaker (e.g., "this is a chair") is absent or extremely weak in the autistic child.

Kanner (1946) further described the speech of autistic children as often metaphorical. Thus, one little girl's mother used to point out to her when she cried that the toy dog or rabbit did not cry. Thereafter, when afraid and about to cry she would say, "Rabbits don't cry; Dogs don't cry; Seals don't cry; Dinosaurs don't cry," etc. The speaking autistic child may engage in *semantic transfers* in which the metaphorical phrase is over-generalized. One boy called a bread basket a "home bakery." This then was his term for a coal basket, a waste basket, and a sewing basket.

THE ROLE OF IMITATION IN FUNCTIONAL SPEECH

Although there remains a great deal of controversy over the role of imitation in speech, we believe that normal children initially acquire words by hearing speech. Perhaps it is not until the child has heard certain sounds over and over again that he will mimic these sounds as others produce them. Schell, Stark and Giddan (1967) approach the area of verbal training from a similar perspective: "Our efforts have been based on the assumption that children first learn to speak by imitation (p. 53)." During normal development, these verbal imitations probably are selectively reinforced in such a manner that a complex verbal repertoire develops. Having accepted this theory as a fundamentally correct view of verbal learning, Lovaas et al. (1966) claim that the first step in creating speech is to establish conditions in which imitation of vocal sounds will be learned. This implies that if a child is to learn to speak, it is necessary not only that he vocalize but also that his vocalizations be brought under the control of the vocal stimuli of others. Risley and Wolf (1967) went one step further by stating that the presence or absence of echolalia (a term applied primarily to autistic children who will consistently mimic the verbal productions of others) is an important predictor of ease of establishing more normal speech.

Clearly related, but more affirmative in nature, is the major theoretical assumption underlying the principals and methods presented here. Not only is imitative verbal behavior considered a prerequisite to functional speech, but functional speech cannot be developed in a nonspeaking child unless that child first imitates the verbal responses of others consistently. Once the child can imitate most words, phrases, and sentences, a diversified topography of verbal behavior can be produced by individual prompting. In accounting for the progress of an autistic child, Wolf, Risley, and Mees (1964) stated:

> Dicky's ability to mimic entire phrases and sentences was apparently crucial to the rapid progress in verbal training . . . without this mimicking behavior a long and arduous handshaping procedure would have been necessary to establish responses of the required topography. (p. 311)

THE FAILURE TO IMITATE

One of the most striking features of the autistic child's behavior is his apparent inability to imitate. While imitation is a prominent response disposition in normal young children, autistic children typically do not imitate other people. An exception, however, applies to those autistic children who rather spontaneously become echolalic usually at or beyond the age of six years.

No clear understanding prevails as to why children imitate or fail to imitate. Some writers (Piaget, 1951; Ritvo and Provence, 1953) seem to hold to the idea that a self-world kind of confusion is the basis for a lack of imitative behavior. Ritvo and Provence hypothesize that the child fails to imitate or imitates less because of a limited self, non-self differentiation. If this is the case, autistic children might profit from an increased emphasis on the exploration of boundaries and limits of their own bodies. One way of doing this is to select imitative responses to be learned that would enhance awareness of self, non-self differentiation (as in *pat-a-cake, bye-bye,* kissing, *so big,* and the words *I* and *yes*).

The nonspeaking autistic child, then, characteristically fails to imitate the behavior of others before the age of five. As a result, he never passes through what appears to be a necessary stage in speech development and thus ends up not using speech by the time he is five years old. This child has a very poor chance of making any sort of *normal* social adjustment.

Stages and Trends in Conditioning Verbal Repertories

The Training Environment

The training environment may vary depending upon the particular stage of conditioning or the needs of the child at the time. At the onset, a room with limited possibilities for distractions is recommended (that is, simple furniture, nonbreakables). Such a setting will usually lower the occurrence of disruptive behavior. One researcher (Hewett, 1965) developed a special isolation booth which, because of its limited size, made disruptive behavior almost impossible. The booth was divided into two sections by a shutter which the clinician could raise and lower. The section for the child contained a chair facing the shutter which, when raised, revealed the section where the clinician sat facing the subject. A light focused on the clinician's side of the booth. When the shutter was lowered, the subject was deprived of light, rewards, and the presence of the clinician.

The Limitation of Disruptive Behavior

The limitation of disruptive behavior becomes particularly important when working with nonspeaking autistic children, who in general tend to be quite disruptive and destructive in their behavior. Some ways of limiting such behavior are suggested here.

One simple method allows the clinician to physically restrain a child by holding the child's legs between his legs while working on verbal behavior.

Lovaas et al. (1966) found a more direct approach to be quite successful. He delivered punishment (spanking and shouting by an adult) for inattentive, self-destructive, and tantrumous behavior which interfered with the training. Most of the undesirable behaviors were thereby suppressed within one week. Incorrect vocal behavior was never punished and should never be punished.

Risley and Wolf (1967) use a technique which they call *time-out from positive reinforcement.* When mild disruptive behavior occurs, the clinician merely looks away from the child. For more disruptive behavior, the time-out procedure involves both extinction of the behavior and removal of the reinforcer—the clinician either leaves the room with the reinforcer or the child is removed to an isolated room.

Turner (1970) reports on the use of time-outs to handle tantrums in a 4½ year old autistic boy, Tommy. She and her co-workers found that relatively short times-outs—not more than five minutes—were more effective. This seemed to lessen the chance of the child's *forgetting* the reason for the time-out. The child was always immediately returned to the situation at the end of the time-out and given another chance to comply. This procedure was highly effective in limiting Tommy's disruptive behavior.

These procedures should not be tried out haphazardly on a particular child. The method chosen should be geared to the child's needs and be used consistently until the child's behavior requires a different approach. An exception, however, applies to general methods of restraint. A clinician may hold the child's legs in his own or in some other manner physically restrict the child's movements while still effectively applying one of the other techniques mentioned.

Milstead, Taylor, and Hall (1972) devised an intriguing method of eliminating off-task behavior during training periods while using engagement in that same behavior as a reinforcement for performance of the task. A seven-year-old autistic girl was seated in a chair, then put under physical restraints at wrists, ankles, and torso. The E also placed his arm across the girl's knees and his assistant held her at the shoulders, making any body movement very difficult. Release from the restraints was contingent on a correct verbal imitation. She was shown a picture of a common household object and prompted verbally ("Cathy, what is this? Cathy, is this a table?"). A correct imitation *earned* her five minutes of free play. Three successful trials were run per session with the number of imitations required for release increasing from one to five.

Whenever any disruptive behavior occurred when the child was tied down to the chair (e.g., crying, spitting), E ignored it by simply looking away until the behavior was discontinued.

This procedure had a dramatic effect on the verbal responses of the child (see Fig. II.1). In order to test that the experimental procedure was the significant factor in increasing the rapidity of her imitations, a reversal period (restraints applied for each correct imitation) was run, followed by a return to the initial contingency (one release per imitation).

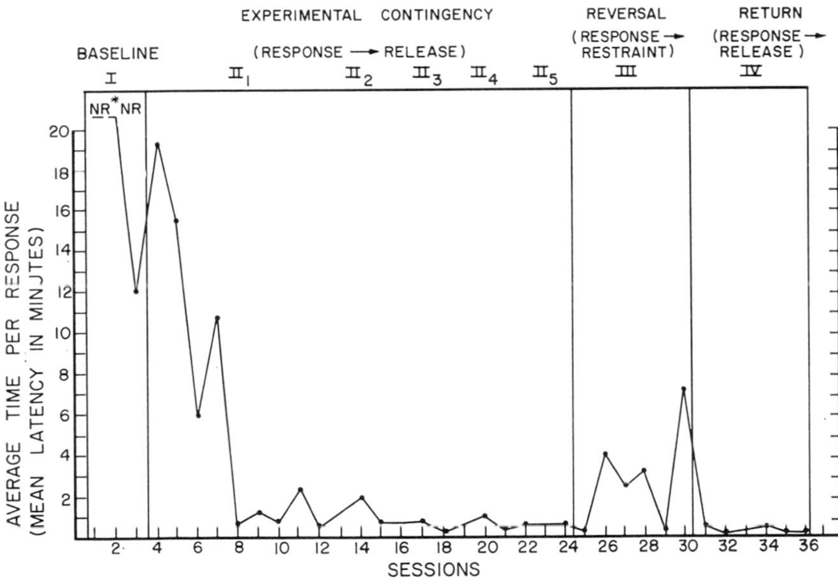

Figure II.1. Escape from physical restraint as a reinforcer for verbal imitation. (Milstead, Taylor & Hall, 1972.)

That procedures to limit disruptive behavior must be fitted to the individual child is beautifully illustrated by the experience of the group at Wisconsin Children's Treatment Center (Turner, 1970). For Tommy, as previously discussed, a time-out room was extremely successful in limiting his temper tantrums. For seven-year-old Wendy, however, placing her in the time-out room merely increased her violent behaviors (head banging, pulling out clumps of hair, biting self on arms or legs). It was decided that electric shock, contingent on violent behavior, was the best course of action. When Wendy next attacked E, she was shocked immediately. Within one session, her disruptive behavior diminished dramatically. After most of her aggressive behavior had stopped, the staff only needed to carry the apparatus with them to limit her behavior.

Risley (1968a) feels that shock as a punisher for undesirable behavior is appropriate if other methods have been tried and have failed. With a six-year-old autistic girl who continuously climbed onto high places, a ten minute time-out contingent on climbing had no effect. When shock was made contingent on climbing, this behavior was eliminated. Risley points out that the aversive method did not (as the conditioned suppression literature suggests) suppress behaviors other than the one being punished, nor did it make S wish to avoid E or the laboratory. In fact, there was an increase in imitative behaviors after shock was introduced. The only change in S's behavior toward E post-shock was an increase in eye contact (both eye contact and imitation were being reinforced with food and praise).

Types of Reinforcers

What reinforcer is used depends to a great extent on the child in question. Autistic children, being so out of contact with others, do not generally respond to social reinforcers such as praise at the beginning of treatment. The most generally effective and most often used reinforcer for these children is food. What food is used depends on the particular child's preference. Candy is typically used because of its almost universal appeal. M&M candies have become legendary in the conditioning field because they are uniform in size, convenient to deposit in the S's mouth, and quickly chewed and swallowed (the human equivalent of the omnipresent food pellet).

Autistic children tend to have unique eating habits and preferences (Rimland, 1964). If the child has a favorite food, this is an excellent reinforcer. Thus, for those children who prefer salty foods to sweets, bits of potato chips are good reinforcers. For the little girl in Risley's (1968a) study, the preferred food was milk. Whatever food is chosen as the reinforcer, however, its consumption should be strictly limited to training sessions.

Occasionally, a child is so uncooperative that snack-type foods are not a sufficient reward. In these cases, a meal may be used for training sessions, with each bite being delivered as a reinforcer for the desired behavior. If necessary, all the S's meals may have to be used as training sessions so that no food is eaten unless desired behavior is elicited. If the response required for reinforcement is made simple enough (e.g., something already in the patient's repertoire, now being brought under stimulus control) it is unlikely that too many meals will be missed. Sherman (1965) found this an effective technique with mute psychotic adults, and it appears to be useful with nonspeaking children as well.

Ferster (1961) used a token system of reinforcement with autistic children. At first they were rewarded with food for performing the desired behavior. Later, they were given coins as reinforcers, a given number of which had to be accumulated in order to exchange them for candy.

Milstead et al.'s (1972) innovative method of release from restraint as a reinforcer has been described earlier in this chapter. Other prized activities such as being spun around in the air, or time with a favorite toy can be used as reinforcers also.

Pairing With a Social Reinforcer

Whenever any primary or unlearned reinforcer such as food is used, it should always be preceded by or paired with a learned social reinforcer, such as praise. Thus, Milstead et al. (1972) always said "Good" and "Good girl," and patted S on the back while removing the restraints. Metz (1965) points out that once the word *good* is established as a reinforcer, it can be instrumental in shaping new behavior—a desired variation in behavior can immediately be reinforced by E from anywhere in the room.

Before giving Wendy the aversive stimulus of electric shock for attacking behavior, Turner (1970) always shouted "no," so that disapproval would come to have S^D properties for her. The effectiveness of this was evidenced later when she cried after being scolded by a staff member.

Schedules of Reinforcement

Another reason to establish social reinforcers while rewarding the child's performance is that one would not wish to go on rewarding with food indefinitely. The whole point of these procedures is to get the child's behavior to approximate as nearly as possible that of a *normal* child. Most children do not have someone shoving an M&M down their throats everytime they do something adults find worthwhile, or shocking them for having temper tantrums. By getting the autistic child to respond to a commonly used reinforcer like praise, you are helping socialize as well as train him.

Not only is food as a reinforcer optimally replaced by praise, high, continuous rates of reinforcement are also replaced by low, intermittent rates of reinforcement. A good example of this is found in Hull and Dokecki (1968). Using candy, verbal praise, and tokens as reinforcers with an autistic, visually-handicapped child, three schedules of reinforcement were employed: 1) continuous reinforcement (CRF) to establish the response; 2) fixed ratio of one reinforcement for every four responses (FR4)—a transitional schedule; and 3) variable ratio (VR) to stabilize the response. Milstead et al. (1972) go from continuous reinforcement to fixed ratios of two, three, four, then five responses required for reinforcement. Since intermittent reinforcement seems to establish the most persistent behaviors (most difficult to extinguish), it is wise to aim for a VR frequency if you wish to establish the strongest response possible.

The importance of changing the reinforcement schedule slowly is emphasized by Dehn (1970). Dehn found that if the schedule is changed abruptly, autistic children will exhibit a marked increase in negative behavior (abrupt change = 26% increase in negative behavior; slow change = 2% rise in negativism). Negativism was defined here as refusal to respond when the child has performed the requested task in the immediate past.

In teaching imitation skills, it has been found that nonrewarded tasks will tend to be imitated if they are imbedded in a series of rewarded tasks (Metz, 1965; Peterson, 1968). This kind of early generalization may lay the groundwork for later generalizations, so once the child is reliably responding, it may be helpful to intermittently include some nonreinforced items.

Conditioning Attention and Eye Contact

Before operant procedures can be utilized satisfactorily, the clinician must have the attention of his subject. Since nonspeaking autistic children are characterized by an unusually limited span of attention, as well as an almost complete failure to attend to other people in general, it is imperative that the clinician first establish some control over this behavior. Imitative behavior appears to be partly contingent upon eye contact and other-directed attention. The child who does not attend adequately to outside cues is incapable of modifying his behavior accordingly and will hardly establish an imitative repertoire leading to the effective use of language.

Risley et al. (1967) maintain the child's attention by having the clinician hold the reinforcer directly in front of his own face. Since the child will tend to look at the reinforcer (in this case food), this procedure ensures that he will be looking toward the clinician's face. To shape eye contact, Risley (1968a) presents the following procedure:

1) Reinforcement given when S looks at cup (with milk in it);

2) Cup moved gradually up toward E's face;

3) Glances at E reinforced;

4) When eye contacts occur at the rate of 6/minute, reinforcement for looking at cup discontinued;

5) Successively longer eye contacts necessary for reinforcement until S gives focussed stare of one second or longer;

6) Concurrent with #5, E gradually moves cup away from face until it is out of sight.

The use of loud noises and manual guidance are more direct and sometimes more effective ways of drawing the child's attention. Slapping a table top loudly or slapping the child's knee seems to draw immediate attention. Yelling or shouting the child's name or some appropriate phrase is also effective. Sometimes the clinician may find it beneficial to yell the word or phrase to be learned. Finally, holding or turning the child's head so that he faces the clinician may be useful.

Blake and Moss (1967), using Hewett's isolation booth, shaped eye contact by first leaving the subject in total darkness. Then, every five seconds, the clinician opened the shutter, put on the lights, and said "Hi, Dolly, look at me!" Rewards were made contingent on the subject's looking in the direction of the clinician. If the subject looked elsewhere, the shutter was dropped for fifteen seconds.

Training Motor Imitation

In reference to the training of autistic children, Goldstein (1959) has said: "These children learn only by doing: through specific movements and activities, they can be brought into contact with a desired task." (p. 549.) Experience with autistic children has shown that, to a large extent, Goldstein seems to be right. For instance, autistic children do appear to learn motor imitations more readily than verbal imitations, especially at the beginning of an operant conditioning program. From such evidence, we argue in favor of conditioning a repertoire of consistent motor imitative behaviors before actually beginning vocal training.

Peterson (1968) suggests beginning with an assessment of the child's current imitative repertoire. This is done by saying to the child "Do this," then making a motor response and repeating this procedure for a variety of motor tasks. With autistic children, this repertoire is likely to be nonexistent, and they will fail to imitate E.

The child will therefore have to be *guided through* the desired behavior at first, the guidance being faded-out as response strength increases. Risley (1968a), for example, used the following procedure to train imitative hand clapping:

1) E clapped his hands and reinforced the child's clapping (a behavior already in her spontaneous repertoire); her clapping did not follow (i.e., imitate) his, however, so he *led her through* the imitation as follows—

2) E clapped his hands, then held S's arms and clapped her hands together;

3) Reinforcement given at first for not struggling, then for slight cooperative movements;

4) E's force faded until he needed only to clap his hands, then touch S's arms and she would clap her hands;

5) Touching S's arms faded, then eliminated.

Metz (1965) gives an elaborate account of conditioning imitative behavior in autistic children. He says that for imitation to occur: 1) the behavior must be similar to and occur on the occasion of example by a model; 2) S must respond to the imitative stimulus differentially. For example, if E touches his toes and S touches his toes, then E touches his head and S touches his toes, he has not learned imitation, but rather has learned the model's behavior (i.e., saying "do this" and making a movement) as a cue for responding only.

Metz (1965) used the following format to condition imitation:

1. Established the word *good* as a reward. Regardless of the S's behavior, E said "good," handed S a token and showed him how to insert token in formboard to receive food. Schedule gradually shifted from CRF to FR-3.

2. Training imitation of three pairs of tasks. Each pair employed the same materials, to assure that S was responding to S^D. E demonstrated task, then physically guided action, then faded-out guidance. A task was considered learned if S imitated it correctly after E's demonstration, without help, six times in a row when it was presented in a series with the five other tasks.

3. Tested for generalized responses. Ten new tasks were presented along with six familiar tasks. If a task was imitated two out of three times, it was considered passed.

4. Eight failed tasks and eight additional tasks were used for a second training period.

The tasks to be used for initial imitation training can be any of innumerable motor behaviors. Metz (1965) lists (among others) stamping a foot, operating a *busy box,* marking with crayon on paper, spinning a top. It is probably a good idea to start off with gross movements such as foot stamping, standing up, and sitting down, introducing the fine motor imitations somewhat later. Still later, the S should be taught facial imitations (sticking out tongue, nodding head, opening mouth) to prime him for the transition to verbal imitation.

Risley (1968b) sometimes incorporates the motor imitations into the verbal training, resulting in what he calls a *complex performance.* For example, the child might be expected to have his arms out to the side, palms of his hands turned back, face frowning, and make the statement "This too shall pass away." The intended result of this type of imitation training was to enable the children to listen to novel language performances and repeat them.

Occasionally a child will fail to generalize imitation training because he has not learned to attend to verbal cues ("Do this"). In such a case, a procedure used by Schell et al. (1967) may be helpful. They trained the S to push a lever when a light went off (visual cue). They then paired an auditory *click* with the dimming of the light. The click was presented alone (auditory S^D); the click was paired with the word *push;* the word *push* was presented alone (verbal S^D).

From Motor to Verbal Imitation

When the subject reaches the level where he imitates almost every new motor performance, vocal training is begun. The clinician now says, "Do this" ("Do this" is used to precede all motor and verbal imitative examples); but instead of making a motor response, he makes a vocal response. If the subject then fails to imitate the vocal response, the vocal response is set into a chain of nonvocal responses, progressively fading out the motor response component.

For example, the clinician might say, "Do this," rise from his chair and walk to the center of the room, turn towards the subject, say a word or syllable, and return to his seat. Such coupling of motor and vocal responses may be maintained for several demonstrations during which time the motor performance is made successively shorter and more economical of motion until finally the clinician can remain in his seat and elicit imitative verbal responses from the subject.

Eliciting Vocalizations

If the child does not make any sounds at all, it may be necessary to shape vocalization. Sherman (1965), working with a mute adult psychotic, started by reinforcing slight lip movements, then required more and more movement for reinforcement until the S was exhibiting a distinct and steady parting of the lips. At this point, his S spontaneously emitted a moan.

If the child does not spontaneously vocalize at this point, however, you can encourage phonation in several ways. You can reinforce imitation of activities which require control of the breath stream such as blowing out a match, blowing the nose, and clearing the throat (Pronovost et al., 1966; Sherman, 1965). Or, once you have the child imitating opening his mouth, you can push in his abdomen to force a vocalization (Schell et al., 1967).

The Systematic Selection of Vocal Responses

Lovaas et al. (1966) list three useful criteria for selecting vocal sounds that the nonspeaking child may readily learn:

1. Vocal sounds may be selected that can be prompted by manually moving the child through the sound. For instance, the clinician might emit the sound [b], holding the child's lips closed with his fingers and quickly removing them when the child exhales

2. The second criterion for the selection of words or sounds centers on their concomitant visual components. Such sounds as those of the labial consonant [m] and front vowels such as [a] are examples. In each case, the clinician should exaggerate their articulation.

3. Those words or sounds that the child already can use (those most frequently used) may be selected for training.

Lovaas et al. (1966) found that children would discriminate words with visual components more easily than those with only auditory components (the consonants [k], [g], [s], and [l] were very difficult for the nonspeaking autistic child and were mastered later than other sounds).

Establishing Control Over Vocal Responses

The assumption that children learn to speak by first imitating the vocal responses of others makes this, then, the most crucial stage in verbal conditioning. The procedure described here comes mainly from the work of Lovaas et al. (1966) with nonspeaking emotionally disturbed children, although the ideas of various other contributors are also included.

Initially, the child should be rewarded for all vocalizations and for visually fixating on the adult's mouth and/or eyes. Even those vocalizations that at first appear meaningless in terms of affecting later verbal behavior should be rewarded. Blake and Moss (1967) demonstrated the significance of reinforcing just such a general type of vocalization. They put a crying child into Hewett's (1965) isolation booth. The child learned that when she stopped crying, pretty colors being presented on a screen would go off. At first the child deliberately cried to reinstate the colors, but slowly the crying shifted to babbling sounds.

The child may now be rewarded only if he emits a sound within the prescribed time after an adult has emitted a sound. Some clinicians favor emitting a sound or word every ten seconds, while other present words more frequently, on the order of one about every four to five seconds. The time allotted for the child to respond is also somewhat arbitrary, although some investigators have followed the policy of progressively shortening the interval between the clinician's vocalization and the child's vocalization as training proceeds.

The next stage requires that the child be rewarded only if the sound he emitted within the prescribed time interval resembled the adult's sound. Most children will require prompting to complete this stage. By holding and guiding the child's lips, the clinician usually can evoke the desired response. The prompting is then gradually faded, first by moving the fingers away from the mouth to the cheek, then by placing them gently on the jaw, and finally by removing them from the child's face altogether. Now the child should be able to reproduce the response without any further prompting. Finally, the child is rewarded only if his vocalizations very closely match the clinician's vocalizations—that is, if the child's response was imitative.

From Sounds to Words

Sherman's (1965) procedure to shape vocalizations is as follows:

1) Teach S to blow out match.
2) Have S *blow out* match without match present.
3) Have S imitate hissing sound;
4) Imitation of aspirate *h;*
5) *ppph* imitated, then *aaa;*
6) *fff, oo,* and *da* imitated (all the components of the word *food*);
7) Sound Chaining: "Say fff (pause while S responds) Say oo," and reinforce.
8) Gradually change instruction to "Say fff (pause while S responds) oo";
9) Change to "Say fffoo";
10) *da* is added to the chain by a procedure similar to #7-10.
11) S should finally be consistently imitating to word *food.* An added feature of this particular example is that the word being shaped *(food)* was reinforced by its proper referent (food). Thus, a form of functional speech was built into the training from the beginning.

Once the child reliably and immediately imitates his first word, a new word may be presented. The two words should then be presented alternately. New words should always be interspersed with old words, since a new response has not been learned (added to the child's vocabulary) until the child can reproduce the word when it its presented again after other words have been learned, and following a passage of time.

The Sudden Emergence of Echolalia

After the child acquires the first word, he may take a great deal more time to imitate the second word. Although such a manner of responding appears to be characteristic at this level of verbal training, it also seems directly related to a rather unsuspected occurrence—the sudden emergence of echolalia. To quote from Risley and Wolf (1967):

> Usually by the second or third word, a general imitative response class will have been established, i.e., the child will then reliably and immediately imitate any new word. (p. 77)

A number of investigators have observed and described this phenomenon in their own studies, but have failed to mention that this pattern also occurs somewhat consistently in other studies. For example, Hewett (1965) reported:

> Once the first two words *go* and *my* were learned, Peter's speech became echolalic and he readily attempted to imitate all words the teachers said. (p. 933)

A study by Isaacs, Thomas, and Goldiamond (1960) reveals that a form of *sudden echolalia* also seems to occur among previously nonspeaking adult schizophrenics:

> At the sixth session (at the end of week six), when the experimenter said, "Say gum, gum," the subject suddenly said, "Gum please." This response was accompanied by reinstatement of other responses of this class, that is, the subject answered questions regarding his name and age. Thereafter, he responded to questions by the experimenter both in individual sessions and in group sessions, but answered to no one else. (p. 9)

Hartung (1970) first observed this phenomenon in the very early stages of a program designed to condition verbal behavior in a nonspeaking autistic boy. Following the accurate and reliable imitation of the word *please,* the subject did not imitate another word for two full months, even under the pressure of excessive prodding. At the end of the two-month period, he finally mimicked the words *potato chip.* Two more weeks were required before he could successfully combine the words *please* and *potato chip* to form the request *please potato chip.* Once this was accomplished, the subject suddenly began to echo almost every word and some short phrases. Generally, all one-syllable words were clearly imitated. Words of two or more syllables were more often imitated crudely, if at all. At first the subject only imitated the therapist, but eventually his imitative response generalized somewhat to other adults. Although he generalized a few words to many people, he continued to reliably and immediately imitate only the therapist.

The Phenomenon of Silent Speech

A number of equally valid explanations can be given to account for the sudden emergence of echolalia. Possibly the autistic child possessed an inner vocabulary all along which he failed to express until he vame echolalic. Such an explanation could account for the sudden acquisition and unusually good pronunciation of words characteristic of the echolalic stage. A closer inspection of the speech characteristics of autistic children suggests that this is a reasonable interpretation.

The speech patterns of autistic children seem to indicate that many of these children develop an unexpressed side of speech but fail to develop the expressive side. A good example of this is the fact that whispering seems to be common among nonspeaking autistic children. The whispering, however, is almost always noncommunicative and unintelligible. The autistic child may initially acquire words silently by hearing them, and it is not until he is willing to imitate the vocalizations of others that his range of words becomes apparent.

Lending further support to this theory is the observation that frequently those autistic children who do not speak are the very ones who had an unusually advanced vocabulary when they were younger. Wolff and Chess (1965) feel that the unusual use of metaphor and symbolic langauge characteristic of both the speaking and the nonspeaking autistic child appears to be the outcome of a relatively advanced level of language development distorted by "repetitive clinging to former modes of expression. . . ."

That nonspeaking autistic children possess a *silent vocabulary* was demonstrated by an autistic child studied by Hartung (1970). All those persons in close daily contact with the child, such as his parents, his teachers, and his clinician, reported having heard his occasional whispering, which they were, however, only infrequently able to understand because of the low volume and idiosyncratic words. The child also displayed unusually good pronunciation once echolalia began. He was able to pronounce well such difficult phrases as *San Francisco* after just one attempt. Soon after echolalia became a prominent feature of the boy's verbal behavior, Hartung found he could count from one to ten. The clarity and rapidity with which he could do this supports the belief that an *unexpressed speech facility* must have been in existence for some time.

The Transition from Imitation to Naming

The following is an integration of the procedures used by Risley and Wolf (1967), Lovaas et al. (1966), and Hartung (1970). Naming is defined as the emission of an appropriate verbal response in the presence of some stimulus object. After imitative responses occur with high probability and short latency following each verbal prompting, stimulus control is shifted from the verbal promptings (imitation) to appropriate objects and pictures (naming).

A picture or object is presented with the verbal prompting, and the child is reinforced for imitating the name. Then the imitative prompting is faded out while the child continues to receive reinforcement for saying the name of the object: (1) the clinician holds up an object (with the reinforcer behind the object) and asks, "What is this?" When the child looks at it, the clinician immediately prompts with the object's name. The child is reinforced for imitating the prompting. When the child is reliably looking at the object without the food being held behind it, the time between the question "What is this?" and the prompting is gradually lengthened to more than five seconds. If after several trials the child continues to wait for the presentation of the verbal prompting, partial prompting is given, for example, "trr" for train. If the correct response does not occur within about three seconds more, the complete prompting is then presented. A correct response results in a bite of food and a social reward such as *right* or *good*. (2) When the child begins saying the name when only the partial prompting is presented, the clinician continues the above procedure but begins to say the partial promptings more softly. (3) Whenever the child inappropriately imitates the question "What is this?" a time-out is programmed, that is, the object is withdrawn and the clinician looks down at the table maintaining about ten seconds of silence.

Stark, Giddan, and Meisel (1968) used a visual shaping procedure to make the transition from imitation to naming. They taught an autistic child to imitate the sounds [m] and [a]. They then presented cards with the letters *m* and *o* and rewarded him for imitating [m] when shown the M card and [a] when shown the O card. The child was finally *reading* the cards. They combined the letters M and O to make *MO* and placed this label under a picture of the S's mother. Later he correctly labeled such items as knee, eye, pie, bow, map.

Answering Questions

Two methods of fading out prompting stimuli are suggested for teaching the child to answer questions. The first method is similar to that used to establish naming. (1) First, teach the child to imitate "How are you? Fine." Then the question is faded by gradually lengthening the time between the question, "How are you?" and the answer, "Fine," to more than five seconds. This procedure does not involve fading in the usually applied sense of that word (as in method two). One advantage of lengthening the time interval between the stimulus question, "How are you?" and the response, "Fine!" is that many children will tend to give an anticipatory response, saying, "Fine" before the clinician prompts that response. Thus, by lengthening the interval between question and answer, the clinician is establishing proper stimulus control of new responses. (2) The child first is given both the question and answer ("How are you? Fine.") for imitation. Gradually the question part is faded by saying it softly and quickly while emphasizing the answer ("How are you? FINE.").[2]

The Establishment of Phrases

The first step in establishing phrases is the same as the procedure used to teach individual words: (1) Mimicking of phrases is reinforced until the phrases are consistently imitated. (2) Then control should be shifted to appropriate circumstances by introducing partial promptings (the first word or two of a phrase), which are gradually faded out. Sentences such as "that's a . . . . . ." or "I want . . . ." may be taught using vocabulary words that the child already knows. (3) Finally, more varied sentences such as "My name is ....," "I live at ....," or "I am .... years old" can be taught.

Conditioning Functional Speech

At this point in verbal training, social and natural reinforcers can be used to maintain the variety of phrases learned. If the child can be shown that his verbal responses change something in his immediate environment, then it is more probable that language will become spontaneous and situationally appropriate. The socially rewarding value of an appropriate response may be taught the child in the following way: The clinician says, "Open the door," when the child wants out. If the child imitates the sentence, the clinician opens the door. Next, the partial prompting "Open" is used for the same procedure. This partial prompting is gradually faded out until the clinician can put his hand on the doorknob, look at the child, and expect the child to respond with, "Open the door." The latter promptings of a hand on the doorknob and looking are also faded out and replaced with, "What do you want?" This is done by mumbling the question softly as the child and the clinician approach the door and then increasing the volume on succeeding trials. Whenever the child inappropriately imitates "What do you want?" the clinician should repeat the question at a lower volume and follow it with a loud partial prompt. (For example, "What do you want? OPEN"). On succeeding trials, the partial prompting "Open," is then decreased in volume until the child responds to the closed door and question with, "Open the door."

The particular likes and dislikes of a child may serve as effective natural reinforcers. For one autistic boy, having a hand placed on the top of his head was aversive. His immediate reaction was to squirm away. The clinician made use of this by placing his hand firmly atop the child's head and simultaneously saying, "Stop it." The child, being echolalic, immediately responded with "Stop it," at which point the clinician quickly removed his hand. Withing thirty minutes, the child no longer needed the clinician's prompt to respond correctly with "Stop it" each time a hand was placed on his head. (The statement "Stop it" occurred spontaneously on one of the trials; fading was not required.) A week passed before the clinician again placed his hand on the child's head. Without prompting, the child immediately shouted, "Stop it!" Elaborations of the phrase were subsequently introduced by adding more words (for example, "Stop it, Jurgen. Please stop it, Jurgen").

Schell et al. (1967) made use of a natural reinforcer, that they discovered accidently, to establish functional speech. They gave the child cereal as a reinforcer instead of the usual candy—he threw the cereal away. The clinician then held the cereal in one hand and the candy in the other, and would open one hand and say "no, no" for the cereal and "Candy, yes" for the candy. Then she would give him the candy. After this, the child began handing the cereal back. When he did this, the clinician would ask "What do you want?", wait until he made a sound, then say "Candy, yes!" while giving him the candy. The child began making a "nana" sound when given cereal and "kiki" when asked "What do you want?"

The Generalization of Appropriate Speech

Newly acquired appropriate speech often will spontaneously generalize to situations outside the specific conditioning environment. Self-initiated speech seems to generalize primarily because of its functional value for the child. The reason imitative verbal behavior generalizes is much less obvious. Baer, Peterson, and Sherman (1967) suggest that imitative behavior eventually develops reinforcing properties of its own. Because the child is consistently rewarded for responding like the adult, the concept of similarity becomes associated with food, and similarity becomes a secondary reinforcer. Thus, a child can provide himself with rewards by imitating adult behavior. Once established, verbal imitations may be maintained by periodic adult reinforcement. Peterson (1968) gives an example which he feels illustrates this phenomenon. A child was required to walk across the room, pick up and put on a fireman's hat and return, in imitation of E. She attempted to grasp it from the top, as did E, although such an exact imitation was not necessary for reinforcement. After several failures to precisely imitate E (her hand was too small), she grabbed the hat by the bill, put it on, and returned to her seat.

These explanations may account for the generalization of verbal behavior in both normal and abnormal children. However, newly acquired words do not spontaneously generalize as readily in non-speaking *emotionally disturbed* children as they do in normal children. It is therefore recommended that the clinician extend generalization systematically. This can be accomplished in a number of ways:

1. Reinforce appropriate speech in a variety of situations such as in the home, in a car, in stores, or out of doors in settings familiar and interesting to the child.

2. Strait (1958) found that generalization was facilitated by gradually bringing other people into the therapy room.

3. Select words for training that have relevance to the child (for example, *cookie* instead of *zebra* or *I am very tired* instead of *This too shall pass*).

4. Make optimal use of the social reinforcers *Good* or *That's right.* Such a verbal statement, besides bridging the gap between the appropriate response and the presentation of the food (making reinforcement contingencies more precise), also favors generalization to verbal reinforcers (social reinforcers).

5. Tramontana and Stimbert (1970) further generalized their autistic S's verbalizations by: writing up his current repertoire and distributing it to other persons involved with the child; having phone conversations with the child on an interoffice system and later at home; training the child's family to extend the technique into the home.

Parents as Therapists

Probably the most effective way of assuring that what the child learns in speech training will generalize into his daily life is to have the parents or caretakers trained in the use of the operant procedures being applied. Patterson, McNeal, Hawkins, and Phelps (1967) point out that many investigators in the area of behavior modification make vague reference to *stimulus generalization,* assuming that this will automatically insure generalization and persistence of the treatment effects. But, ". . . the members of the child's social environment are the final arbiters in determining the practical outcomes of intervention programmes (p. 181)."

The little girl to whom Risley (1968a) applied electric shock to stop her dangerous climbing behavior was later given shock by her mother for the same behavior in the home. Within four days climbing was reduced from 29/day to 2/day, then went to zero. On the fifty-first day of the in-home program, the shock device was removed and the mother was instructed to spank the child for climbing. But the mother felt this was a more brutal punishment, so another technique had to be devised. Using shock as a threat, the girl was taught to sit in a chair when told to do so. Starting on the seventy-sixth day, the girl was made to sit in a chair for a ten-minute time-out when she climbed. If she did not go to or stay in the chair, she was shocked. This technique was not quite as effective as direct shock, but it was retained because *it approximated normal child-rearing procedures.* The mother started using this time-out/shock technique for limiting other disruptive behavior as well as teaching her child five new imitations in the home.

The Wisconsin Children's Treatment Center (Turner, 1970)[3] uses the parents as "an integral part of the treatment team (p. 2148)." Attendance of parents at least once a week is required from the very beginning of treatment. Initially, the parents have a conference with a psychologist and a social worker who explain to them techniques for teaching their child more appropriate behaviors. The parents are then observed in short play periods with their children to assess how they reinforce desirable behavior. This data is then discussed with the parents. Next, a staff member monitors a session between parent and child. Staff participation is gradually faded out as the parent gains more control of the child's behavior. Parental involvement is then generalized to mealtime shaping, bathroom routines, and general play periods. The child's siblings are next brought into treatment to teach them more effective ways of interacting with S. For increased generalization, the child makes short trips with the family. Next he makes visits home, at first with a staff member along, later with his family alone. All trips and visits are discussed by the family and staff afterward.

Another method of parent training would be to have the

mother watch all training sessions through a one-way mirror. If an assistant E is available, he can explain the procedure to the mother while she is watching. This will serve two functions which will help the parent when she takes over training later on. First, she will learn the necessary principles of behavior modification. And second, she will see the effect of such procedures on her child over a span of time (*faith* in your technique is an important part of successful therapy).

The reader is again reminded that these procedures should not be taken as fixed and unchanging. One of the advantages of a behavioral technique lies in the possibilities of refining its procedures and adapting them to specific human problems.

REFERENCES

Baer, D., Peterson, R., and Sherman, J.: The development of imitation by reinforcing behavioral similarity as a model. *J. Exp. Anal. Behav., 10*: 405-416, 1967.

Blake, P., and Moss, T.: The development of socialization skills in an electively mute child. *Behav. Res. Ther., 5*:349-356, 1967.

Cunningham, M. A.: A five-year study of the language of an autistic child. *Journal of Child Psychology and Psychiatry, 7*:143-154, 1966.

Dehn, J. K.: An investigation of the development and maintenance of the negative behavior of autistic children. Unpublished doctoral dissertation, Washington University, 1970. *Diss. Abstr. Int., 31*: (4A) , 1902-1903, 1970.

Eisenberg, L.: The autistic child in adolescence. *Amer. J. Psychiat., 112*: 607-612, 1956.

Ferster, C. B.: Positive reinforcement and behavioral deficits of autistic children. *Child Development, 32*:437-456, 1961.

Goldstein, K.: Abnormal mental conditions in infancy. *J. Nerv. Ment. Dis., 48*:538-557, 1959.

Hartung, J. R.: A review of procedures of increase verbal imitation skills and functional speech in autistic children. *Journal of Speech and Hearing Disorders, 35*:203-217, 1970.

Hewett, F.: Teaching speech in an autistic child through operant conditioning. *Amer. J. Orthopsychiat., 35*:927-936, 1965.

Hull, H., and Dokecki, P.: Modification of the behavior of an autistic visually limited child: an experimental-clinical case study. Paper presented to the Annual Meeting of the Southwestern Psychological Association: New Orleans, Louisiana, April 18-20, 1968.

Isaacs, W., Thomas, J., and Goldiamond, I.: Application of operant conditioning to reinstate verbal behavior in psychotics. *J. Speech Hearing Dis., 25*:8-12, 1960) .

Kanner, L.: Austistic disturbances of affective contact. *The Nervous Child,*

2:217-250, 1943. Cited by L. Kanner: Irrelevant and methaphorical language in early infantile autism. *American Journal of Pediatrics, 103*:242-246, 1946.

Kanner, L.: Early infantile autism. *Journal of Pediatrics, 25*:211-217, 1944. Cited by L. Kanner: Irrelevant and metaphorical language in early infantile autism. *American Journal of Psychiatry, 103*:242-246, 1946.

Kanner, L.: Irrelevant and metaphorical language in early infantile autism. *American Journal of Psychiatry, 103*:242-246, 1946.

Kanner, L., and Eisenberg, L.: Notes on the follow-up studies of autistic children. In P. Hoch and J. Zubin (Eds.): *Psychopathology of Childhood*, New York, Grune and Stratton, 1955.

Kozloff, M. A.: Social and behavioral change in families of autistic children. Unpublished doctoral dissertation, Washington University, 1969. *Diss. Abst. Int., 30*: (12-A), 5543, 1970.

Lovaas, I., Berberich, J., Perloff, B., and Schaefter, B.: Acquisition of imitative speech by schizophrenic children. *Science, 151*:705-707, 1966.

Lovaas, I.: A program for the establishment of speech in psychotic children. In H. Sloane and B. MacAulay (Eds.) : *Operant Procedures in Remedial Speech and Language Training*. Boston, Houghton Mifflin, 1968.

Lovaas, I., Schreibman, L., Koegel, R., and Rehm, R.: Selective responding by autistic children to multiple sensory input. *Journal of Abnormal Psychology, 77*:211-222, 1971.

Metz, J. R.: Conditioning generalized imitation in autistic children. *Journal of Experimental Child Psychology, 2*:389-399, 1965.

Milstead, J., Taylor, D., and Hall, J.: Escape from physical restraint as a reinforcer for verbal imitation in an autistic child. Unpublished manuscript, Southwest Texas State University, 1972.

Patterson, B. R., McNeal, S., Hawkins, N., and Phelps, R.: Reprograming the social environment. *Journal of Child Psychology and Psychiatry and Allied Disciplines, 8*:181-195, 1967.

Peterson, R.: Imitation: A basic behavioral mechanism. In H. Sloane and B. MacAulay (Eds.) : *Operant Procedures in Remedial Speech and Language Training*, Boston, Houghton Mifflin, 1968, pp. 61-74.

Piaget, J.: *Play, Dreams and Imitation in Childhood*. New York, W. W. Norton, 1951, pp. 73-74.

Pronovost, W., Wakstein, M. P., and Wakstein, J. J.: A longitudinal study of the speech behavior and language comprehension of fourteen children diagnosed atypical or autistic. *Exceptional Children, 33*:19-26, 1966.

Rimland, B.: *Infantile Autism*. New York, Appleton-Century-Crofts, 1964.

Risley, T., and Wolf, M.: Establishing functional speech in echolalic children. *Behav. Res. Ther., 5*:73-88, 1967.

Risley, T.: The effects and side effects of punishing the autistic behaviors of a deviant child. *Journal of Applied Behavior Analysis, 1*:21-35, 1968a.

Risley, T.: Learning and lollipops. *Psychology Today*, January, 1968b.

Ritvo, S., and Provence, S.: Form perception and imitation in some autistic children: Diagnostic findings and their contextural interpretation. *Psychoanal. Stud. Child.*, *8*:155-161, 1953.

Schell, R. E., Stark, J., and Giddan, J. J.: Development of language behavior in an autistic child. *Journal of Speech and Hearing Disorders, 32*:51-64, 1967.

Sherman, J. A.: Use of reinforcement and imitation to reinstate verbal behavior in mute psychotics. *Journal of Abnormal Psychology, 70*:155-164, 1965.

Stark, J., Giddan, J. J., and Meisel, J.: Increasing verbal behavior in an autistic child. *Journal of Speech and Hearing Disorders, 33*:42-48, 1968.

Strait, R.: A child who was speechless in school and social life. *J. Speech Hearing Dis., 23*:253-254, 1968.

Tramontana, J. and Stimbert, V. E.: Some techniques of behavior modification with an autistic child. *Psychological Reports, 27*:498, 1970.

Turner, R.: A method of working with disturbed children. *American Journal of Nursing, 70*:2146-2151, 1970.

Wolf, M., Risley, T., and Mees, H.: Application of operant conditioning procedures to the behavior problems of an autistic child. *Behav. Res. Ther., 1*:305-312, 1964.

Wolff, S., and Chess, S.: An analysis of the language of fourteen schizophrenic children. *J. Child Psychol. Psychiat., 6*:29-41, 1965.

FOOTNOTES

1. This paper is a revision and expansion of a paper first appearing in the *Journal of Speech and Hearing Disorders,* 35, 1970. Sections reprinted by permission.

2. This method also can be used effectively to establish *naming* (for example, "What is this? DOG!") .

3. Both the children reported in this article, Tommy and Wendy, were severely disturbed and showed typical signs of autism

CHAPTER III

STUTTERING

Richard Martin and Roger Ingham

As DISCUSSED in the Introduction, two principles of learning are of special interest in this text: operant learning and imitative learning. To date, little work has been reported involving application of an imitative or modeling paradigm to the modification of stuttering. Over the past ten to fifteen years, however, stuttering has been the focus of considerable behavior modification experimentation stemming from an operant learning framework. Most of this work has been in the form of controlled laboratory studies designed to explore those variables that determine the extent and manner by which environmental consequences influence stuttering frequency. Relatively little work has been reported where an attempt was made to execute and evaluate systematic response contingent therapy programs.

In the first section of this chapter, laboratory experiments of stuttering involving response contingent consequences will be considered. Operant behavior modification experiments explicitly involving a therapeutic procedure will be treated in the second section.

EXPERIMENTAL STUDIES

Studies Using Response Contingent Noise, Shock, and Verbal Statements

It is generally agreed that Flanagan, Goldiamond, and Azrin (1958) reported the first *operant* study in stuttering. An earlier experiment by Sheehan (1951) yielded data germane to the modification of stuttering through response contingent consequences, although the study was not framed within the operant paradigm.

Sheehan had twenty adult stutterers read a two hundred-word passage seven times. For the first five readings, when subjects were in the control condition they simply read aloud. In the experimental condition, however, the subjects were required to repeat a stuttered word until they said it fluently before they could continue reading. In the sixth reading, the subjects read without repeating stuttered words. The seventh reading was the same as the sixth, but thirty minutes later. This experiment clearly demonstrated that when the environmental consequence of repeating the word until fluent was made contingent on each stuttering, the frequency of stuttering decreased.

Flanagan, Goldiamond and Azrin (1958) had three stutterers read orally. Each subject read for two ninety-minute sessions. In the aversive session, the subjects simply read for approximately the first thirty minutes (baserate). For the next thirty minutes (treatment), each stuttering was followed by a one-second blast of 105 decibels of white noise in the subjects' earphones. For the last thirty minutes (extinction), the noise was turned off. For all three subjects, stuttering frequency decreased during the noise period and increased again during extinction. In the escape session, the same procedures were followed except during the treatment period. In the thirty-minute treatment period, the white noise was on continuously, and each stuttering was followed by a five-second period of no noise. Stuttering frequency increased during treatment and decreased again in extinction. Not only was the Flanagan et al. study a pioneer experiment in the exercise of operant control of stuttering, but the study also incorporated the desirable feature of demonstrating that stuttering frequency could be increased or decreased, depending on the nature of the environmental consequences.

One question about the Flanagan et al. study concerns the relatively short baserate period (approximately thirty minutes). The researchers reported their data in the form of cumulative recordings. It is entirely possible that the stuttering frequency of one or more subjects may have been decreasing slightly, but systematically, over the baserate period. However, the cumulative recording might not have been sensitive enough to show this reduction in such a short period of time.

In a second study conducted by the same authors (Flanagan, Goldiamond and Azrin, 1959), stuttering frequency in normal speakers was recorded in baserate and in a treatment condition where each stuttering occasioned a ten-second termination of a continuous (ten shocks per second) electric shock. In this condition, if a subject emitted a stuttering each ten seconds or less, he could avoid shock entirely. Stuttering frequency increased markedly above baserate level during the shock avoidance condition. Removal of the shock condition entirely (extinction) resulted in a decrease in stuttering, but this decrease was relatively slow. Flanagan et al. defined stuttering as "any hesitation, stoppage, repetition or prolongation in the rhythmic flow of verbal behavior" (p. 980). There exists little question that the results of the Flanagan et al. experiment are important with respect to disfluencies in the speech of normal speakers. However, all the data are not in yet concerning the extent to which these findings can be generalized to the speech of stutterers.

Wingate (1959) conducted an experiment that involved the presentation of certain stimuli contingent on stuttering. Eighteen adult stutterers read a set of questions over a microphone to an experimenter in another room. Each subject read the directions eight times in each of three conditions. In the control condition, the subject simply read the directions. In the *interrupted* condition, each subject was signalled when he stuttered and was not allowed to continue until he said the word fluently, in the *reminded* condition, the subject was reminded of each stuttering by a counter registering, but he was allowed to continue speaking. In all eight readings, subjects stuttered significantly less in the two experimental conditions (interrupted and reminded) than in the control condition. The Wingate study was not designed as a typical single-subject experiment in which the response contingent treatment is preceded by a stable response baserate and followed by a period of extinction. However, the findings of this study indicate that "calling attention to stuttering" by either interrupting or signalling operates as a punishment in that it reduces the frequency of stuttering. One aspect of Wingate's design makes the data difficult to interpret. The subjects were requested "to speak as fluently as possible" in the experimental conditions, but were told to speak in their "usual manner" in the control condition. It is possible, of course, that the request to speak as fluently as possible may have accounted for the reduced stuttering in the experimental conditions. This is especially problematic because the experimental conditions always followed the control conditions.

Beginning in the late 1950's, Goldiamond undertook a research program designed to explore the effects of delayed auditory feedback on stuttering. In his initial study, Goldiamond (1962) made five seconds of delayed auditory feedback contingent upon stuttering (punishment). He then presented continuous delayed feedback and each stuttering occasioned a ten-second period of no delayed feedback (escape). At this point, Goldiamond concluded that delayed feedback functioned as an aversive stimulus in the same way that noise and shock had done previously. In later sessions, however, Goldiamond (1965) observed that for some subjects stuttering frequency reduced in the escape condition with delayed feedback. This finding was unexpected from an operant learning paradigm, and led Goldiamond to hypothesize that a *new pattern* of speech was learned. This new speech was controlled by different stimuli from those that controlled the *old* (stuttered) speech. To date, Goldiamond has presented no data relative to the development of a new speech pattern. However, he has developed and disseminated a treatment program utilizing the empirical data that evolved from the delayed feedback work.

In 1966, Martin and his colleagues at the University of Minnesota reported the first in a series of studies designed to explore the effects of presenting various stimuli contingent on stuttering. Martin and Siegel (1966a) had three adult stutterers speak spontaneously until their stuttering frequencies stabilized. Next, each subject was presented electric shock contingent upon each stuttering. For one subject, shock was contingent on *nose wrinkling*, and later on emission of a vocalized "uh-uh-uh." For a second subject, the contingency was tongue protrusion, and later, emission of [s]-prolongation. For a third subject, shock was presented contingent upon a moment of stuttering. For all subjects, introduction of response contingent shock resulted in a marked reduction in the frequency of the particular stuttering behavior, and cessation of shock was followed by an increase in stuttering frequency to near baserate level. In addition, the researchers demonstrated that stuttering could be brought under discriminative stimulus control —in one instance a wristband; in another, a blue light. The Martin and Siegel (1966a) study extended the findings of Flanagan et al. (1958) in several ways. (1) Spontaneous speech was employed. (2) A lengthy, stable baserate was achieved before treatment was introduced. (3) Both specific behaviors and a moment of stuttering were shown to be reliable, manipulable response classes. (4) Stuttering behavior was brought under discriminative stimulus control.

Daly and Cooper (1967) undertook a contingent shock experiment in which they had eighteen stutterers read a passage five times under three experimental conditions. In the contingent shock condition each subject was shocked as soon as the investigator perceived a stuttering. In the *following* condition the subject was shocked immediately following each stuttering. In the control condition the electrodes were attached to the subject, but no shock was delivered.

Stuttering frequency reduced from reading to reading in all three conditions. However, in all five readings less stuttering occurred in the following condition than in the control condition, and less stuttering occurred in the contingent condition than in the following condition. In spite of some methodological problems, the Daly and Cooper study clearly indicated that when shock was presented contingent on stuttering it occasioned a reduction in the frequency of that response.

The difference in stuttering frequency between the contingent and following conditions is difficult to evaluate. The authors report that the experimenter was a reliable observer of stuttering, but they do not report any data to suggest that the observer was sufficiently perceptive and rapid to present the shock differentially during a stuttering and following a stuttering.

The experimental procedure employed by Daly and Cooper poses a problem that has plagued research in stuttering for years. When subjects read a given passage five times in control and five times in experimental conditions, it generally happens that stuttering frequency decreases with each reading even if no treatment is introduced. Treatment effects can be *teased out* of such a design only by observing variations in adaptation corresponding to introduction and cessation of treatment. However, the data from such a design always are confounded by the so-called *adaptation effect* and by the possible interaction of this effect with the treatment effect.

In a second study by Martin and Siegel (1966b), the effects of punishing stuttering and reinforcing fluency were considered. Two adult stutterers read orally for eight sessions, and stuttering frequency was recorded continuously. After stuttering frequency stabilized, the experimenter said "not good" after each stuttering and "good" after each thirty-second interval in which no stuttering occurred. For two sessions, a wrist strap was attached during the time the verbal stimuli were presented. In subsequent sessions, the strap was attached but no verbal stimuli were presented. Instructions to read carefully and say each word fluently were given at the beginning of certain sessions. Results of the Martin and Siegel (1966b) study were several. (1) Response contingent presentations of the verbal stimuli occasioned a marked reduction in baserate stuttering frequency. Clearly, however, the effects of the "good" for not stuttering and "not good" for stuttering were confounded. (2) Stuttering frequency was brought under the discriminative stimulus control of the wrist strap. Unfortunately, however, the effect of the wrist strap alone on stuttering frequency was not assessed. (3) In one session the presentation of instructions alone occasioned a reduction in stuttering frequency from baserate. However, this reduction was transitory, and by the end of twenty minutes stuttering frequency had returned to baserate level.

Quist and Martin (1967) studied the effects of response contingent *wrong* on stuttering in three adult male stutterers. Each subject's stuttering baserate was obtained, then the word *wrong* was presented via earphones contingent on each stuttering. For two subjects, *wrong* occasioned only a 30% to 40% reduction in stuttering after several sessions of contingent *wrong*. For a third subject, *wrong* produced almost total suppression of stuttering, removal of *wrong* was followed by a return to baserate stuttering frequency, and reintroduction of *wrong* occasioned an immediate and dramatic reduction in stuttering.

Studies Using Response Contingent *Time-Out*

Beginning in 1968, Martin and his colleagues conducted a series of studies in which a period of time-out from speaking was made contingent on each stuttering. The rationale for the use of time-out was that, presumably, the various responses in a complex speech chain produce internal stimulation. When a speech unit is reinforced, the response-produced stimuli are paired with the reinforcement and take on reinforcing properties of their own. Subsequently, presence of the response-produced stimuli alone is sufficient self-reinforcement to maintain the speech chain. Assuming this self-reinforcement hypothesis is correct, exposing a human subject to periods of time-out from speaking might be an aversive event. If so, then arranging an experimental situation in such a way that time-out from speaking is made contingent upon a stuttering behavior should result in a decrement in stuttering frequency. The initial time-out study was conducted by Haroldson, Martin and Starr (1968). These researchers had four adult stutterers speak spontaneously for fifteen sixty-minute sessions. During the time-out treatment, a red light was activated and remained on for ten seconds contingent on each stuttering. Subjects were instructed to cease speaking when the light came on and to remain silent for as long as the light was on. The first two sessions were baserate sessions. In sessions three through seven, the subjects received time-out contingent on stuttering for the first forty minutes and no time-out (extinction) for the last twenty minutes of each session. In sessions eight through thirteen, subjects received time-out for the entire session. The final two sessions were extinction sessions. Stuttering was relatively stable across the two baserate sessions. In sessions three through thirteen, stuttering frequency of all subjects decreased during time-out and increased in extinction. Three of the four subjects stuttered on less than 1% of the spoken words in sessions eight through thirteen. The Haroldson et al. study demonstrated that time-out from speaking operates as an aversive stimulus when made contingent on stuttering.

In a subsequent study, Martin and Haroldson (1969) compared the performance of two groups of ten adult stutterers under two treatment procedures. In one condition the subjects were exposed to pre-treatment speaking tasks and attitude questionnaires, to eight sessions of traditional *information-attitude* therapy, and to post-treatment speaking tasks and attitude questionnaires. In a second condition, the same pre- and post-treatment measures were obtained. However, these subjects were given eight sessions of the same ten-second time-out procedure used by Haroldson et al. (1958). In general, for neither information-attitude group nor time-out group subjects were there significant differences between pre- and post-attitude scale scores. The information-attitude subjects' stuttering frequencies changed very little during the course of the eight treatment sessions. By contrast, all ten time-out group subjects experienced a marked reduction in stuttering frequency during the eight time-out sessions. However, the reduction in stuttering frequency observed during the time-out sessions extinguished during the post-treatment speaking task.

Martin and Haroldson (1971) conducted an experiment designed to study the effects of time-out on stuttering during conversation. Four adult stutterers were divided into two pairs. Each pair was placed in a conversational speech situation. In baserate I (BR I), the subjects conversed and the experimenters (one for each subject) tallied stutterings. In baserate II (BR II), the conditions remained unchanged, but each subject was given a handswitch and instructed to press it whenever the other subject stuttered. In the first treatment condition (COND I), each depression of either subject's handswitch occasioned a ten-second time-out for both subjects. In the second treatment phase (COND II), the procedures were the same except that now depression of the experimenters' handswitches also occasioned a time-out. During extinction (EXT), no time-out was administered. In a post-extinction period (COND IA), the same procedures as those employed during COND I were reinstated. The results for both pairs of subjects were similar. Stuttering frequency for both subjects did not increase or decrease in any systematic way during the two baserate periods. In COND I, the stuttering frequencies of both subjects decreased, albeit sporadically. In COND II, however, the stuttering frequencies of both subjects reduced essentially to zero. During EXT, the stuttering frequencies of both subjects increased. Reintroduction of time-out by the experimenters occasioned a dramatic reduction in stuttering for one subject, but much less of a reduction in the other subject. Interestingly, the four stutterers depressed their handswitches very infrequently in COND I. In no instance did a subject push his handswitch on more than 2% of his partner's stutterings.

Martin and Berndt (1970) had a twelve-year-old stuttering boy read orally for fifteen forty-minute sessions. The first four sessions were baserate sessions in which the boy simply read and the experimenter tallied stutterings. During sessions five through eleven, a ten-second time-out was presented contingent on each stuttering. Sessions twelve through fifteen were baserate. The subject's stuttering was stable during baserate sessions, decreased essentially to zero during time-out sessions, and increased only slightly during extinction sessions.

Adams and Popelka (1971) reported a time-out study in which eight adult stutterers read three hundred-word passages in two conditions. In the control condition, the subjects read one passage five times in succession. In the experimental condition, the subjects read the other passage five times in succession, but were presented a ten-second time-out contingent on each stuttering. In all five readings, subjects who received time-out had fewer stutterings. The Adams and Popelka study suffers the same possible confounding by the adaptation effect as discussed in the Daly and Cooper (1967) experiment. Adams and Popelka also questioned subjects about their reactions to time-out. Some subjects indicated that time-out *alerted* them; some felt time-out *punished* them; some felt time-out *relaxed* them. These findings appear to reflect the current state of affairs relative to time-out; namely, making a period of time-out from speaking contingent upon a stuttering reduces the frequency of stuttering in a large number of subjects. Why this occurs, however, is far from clear.

Egolf, Shames and Seltzer (1971) reported an experiment involving a variation on the time-out procedure. Ten adult stutterers met for a ninety-minute group therapy session each week for five weeks. During each of the five sessions either a control or experimental *run* was conducted. In the first control run (session one) each stutterer talked for five minutes. In the first experimental run (session two) each subject was told that he could talk until he stuttered, at which time he was required to *relinquish* the floor. In the second control run (session three) the same situation obtained as in the first control run. In the second experimental run (session four) the same situation existed as in the first experimental run. The last control run (session five) was the same as the first and second control runs.

For each subject in each run, calculations were made of the time elapsed until the first stuttering and the number of words spoken until the first stuttering. In general, the results followed a predictable pattern. Both the number of words spoken and the length of time elapsed before the first stuttering increased between the first control run and the first experimental run, decreased between the first experimental run and the second control run, increased again between the second control run and the second experimental run, and decreased again between the second experimental run and the third control run.

Studies Using Response Contingent *Response-Cost*

Halvorson (1971) conducted an experiment in which he explored the effects of response-cost contingent on stuttering. Subjects spoke spontaneously and were instructed that their task was to earn as many points as possible. In baserate sessions, no response contingent stimuli were introduced. In punishment sessions, each stuttering caused a reduction of one point on a counter in front of the subject. In pairing sessions, each stuttering produced subtraction of a point; if the next word was spoken fluently, ten points were added. In extinction sessions, no points were added or subtracted. In a second series of punishment sessions, the same procedures as those used in the initial punishment sessions were reintroduced.

As Halvorson indicated, "response cost can be added to the array of already 'effective' punishers for stuttering" (p. 362). Halvorson postulated that the reason stuttering frequency increased during pairing was because the punishment (point loss) for stuttering served as a discriminative stimulus for positive reinforcement of the next fluent word. However, there may be an alternative explanation for Halvorson's data. The Adams and

Popelka (1971) study provided a partial demonstration that when a response contingent stimulus is presented for stuttering during ongoing speech, it often happens that the stimulus presentation coincides temporally with the next word or two after the stuttered word. The fact that stuttering frequency reduces even when some latitude exists in the temporal contiguity between stuttering and contingent stimulus suggests that Halvorson's subjects may not have differentiated between a stuttered word and the next fluent word. Rather, the subjects simply may have concluded that they lost one point and gained ten points whenever they stuttered. This, of course, would result in an increase in stuttering frequency during pairing sessions.

Studies Concerning Characteristics of the Response Contingent Stimulus

Certain characteristics of the response contingent stimulus situation have been explored in several experiments. Cooper, Cady and Robbins (1970) had fourteen adult stutterers and fourteen nonstutterers read aloud in three conditions. In the *right* condition a subject read for seven minutes without treatment, read for seven minutes during which the word *right* was presented for each disfluency, and then read for seven minutes under no treatment. In the *wrong* condition the same procedures were followed except that *wrong* was presented for each disfluency. In the third condition, *tree* was presented for each disfluency.

Presentation of the verbal stimulus during the middle seven-minute segment of each condition resulted in a significant decrease in the number of disfluencies. However, the amounts of reduction were not significantly different in conditions that employed the words *right, wrong,* or *tree* as the contingent stimulus. Cooper et al. concluded that because the presumably neutral stimulus word *tree* resulted in a decrease in disfluencies, it is entirely possible that any contingent stimulus which serves to call the stutterer's attention to his stuttering will occasion a reduction in stuttering. If this proves to be the case, then it renders traditional *learning theory* explanations for the results of response contingent studies somewhat tenuous.

Another characteristic of the reinforcement/punishment stimulus situation which has been explored experimentally involves the stimulus-response contingency. Biggs and Sheehan (1969) had six stutterers read orally under three conditions. The conditions were randomized across three sessions, and the subject read the same passage throughout an entire session. In the *aversive* condition each subject read for approximately fifteen minutes with no treatment. During the next twenty-minute period the subject received a loud tone contingent on each stuttering. In the extinction period the subject read for an additional twenty minutes, but no tone was presented. The same procedures were followed in the *escape* condition except that during treatment a continuous 4,000 Hz, 108 decibel tone was terminated for five seconds contingent on each stuttering. Again, the same procedures were followed in the *random* condition except that tone bursts were presented randomly during the twenty-minute treatment period. The authors conducted a statistical analysis which revealed that stuttering frequency decreased significantly between the pre-treatment and treatment period. However, no significant differences in stuttering frequencies were observed among the various treatment conditions. Biggs and Sheehan concluded from their data that because stuttering frequency reduced under the random condition, the most parsimonious explanation of the results obtained in all three conditions was that the tone functioned as a distraction rather than a response contingent punishing stimulus.

The Biggs and Sheehan study leveled a serious charge against all response contingent behavior modification experiments. The validity of the charge is difficult to assess because a metholodogical error in the design of the study raises a serious question about the reliability of the data. In fourteen of the eighteen sessions (six subjects by three conditions), stuttering frequency decreased from pre-treatment to treatment, and decreased even more from treatment to post-treatment. Obviously, the same results might have been achieved had the subjects simply read for the same length of time with no tone present at all.

In an attempt to clarify the contingency question, Martin and Haroldson in an unpublished study had two adult stutterers speak spontaneously in twenty-one forty-minute sessions. The first four sessions were baserate. For the next seven sessions, the subjects were given ten seconds of time-out on a random schedule. The same number of time-outs was given in each session as the subject experienced stutterings in the average baserate sessions. For the next eight sessions, each subject received a ten-second time-out contingent on each stuttering. In sessions twenty and twenty-one (extinction), the same procedures were followed as in baserate.

Results for one subject in the Martin and Haroldson study are shown graphically in Figure III.1. As the curves indicate, the introduction of random time-out occasioned a slight reduction in stuttering frequency, but a marked decrease in word output. As a consequence, the percent words stuttered increased in the random time-out condition. In the contingent time-out condition the frequency of stuttering decreased, but the word output increased back to baserate level. As a result, the percent words stuttered decreased markedly during the contingent time-out condition. Both stuttering frequency and word output returned to near baserate levels during extinction.

The second subject followed essentially the same pattern. Results of the Martin and Haroldson experiment indicate that the

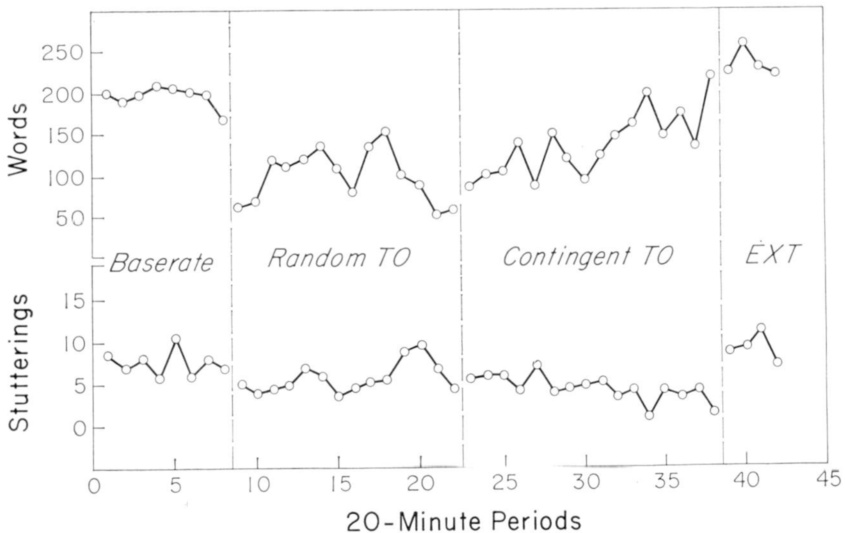

Figure III.1. Mean numbers of words and stutterings per two minutes for each twenty-minute period during baserate (Baserate), random time-out (Random TO), contingent time-out (Contingent TO), and extinction (EXT).

time-out stimulus needs to be contingent before a substantial reduction in stuttering percent is observed. The ambiguous notion of distraction is not sufficient to account for the Martin and Haroldson results.

One feature of the response contingent stimulus situation that has been investigated only tangentially concerns other speech variables. That is, to what extent, if any, are speech parameters such as rate, pitch, inflection and loudness modified when environmental consequences are made contingent upon a *moment of stuttering?* In no experiments to date have the researchers reported data on pitch, inflection and loudness. Goldiamond (1965) stated that his subjects learned a *new pattern* of speech, but he presented no data to indicate what speech parameters were changed and by how much.

Several experimenters have reported data relative to word output. In the Martin and Berndt (1970) study, for example, the authors included a graph showing the number of stutterings and the number of words read each session. This allows the reader to determine the effects of the contingent stimulus on more than just stuttering frequency. On the other hand, Cooper, Cady and Robbins (1970) had their subjects read in three successive seven-minute conditions and the researchers simply presented the number of disfluencies in each condition. No data were reported relative to the number of words read. The problem with this procedure is that the particular treatment employed might result in a marked reduction in reading rate. This could result in a decrease in the number of disfluencies or stutterings, but the percent of words stuttered might actually increase during the same time.

Studies Using Expectation as the Response Class

Three experiments have been reported in which the response class was not stuttering as observed by the experimenter, but rather the expectation or anticipation by the subject that he was going to stutter. Curlee and Perkins (1968) found that frequencies of both expectancy and stuttering decreased when shock was presented contingent on signaled expectancies. Daly and Frick (1970) also delivered electric shock contingent on expectancy responses and contingent on stuttering. They found that shock for signaled expectancies produced a moderate reduction in expectancies, shock for stuttering produced a marked reduction in stuttering, and shock for both expectancies and stutterings produced a marked reduction in both responses. Harris, Martin and Haroldson in an unpublished study reported that for one subject, punishing (time-out) expectancy responses decreased the frequency of expectancy responses, but decreased stuttering very little. For a second subject, simply depressing a handswitch contingent upon each expectancy response (with no time-out administered) produced a reduction in both expectancy and stuttering. For a third subject, punishing expectancy responses resulted in a marked reduction in stuttering, but a much smaller decrease in expectancy responses.

THERAPY STUDIES

The experimental studies reviewed in the preceding pages clearly indicate that a number of different response contingent events or stimuli occasion a change in the frequency of stuttering. Only in the last few years, however, have any attempts been made to incorporate these operant procedures and findings into the clinical management programs of stutterers. The few studies of this type that have been reported will be discussed in the following pages. An experiment will be included only if the author specifically claims that the study is therapeutic in nature.

Studies Using Response Contingent Positive Reinforcement

Rickard and Mundy (1965) treated a nine-year-old boy whose stuttering was *characterized by repetition and blockage*. The child was reinforced (*good, excellent,* etc.) for fluency as he said phrases, then sentences, then paragraphs, and then stories. Finally, he conversed with the clinician. In a *generalization* phase, the parents reinforced the boy for fluent speech.

According to Rickard and Mundy, the boy's stuttering frequency reduced essentially to zero during the treatment phase. However it is difficult to determine precisely what responses were manipulated. The authors stated that "stuttering behavior was defined by repetition errors per task unit ('g-g-g-going' as a one word task unit would yield a score of three repetition errors). Blocking, flushing, and other concomitants of stuttering were not recorded" (p. 270). Although there was a reduction in the frequency of repetition errors, changes in other features of the stuttering (*blockages,* for example) were not considered. This use of a very narrow response class might explain why a relapse was observed when the boy was interviewed six months after therapy.

Russell, Clark and van Sommers (1968) reported a study that involved essentially four experiments with a particular reinforcement procedure. The first three studies were done with one adult stutterer. In the first experiment, the subject ostensibly was reinforced by a flashing light and buzzer after fluently reading an average of five words, phrases, or sentences that were machine-projected on a screen. Stuttering frequency decreased with this treatment. Although the authors don't mention it, there exists the possibility that the subject also was punished. That is, when the subject "stammered, the slide was exposed for five seconds before a new slide was presented" (p. 448). When the subject read without the machine or reinforcement, the frequency of stuttering returned to baserate level.

In a second experiment, the machine reading (including reinforcement) was placed on an intermittant schedule. Stuttering percent reduced by one-half under this condition. In a third experiment with the same subject, machine reading was used, but the reinforcers (green light, buzzer, etc.) were presented, removed, and reintroduced. The results indicated that presence of the reinforcers resulted in over a 50% reduction in stuttering. In a fourth experiment, two new subjects were exposed to the machine reading procedure and their stuttering frequency reduced markedly.

Several aspects of the Russell, Clark and van Sommers therapy experiment make the data and conclusions suspect. (1) No data were reported relative to follow-up or carry-over. (2) No reliability data were reported. (3) No data relative to the rate of speech during treatment were reported. (4) As mentioned previously, data from time-out experiments suggest that requiring the subject to wait five seconds for the next slide each time he stuttered may have been sufficient to account for the results of this study. At any rate, the data from the study don't support the Russell et al. statement that, "The results point towards positive reinforcement as a better choice of conditioning procedure than aversive therapy" (p. 453).

Leach (1969) used a fluency reinforcement procedure with a twelve-year-old boy. The boy conversed with the examiner for thirty-minute sessions. Beginning with the seventh session, during the first fifteen minutes the boy was paid two cents per minute for conversing with the examiner. During the second half, he received an additional penny for each fifteen-second period of fluent speech. Leach reported that the *mean block rate* for the first fifteen-minute periods reduced across sessions to less than one per minute. Unfortunately, Leach did not report data for the second fifteen-minute periods of each session. Consequently, it is not possible to determine if the reinforcement of fifteen seconds of fluency had anything to do with this boy's reduction in *blocks*. In addition, Leach reported no reliability data and only casual, unsystematic observational data regarding carry-over. Leach observed a partial return of the boy's *disfluent speech behavior* during a two-month follow-up session, but presented no data.

Browning (1967) conducted a treatment program with a nine-year-old schizophrenic boy who stuttered. Initially, stuttering baserate was established. Then the boy was exposed to *reciprocal inhibition* relaxation sessions. In the next sessions, a complex of procedures was involved, but the boy received both tokens and verbal reinforcers from the experimenter for fluent speech. This was followed by several extinction sessions. Finally, the boy was put on the reinforcement regimen a second time, but with the hospital staff as the reinforcing agents. At the end of 140 sessions, the boy's stuttering frequency was markedly reduced. Unfortunately, the number and order of the different procedures to which the subject was involved make it difficult to evaluate the treatment. As Browning states, "Precise information on the relative effectiveness of each technique was not established" (p. 34). Additional problems with the Browning study are the lack of demonstrated reliability relative to identifying stuttering, the absence of data concerning carry-over and follow-up, and the absence of data about the rate of speech.

Bar (1971) claimed to have produced fluency in forty-four of fifty-nine stuttering children between the ages of two and six.

Presumably, this was achieved by reinforcing with positive verbal statements, and hence calling attention to, fluent speech. Considering the difficulties with stuttering therapy in general, it is perhaps unfortunate when such extravagant claims are not supported by data.

Studies Using Response Contingent Punishment

In spite of a substantial body of experimental literature demonstrating the efficacy of punishment in reducing stuttering, only a few attempts have been made to use such procedures clinically. McDermott (1971) used a time-out procedure with a nine-year-old boy. Initially, a ten-second time-out interval contingent on stuttering resulted in increased fluency with the therapist. Rewarding fluency and increasing the number of listeners were then added. Subsequently, a click on the counter replaced time-out. McDermott reported that in eleven twenty-four-minute sessions spanning seven weeks, stuttering was reduced from around 14% essentially to zero. Follow-up fifteen weeks later revealed 3.4% words stuttered. The author reported no data relative to reliability or word output.

Curlee and Perkins (1969) reported a clinical procedure they termed conversational rate control therapy. In this program, the main treatment technique was delayed auditory feedback. At one point in the program, however, the stutterers were timed-out for each stuttering; that is, the room lights were extinguished and the subject was not allowed to speak. Curlee and Perkins stated that subjects improved as a result of conversational rate control therapy, but only group average data were presented. No reliability, carry-over, or follow-up data were reported.

A variation of the time-out procedure was conducted in an unpublished study by Martin, Kuhl and Haroldson. These experimenters constructed a *talking* puppet apparatus in which the puppet could be made to disappear by extinguishing the stage lights. The puppet and stage were not available to the subject, but were located behind a two-way glass. The experimenter served as the *voice of the puppet* over an intercom system. Experimentally, the apparatus was employed in the following way. A young child who stuttered was placed in the experimental room and allowed to talk with the puppet. No other people were in the room. During the conversation, the experimenter serving as the puppet could stop talking and turn off the stage lights (*time-out* from the puppet) for a predetermined period of time whenever the child stuttered.

The first subject (JC) was a 3½-year-old child whose moments of stuttering sometimes exceeded fifteen seconds. JC was placed alone in the experimental room and allowed to talk with the puppet for one twenty-minute session each week. The general design and resulting data are shown in Figure III.2. In the initial baserate sessions, JC simply talked with the puppet. After the first ten minutes of session four, time-out was initiated. Each time JC stuttered, the experimenter stopped talking and extinguished the stage lights for ten seconds. Because JC stuttered so frequently, the response class used during the early time-out sessions was defined as a stuttering *episode* of at least two seconds in duration. Beginning with session seventeen and continuing through session thirty-one,

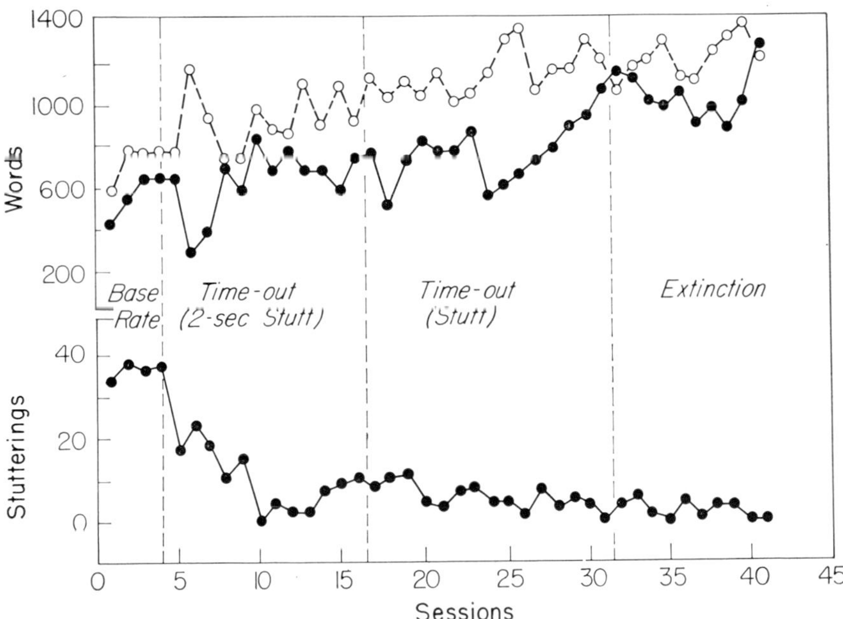

Figure III.2. Numbers of words spoken by JC (top closed circles) and puppet (open circles), and number of stutterings by JC (bottom closed circles) each treatment session.

JC was timed-out for each stuttering regardless of duration. Beginning with session thirty-two, time-out was discontinued. The number of stutterings and words emitted by JC each session, and the number of words spoken by the puppet each session, are given in Figure III.2. The number of words spoken by both the puppet and the child increased across sessions. JC's stuttering frequency decreased markedly coincident with the beginning of time-out.

In order to determine the extent to which any changes in stuttering observed during the time-out sessions generalized to other speaking situations, monthly *probe* sessions were conducted. Each month JC spoke with a different experimenter for twenty minutes in a different room from the one in which the puppet

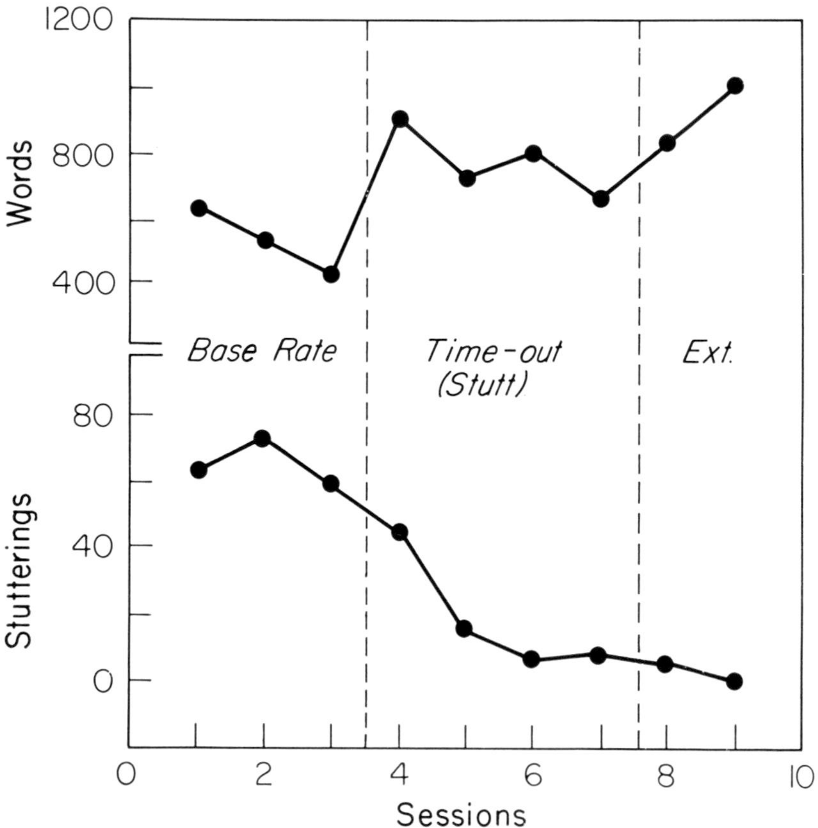

Figure III.3. Numbers of words and stutterings by JC each probe session.

TABLE III.I

NUMBER OF STUTTERINGS AND NUMBER OF WORDS EMITTED BY JC IN CONVERSATIONS OUTSIDE THE LABORATORY

Situation	*Minutes*	*Words*	*Stuttering*
JC with family at dinner	28	481	0
JC with family in living room	26	664	2
JC with family (except father) in living room	28	266	1
JC with family at lunch	32	735	3

sessions were conducted. The numbers of stutterings and words for each generalization session are shown in Figure III.3. No time-out treatment was employed during the probe sessions, but the graph in Figure III.3 is divided into baserate, time-out and extinction according to what was taking place in the puppet session on any given probe session date.

After JC completed all puppet sessions and all probe sessions, tape recordings were obtained of four home speaking situations. In each of these, the recorder and microphone were disguised in order to keep the client unaware that he was being recorded. Data from the home tapes appear in Table III.I.

Approximately eleven months after the final puppet session, JC returned for a follow up session. A tape recording was made of JC talking with an experimenter—not the experimenter who who was the puppet voice. During the first ten minutes, JC spoke 431 words and stuttered three times (.7%); in the second ten minutes, the child spoke 423 words and emitted four stutterings (.95%).

The second subject (SS) was a 4½-year-old boy who stuttered. SS was run in treatment sessions with the puppet in much the same way as JC. The data for the treatment sessions are shown in Figure III.4.

Generalization of treatment effects was assessed as follows. Immediately after each puppet session, SS was taken to a different room where he conversed with his mother for twenty minutes. Data from the probe sessions are given in Figure III.5.

To check for carry-over, tape recordings were obtained of four *outside* conversations. The recorder and microphone were dis-

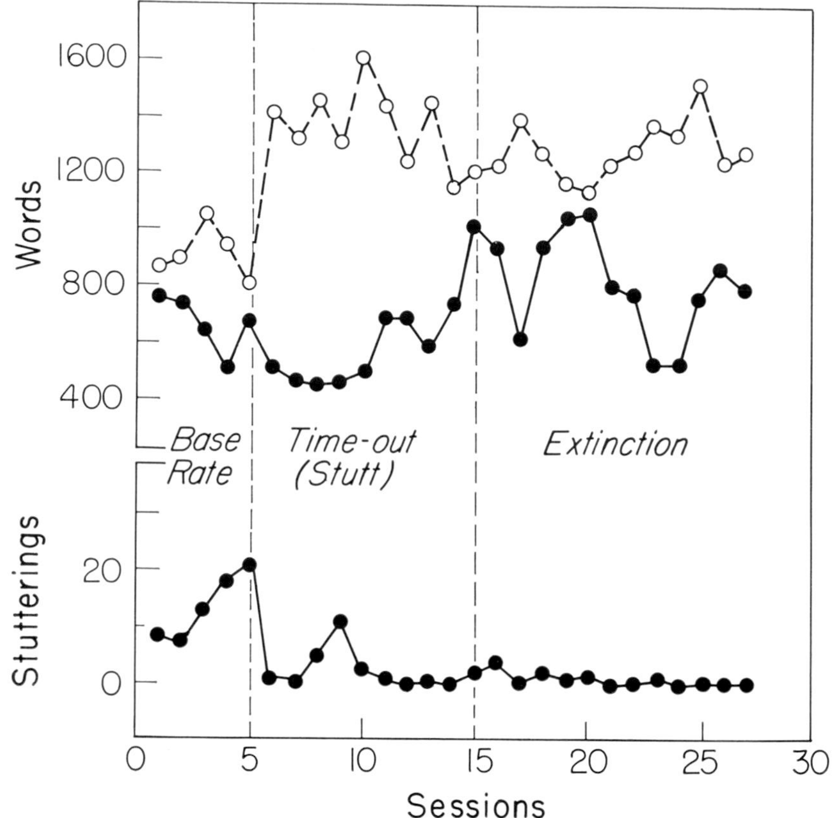

Figure III.4. Numbers of words spoken by SS (top closed circles) and puppet (open circles), and number of stutterings by SS (bottom closed circles) each treatment session.

TABLE III.II

NUMBER OF STUTTERINGS AND THE NUMBER OF WORDS EMITTED BY SS IN CONVERSATIONS OUTSIDE THE LABORATORY

Situation	*Minutes*	*Words*	*Stutterings*
SS with mother at breakfast	10	89	0
SS with mother and aunt at dinner	10	147	0
SS with father in workshop	40	1018	0
SS with mother and Experimenter in car . .	15	164	0

guised. Data for the carry-over situations are shown in Table III.II.

Approximately thirteen months after the final puppet session, SS was run in a follow-up session. A tape recording was made of the child talking with a speech clinician. During the first ten minutes, SS spoke 392 words and emitted three stutterings (.76%); in the second ten minutes, he spoke 330 words and stuttered once (.30%).

In order to assess experimenter reliability, twelve ten-minute segments were selected randomly from the tape recordings of all baseline and extinction puppet treatment sessions for both JC

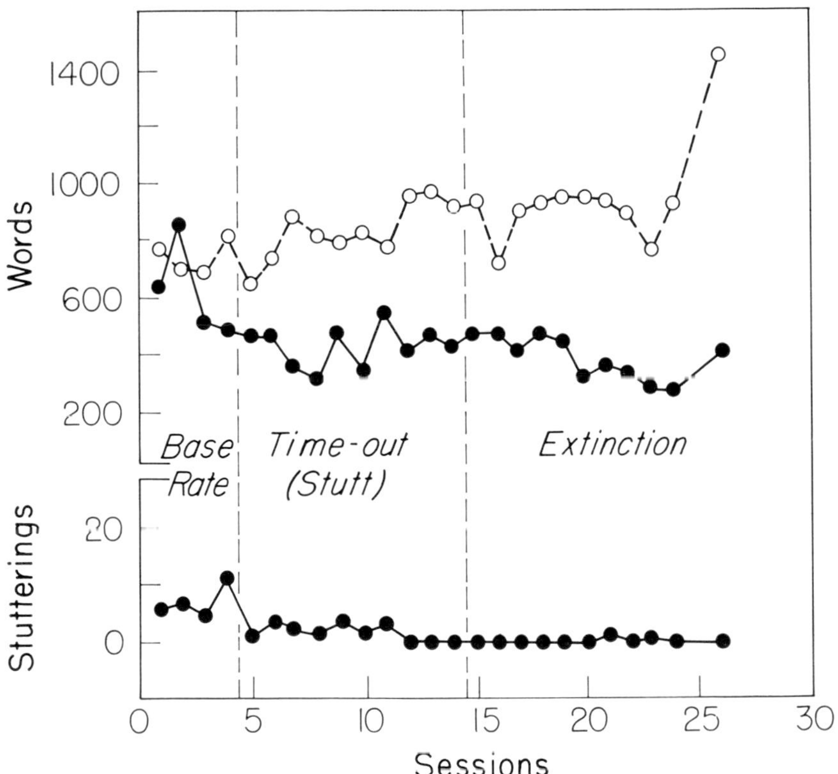

Figure III.5. Numbers of words spoken by SS (top closed circles) and mother (open circles), and number of stutterings by SS (bottom closed circles) each probe session.

and SS. These twelve segments were dubbed, in random order, onto a master tape. An independent observer counted the number of words and stutterings for each ten-minute segment. Figures III.6 and III.7 give the number of words and stutterings produced by JC and SS as counted by the experimenter and the independent observer.

Ryan (1971) reported a study in which four children were treated in a program involving reinforcement of fluency and punishment of stuttering. The programs were too complex to discuss in detail, but the children were either praised or awarded points

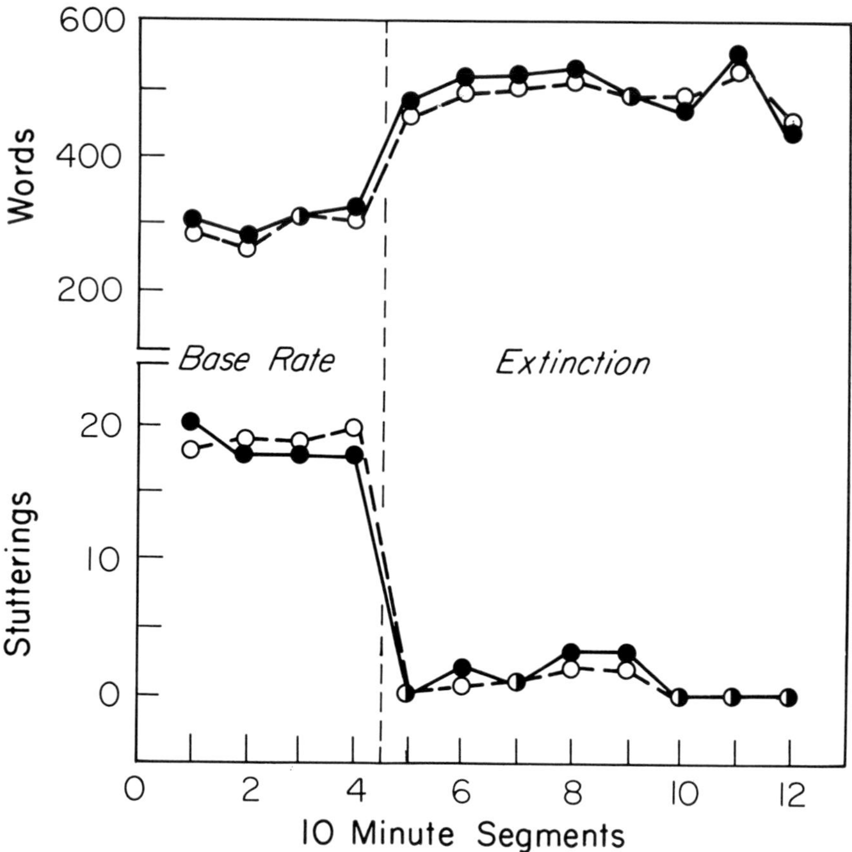

Figure III.6. Numbers of stutterings and words counted by experimenter (closed circles) and independent observer (open circles) for random segments of JC.

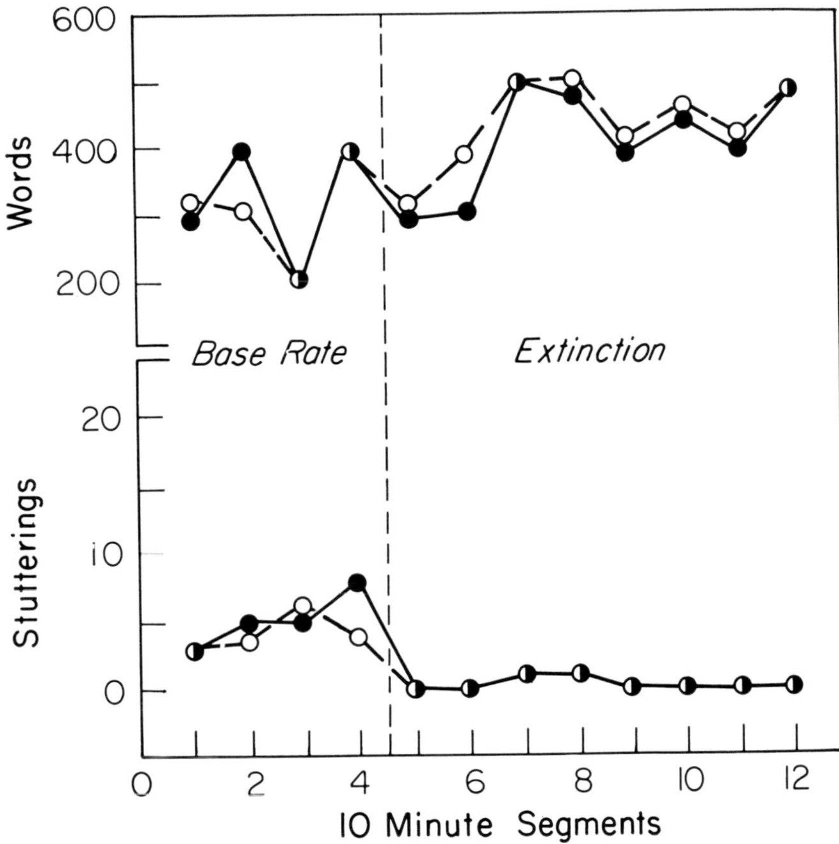

Figure III.7. Numbers of stutterings and words counted by experimenter (closed circles) and independent observer (open circles) for random segments of SS.

(exchangeable for toys) for fluent utterances. In three subjects, stuttering was contingently punished by repeating each stuttered word, counting stutterings with a hand counter during conversation, or deducting points for each stuttering. Each child was treated individually, and for three of the children a maintenance program of reinforcement and punishment was conducted in the home by the parents.

In general, Ryan found that stuttered words per minute decreased essentially to zero in the clinical situation. However, no data were presented to indicate if the subjects' speech rates increased, decreased, or remained the same during treatment. Also, no information was reported as to how stutterings were identified and whether or not they were scored reliably.

Ryan obtained follow-up data in the clinic at around three months after treatment, and these data indicated that the reduced stuttering frequency was maintained. The author also stated that the children remained fluent in the home, classroom, and other situations outside of the clinic. Unfortunately, no data was presented to substantiate these claims.

Studies Combining Traditional Therapy and Response Contingent Procedures

Shames and his colleagues at the University of Pittsburgh have reported a series of experiments directed toward the integration of traditional therapy procedures into the operant model. In an initial study, Shames (1969) attempted to modify a stutterer's verbal content by reinforcing (*good, right,* etc.) desired statements and presumably punishing (silence by clinician) undesired statements. The result was a marked increase in desired responses across the seventeen therapy sessions. Also noted was a decrease in certain stuttering behaviors across sessions, although these stuttering behaviors were not the focus of any response contingent stimuli. With a second subject, Shames attempted to modify the *overt stuttering behavior* directly. The stutterer's baserate was determined. Then he was trained to identify his stutterings at 80% accuracy. Following this, he was trained in eight types of stuttering modification following generally a Van Riper program. The subject moved from one type of modification to the next when he was able to emit the appropriate behavior 80% of the time. Appropriate responses were followed by verbal praise; inappropriate responses by *no.* Stuttering frequency reduced steadily across sessions and was at zero by the end of treatment. With regard to follow-up, Shames reported that, "In school, at home, and with friends, this client's stuttering has remained at a very low, if nonexistent, frequency level" (p. 112). However, no data were presented to substantiate this claim. In addition, no reliability data were reported.

Shames, Egolf and Rhodes (1969) described a series of refinements on the Shames procedure in which the direct stuttering modification program was reduced to four steps and the criterion for moving from one step to the next was increased to 90% correct responses on stuttered words. In addition, three *Thematic Content Modification Programs* (TCMP) were employed. In TCMP 1, the clinician responded either positively or negatively to appropriate themes in the subject's conversation. The clinician also made noncontingent responses ("tell me more," "Is there anything else?"). In TCMP 2, only *positive* statements were reinforced. In TCMP 3, the noncontingent clinician responses were omitted from the TCMP 1 schedule. Shames et al. provided only preliminary within-therapy data for four stutterers as illustrative of the various programs.

The one subject treated by the four-phase behavior modification program decreased in stuttering frequency from fourteen percent stuttering in the first session to two percent stuttering in the sixth session. The subjects exposed to TCMP 1 and TCMP 3 procedures showed increases in *positive language responses* and decreases in *negative language responses*. At the same time, these two subjects reduced markedly in percent stuttering. The subject that received TCMP 2 increased his *positive language responses* very little. At the same time, this subject's stuttering frequency decreased only slightly after the first three sessions. Shames, Egolf and Rhodes reported no data relative to carry-over, follow-up or reliability.

Egolf, Shames and Blind (1971) described a further variation on the stuttering modification procedure with an adult female stutterer. In the first stage of treatment the client was told "look at me" each time she was talking and not looking at the clinician. At the end of this phase, eye-contact frequency was higher and stuttering frequency was lower. In the next stage, the client was exposed to the same TCMP 3 program outlined by Shames, Egolf and Rhodes (1969). Stuttering frequency reduced even more in this phase. In the third phase, the same procedures were in effect, except that now statements that reported avoidance behaviors were reinforced. Stuttering frequency continued to decrease in this third phase. At a six-month follow-up, the client stuttered on fewer words than at the end of treatment. At a year follow-up, stuttering frequency was zero.

The Egolf, Shames and Blind study is noteworthy in that the authors reported carefully collected data on reliability of the various response classes. On the other hand, this study suffers a serious methodological shortcoming. It is entirely possible that the reduction in stuttering frequency was independent of any of the three treatments. This is particularly problematic because the stuttering frequency reduced across sessions irrespective of treatment.

Another amalgamation of the operant paradigm with a *traditional* stuttering therapy procedure has been conducted by Ingham and Andrews in Australia. Originally, this program combined a token system with a syllable-timed speech technique (Andrews and Harris, 1964). Subjects were treated in groups of ten for two weeks under outpatient conditions in a hospital. This was followed by a once-weekly, nine-month follow-up treatment program. Subsequently, this program was modified to an inpatient program for groups of four adult subjects who lived together under controlled token economy conditions for three weeks. The outcome of therapy was then evaluated over the following nine months.

A central feature of the three week treatment process was the rating session. This was a forty-five-minute period in which subjects were required to speak (in conversation) a specified number of syllables. Each syllable was rated, *on-line,* by two speech therapists as either stuttered or fluent. At the end of a rating session, subjects earned or lost tokens according to their percent syllables stuttered, and relative to the baseline percent syllables stuttered for each subject. With improvement, a subject's baseline percent syllables stuttered was lowered and token earning or loss levels adjusted accordingly. When the subject's token schedule reached zero percent syllables stuttered, increases in syllable per minute rate were integrated with the schedule. The *target behavior* towards which this schedule shaped speech behavior was zero percent syllables stuttered at a speaking rate of between 180 and 220 syllables per minute.

Each subject in a treatment group was issued individually

colored tokens so that spending and saving activity could be recorded. Subjects also agreed to abide by the rule that tokens were the only means by which food, drink, or any luxury item (magazines, cigarettes, etc.) could be obtained while in the hospital. The token was valued at five cents (Australian) and was therefore convertible to the currency price of all items within the hospital.

The twenty-day treatment process included 160 rating sessions scheduled at regular intervals throughout the 7:00 A.M. to 10:00 P.M. treatment day. At the end of the treatment day, subjects also recorded a thirty-minute conversation which was not observed by other than group members. This was used as a *probe* measure of therapy progress. The treatment period was divided into three stages, each involving a different procedure. In Stage A, subjects were treated by the token system only. Stage B involved the introduction of either syllable-timed speech or delayed auditory feedback in association with the token system. When subjects reached a criterion of zero percent syllables stuttered at between 180 and 220 syllables per minute for four consecutive rating sessions in Stage B, they passed into the final stage.

Stage C included a hierarchy of speech situations ranked for *stuttering difficulty* by subjects before treatment. There were four levels in the hierarchy ranked according to majority judgment. At the lowest level, subjects obtained tape recordings of conversations between themselves and hospital patients. At a higher level, subjects conversed with salesmen or personnel interviewers (for a position). Finally, subjects either conversed with *ladies of pleasure* in a well known locality of Sydney or participated in a talk-back radio program. Passage through each level was contingent upon a subject obtaining a sequence of two stuttering-free samples of 1,000 syllables of speech (at above 160 syllables per minute) on a concealed cassette recorder.

Concurrently with Stage C of the treatment process, subjects were response contingently penalized one token for a moment of stuttering and one token for an observed period of five seconds silence in the intervals between rating sessions. During the same intervals, subjects also were required to complete regular telephone tasks. These were 400-syllable conversations which also were token rewarded or penalized according to a separate token schedule. Therefore, during almost the last half of treatment, subjects were conversing under token control conditions for most of their waking hours.

A number of experiments were conducted within each stage of the treatment process. These included an experiment designed to assess the treatment effect of some of the components of the token system. An ABAB experimental design was used on three sets of groups over all rating sessions of Stage A in the treatment program. It was found that a combined reward and penalty schedule increased rate of performance when compared with the use of the reward schedule only. It also was found that doubling the number of tokens that could be earned on the reward schedule increased rate of improvement, as did the introduction of the *normal* token schedule following a period of use of a noncontingent schedule. Figure III.8 gives the data for the contingent-noncontingent experiment.

In Stage B of the treatment program, approximately half of the subjects were treated by a modification of Curlee and Perkins' (1969) graded delayed auditory feedback (G.D.A.F.) therapy pro-

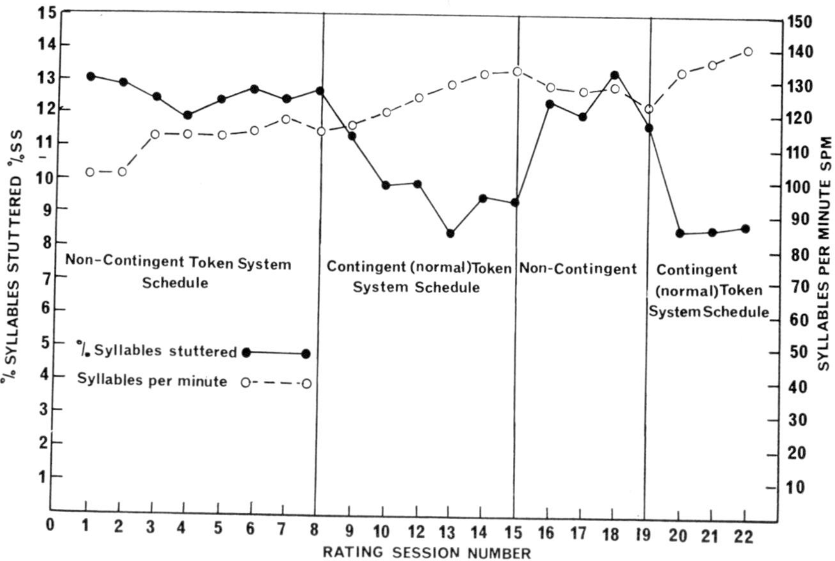

Figure III.8. Mean percent syllables stuttered and syllables spoken per minute in contingent token and non-contingent token sessions of Stage A.

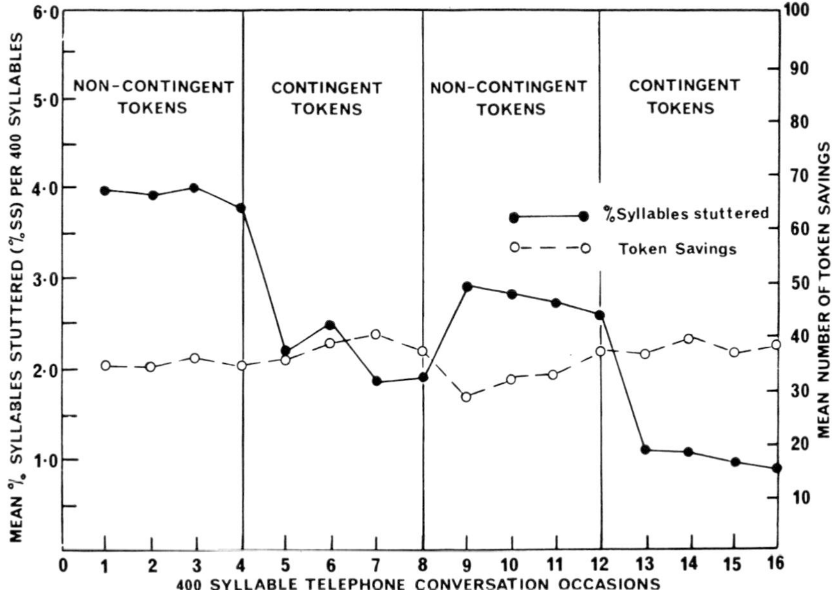

Figure III.9. Mean percent syllables stuttered and mean tokens saved in each 400-syllable telephone conversation. Figure shows mean token savings immediately before telephone task.

cedure. The G.D.A.F. schedule varied from Curlee and Perkins insofar as subjects were required only to obtain fluency within each delay level before passing to the next level. Also, ranges of speaking rate were prescribed for each delay level and integrated within a token schedule. In the *contingent* token schedule, subjects were penalized for departives from the prescribed syllable per minute rate, and for moments of stuttering. This schedule excluded prolongations from *moments of stuttering* until the 50 msec. delay level was reached. Then, to shape fluency, prolongations were penalized. In the *noncontingent* token schedule, which was used with half of the G.D.A.F.-treated subjects, tokens were earned for completing the requisite syllables for the rating session. A comparison of the number of rating sessions required to complete the G.D.A.F. program revealed that the contingent token schedule group took significantly fewer sessions to complete the program.

The final treatment process stage included an evaluation of the effects of G.D.A.F. and syllable-timed speech on *quality of fluency* (Ingham and Andrews, 1971). The G.D.A.F. group was not as limited in conversation syllables per minute rate as was the syllable-timed group towards the end of the treatment process period. Moreover, the remaining *residual* stutterings were equivalent in both groups, but were characterized by a much greater percent of *blocks* and *prolongations* in the syllable-time group then in the G.D.A.F. group.

An attempt was made to determine the role of token savings in the operation of the therapy program. Figure III.9 shows the effect of introducing and removing the contingent token schedule that accompanied the 400-syllable telephone conversations in Stage C. The figure shows that token savings of the subjects as a group remained relatively constant throughout the period. Within this group, however, there were two groups whose token savings were either relatively *high* or *low* during the contingent tokens period.

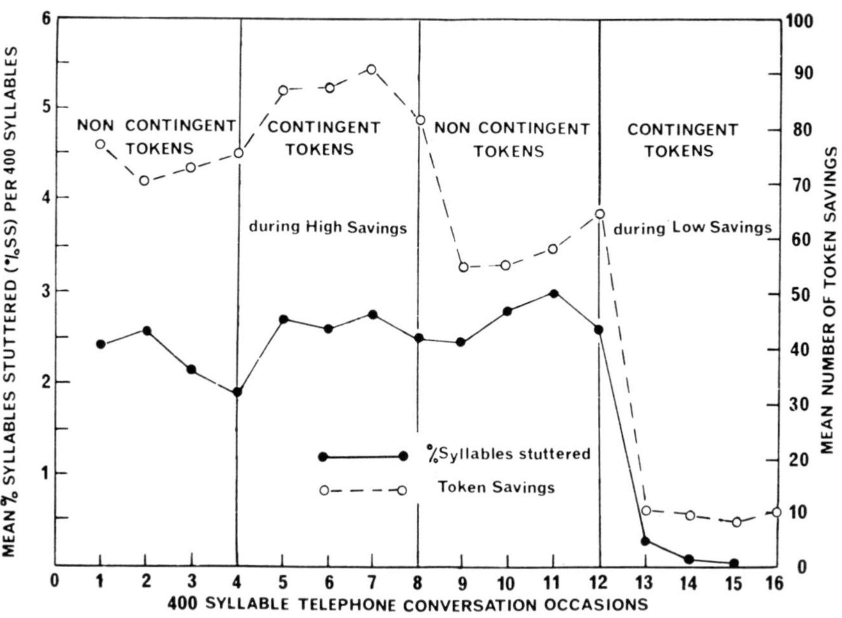

Figure III.10. Mean percent syllables stuttered in each 400-syllable telephone conversation by subjects who had *high* followed by *low* token savings during contingent token schedule.

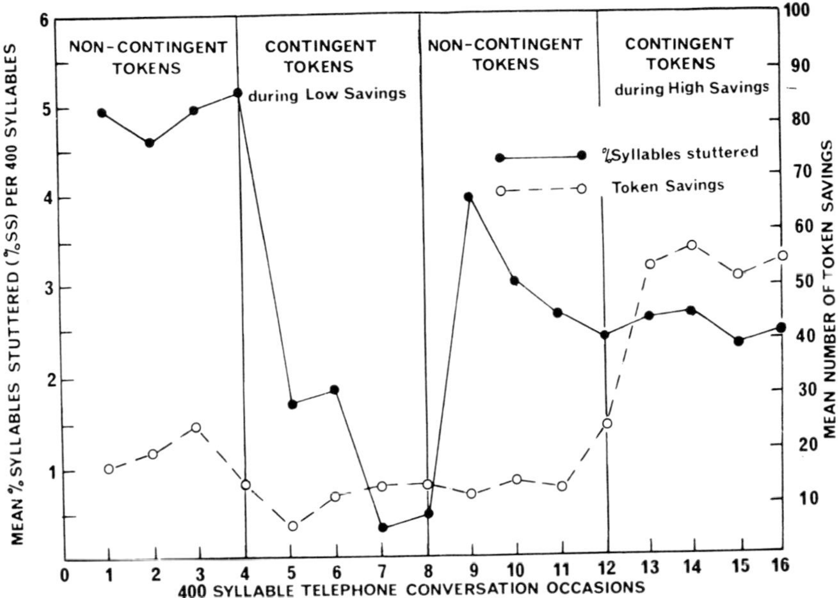

Figure III.11. Mean percent syllables stuttered in each 400-syllable telephone conversation by subjects who had *low* followed by *high* token savings during contingent token schedule.

The trend of percent syllables stuttered for both groups is shown in Figures III.10 and III.11. Apparently, the contingent tokens *treatment effect* was negated by the appearance of *high* savings within a token system.

Evaluation of the outcome of the three-week, in-hospital treatment program involved the administration of an assessment battery to all subjects on six assessment occasions: six months before treatment, immediately before treatment, immediately after treatment, three months after treatment, six months after treatment, and nine months post treatment. The assessment battery was composed of a group and individual version of the Iowa Job Task (Johnson, Darley and Spriestersbach, 1963) and the Stutterers Self Rating of Reactions to Speech Situations Scale (Johnson, et al., 1963). Three personality tests also were administered: E.P.I. (Eysenck and Eysenck, 1963), N.S.Q. (Scheier and Cattell, 1961), and I.P.A.T. Self Analysis Anxiety Scale (Cattell, 1964). From this battery, evaluations were made on speech performance and the association between speech and personality variables over the six assessment occasions. A three-mode factor analysis procedure conducted on *persons, measures,* and *occasions* yielded four major factors: Fluency Factor (Fl), Anxiety Factor (F2), Depression Factor (F3), Sensitivity Factor (F4). Factor scores were then derived for each subject on each factor, and the trend of group scores is shown in Figure III.12. The treatment process produced a marked change in the Fluency Factor (Fl), but this was not paralleled by any significant change in the three personality factors. Thus, there was no evidence that the treatment process affected changes in personality characteristics that were measured by the assessment battery.

A further evaluation of outcome performance was made by comparing the Job Task scores of a matched group of G.D.A.F. and syllable-timed speech treated subjects over the assessment

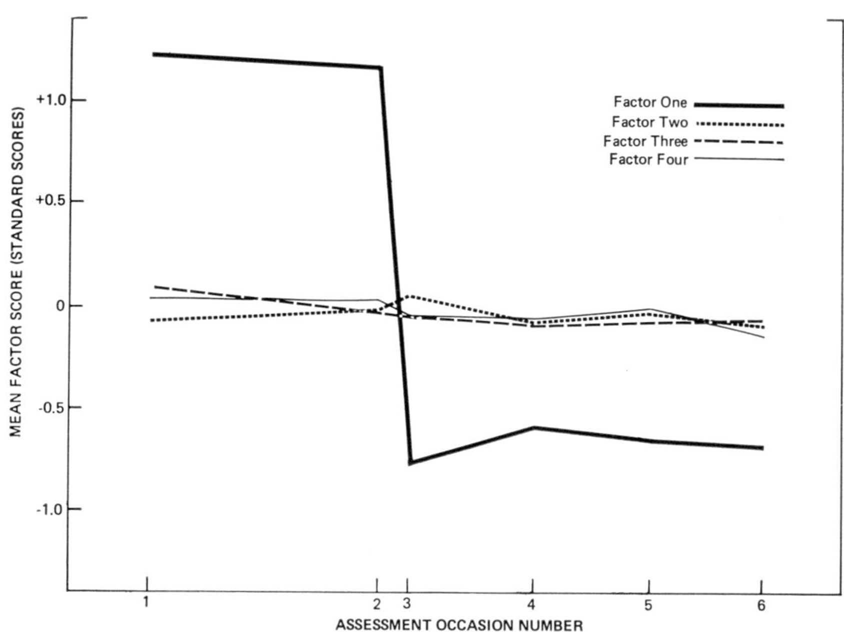

Figure III.12. Mean factor scores for all subjects in each assessment occasion. Factor One (Fluency Factor), Factor Two (Anxiety Factor), Factor Three (Depression Factor), Factor Four (Sensitivity Factor).

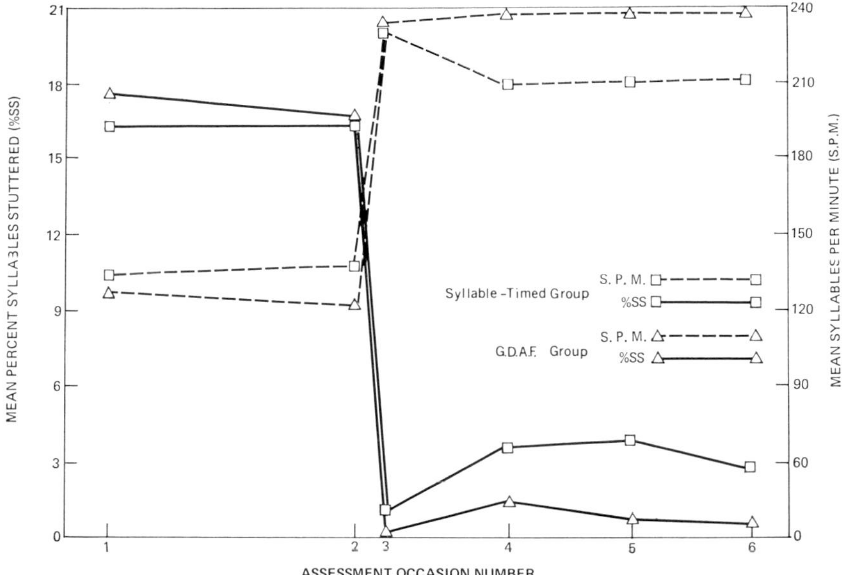

Figure III.13. Mean percent syllables stuttered and syllables spoken per minute on Iowa Job Task in each assessment occasion for subjects treated by syllable-timed speech and subjects treated by G.D.A.F. in Stage B.

occasions. The mean percent syllables stuttered and syllables per minute are shown in Figure III.13. An analysis of these scores revealed no significant difference between the syllable-timed speech and G.D.A.F. groups with respect to percent syllables stuttered. However, the G.D.A.F. group spoke significantly more syllabes per minute in the post-treatment evaluation periods.

The reliability with which percent syllables stuttered and stutterings per minute were scored was assessed by rerating randomly selected rating sessions. For the two raters, the reliability correlation coefficients were .97 and .98 for percent syllables stuttered, and .98 and .99 for speech rate.

Eighteen months after completion of the treatment process, and nine months after the last assessment battery was administered, subjects in the G.D.A.F. group were visited by a female student who sought their assistance in a class project. Unknown to the subjects, she recorded their performance on a T.A.T. test and in a conversation. The result showed that the G.D.A.F. group had relapsed to a mean of 7.8 percent syllables stuttered at 152 syllables per minute. This was superior to the pretreatment mean of 16.4 percent at 91.3 syllables per minute, but vastly inferior to the nine-month Job Task score of 0.50 percent syllables stuttered at 205 syllables per minute.

SUMMARY

The experimental data obtained in the laboratory convincingly indicate that stuttering frequency can be manipulated through a variety of response contingent consequences. The quality and rigor of these laboratory studies are sufficient to warrant optimism that future research will isolate some of the important variables in the modification process. Unfortunately, there is less reason for optimism about the extent to which the experimental work will have any significant impact on explaining the nature of stuttering, especially the onset. There is also some question about whether the experimental work will lead to the development of reliable treatment procedures.

The empirical demonstration that stuttering frequency can be modified by response contingent consequences does not necessarily mean that stuttering is an operant behavior. Nor does it mean that the onset and development of stuttering are best explained in terms of environmental consequences. Whether research stemming from the operant model can make any significant contribution to the understanding of stuttering is a moot point at the present time.

The extent to which the laboratory data can be used to develop reliable therapeutic procedures for stutterers is more encouraging, but considerable work remains to be done. The reports of response contingent stuttering therapy programs or techniques reviewed above are far from satisfactory. There is evidence that the procedures may affect changes within some therapy programs, but the data are difficult to evaluate. Most reports are premature and do not include carefully obtained carry-over or follow-up data. Most reports contain no information at all about the reliability of the observers. Many reports do not employ a carefully specified and unambiguous stuttering response class. Many reports do not make it clear that the treatment variable under study is in fact responsible for the change in stuttering. Most reports contain no data about the extent to which speech parameters other than fluency are modified. Hopefully, future clinical studies will take account of these shortcomings, even though it may be expensive. In the interim, there is little reliable evidence to support the use of response contingent treatment procedures in stuttering therapy.

REFERENCES

Adams, M. R. and Popelka, G.: The influence of "time-out" on stutterers and their disfluency. *Behav. Ther., 2*:334-339, 1971.

Andrews, G. and Harris, M.: *The Syndrome of Stuttering*. Clinics in Developmental Medicine No. 17. London, Heinemann, 1964.

Bar, A.: The shaping of fluency not the modification of stuttering. *J. Commun. Disord., 4*:1-8, 1971.

Biggs, B. and Sheehan, J. G.: Punishment or distraction? Operant stuttering revisited. *J. Abnorm. Psychol., 74*:256-262, 1969.

Browning, R. M.: Behavior therapy for stuttering in a schizophrenic child. *Behav. Res. Ther., 5*:27-35, 1967.

Cattell, R. B.: *I.P.A.T. Self Analysis Scale,* Champaign, Institute for Personality and Ability Testing, 1964.

Cooper, E. B.; Cady, B. B., and Robbins, C. J.: The effect of the verbal stimulus words "wrong," "right," and "tree" on the disfluency rates of stutterers and nonstutters. *J. Speech Hear. Res., 13*:239-244, 1970.

Curlee, R. F. and Perkins, W. H.: Conversational rate control therapy for stuttering. *J. Speech Hear. Disord., 34*:245-250, 1969.

Curlee, R. F. and Perkins, W. H.: The effect of punishment of expectancy to stutter on the frequencies of subsequent expectancies and stutterings. *J. Speech Hear. Res., 11*:787-795, 1968.

Daly, D. A. and Cooper, E. B.: Rate of stuttering adaptation under two electroshock conditions. *Behav. Res. Ther., 5*:49-54, 1967.

Daly, D. A. and Frick, J. V.: The effects of punishing stuttering expectations and stuttering utterances: a comparative study. *Behav. Ther., 1*:228-239, 1970.

Egolf, D. B.; Shames, G. H., and Blind, J. J.: The combined use of operant procedures and theoretical concepts in the treatment of an adult female stutterer. *J. Speech Hear. Disord., 36*:414-421, 1971.

Egolf, D. B.; Shames, G. H., and Seltzer, H. N.: The effects of time-out on the fluency of stutterers in group therapy. *J. Commun. Disord., 4*:111-118, 1971.

Eysenck, H. J. and Eysenck, S. B. G.: *Eysenck Personality Inventory*. London, University of London Press, 1963.

Flanagan, B.; Goldiamond, I., and Azrin, N. H.: Instatement of stuttering in normally fluent individuals through operant procedures. *Science, 130*:979-981, 1959.

Flanagan, B.; Goldiamond, I., and Azrin, N. H.: Operant stuttering: the control of stuttering behavior through response contingent consequences. *J. Exp. Anal. Behav., 1*:173-177, 1958.

Goldiamond, I.: Stuttering and fluency as manipulatable operant response classes. Chapter VI in L. Krasner and L. Ullmann (Eds.) : *Research in Behavior Modification.* New York, Holt, Rinehart and Winston, 1965.

Goldiamond, I.: The maintenance of ongoing fluent verbal behavior and stuttering. *J. Mathetics, 1*:57-95, 1962.

Halvorson, J. A.: The effects on stuttering frequency of pairing punishment (response cost) with reinforcement. *J. Speech Hear. Res., 14*:356-364, 1971.

Haroldson, S. K.; Martin, R. R., and Starr, C. D.: Time-out as a punishment for stuttering. *J. Speech Hear. Res., 11*:560-566, 1968.

Ingham, R. J. and Andrews, G.: Stuttering: the quality of fluency after treatment. *J. Commun. Disord., 4*:279-288, 1971.

Johnson, W.; Darley, F. L., and Spriestersbach, D. C.: *Diagnostic Methods in Speech Pathology.* New York, Harper and Row, 1963.

Leach, E.: Stuttering: clinical application of response-contingent procedures. Chapter XI in B. Gray and G. England (Eds.) : *Stuttering and the Conditioning Therapies.* Monterey, California, Monterey Institute for Speech and Hearing, 1969.

Martin, R. R. and Berndt, L. A.: The effects of time-out on stuttering in a 12 year old boy. *Exceptional Child, 37*:303-304, 1970.

Martin, R. R. and Haroldson, S. K.: The effects of two treatment procedures on stuttering. *J. Commun. Disord., 2*:115-125, 1969.

Martin, R. R. and Haroldson, S. K.: Time-out as a punishment for stuttering during conversation. *J. Commun. Disord., 4*:15-19, 1971.

Martin, R. R. and Siegel, G. M.: The effects of response-contingent shock on stuttering. *J. Speech Hear. Res., 9*:340-352, 1966a.

Martin, R. R. and Siegel, G. M.: The effects of simultaneously punishing stuttering and rewarding fluency. *J. Speech Hear. Res., 9*:466-475, 1966b.

McDermott, L. D.: Clinical management of stuttering behavior. *Feedback, 4*:6-7, 1971.

Quist, R. W. and Martin, R. R.: The effects of response contingent verbal punishment on stuttering. *J. Speech Hear. Res., 10*:795-800, 1967.

Rickard, H. C. and Mundy, M. B.: Direct manipulation of stuttering behavior: an experimental-clinical approach. Chapter 30 in L. Ullmann and L. Krasner (Eds.) : *Case Studies in Behavior Modification.* New York, Holt, Rinehart and Winston, 1965.

Russell, J. C.; Clark, A. W., and van Sommers, P.: Treatment of stammering by reinforcement of fluent speech. *Behav. Res. Ther., 6*:447-453, 1968.

Ryan, B. P.: Operant procedures applied to stuttering therapy for children. *J. Speech Hear. Disord., 36*:264-280, 1971.

Scheier, I. H. and Cattell, R. B.: *Neuroticism Scale Questionnaire.* Champaign, Institute for Personality and Ability Testing, 1961.

Shames, G. H.: Verbal reinforcement during therapy interviews with stutterers. Chapter X in B. Gray and G. England (Eds.): *Stuttering and the Conditioning Therapies.* Monterey, Monterey Institute for Speech and Hearing, 1969.

Shames, G. H.; Egolf, D. B., and Rhodes, R. C.: Experimental programs in stuttering therapy. *J. Speech Hear. Disord., 34*:30-47, 1969.

Sheehan, J. G.: The modification of stuttering through non-reinforcement. *J. Abnormal. Soc. Psychol., 46*:51-63, 1951.

Wingate, M. E.: Calling attention to stuttering. *J. Speech Hear. Res., 2*:326-335, 1959.

ACKNOWLEDGMENT

Preparation of this manuscript was supported in part by the U. S. Office of Education Research, Development and Demonstration Center in Education of Handicapped Children, OEG-0-9-332189-4533 (607), and by Public Health Service Research Grant No. MH-08743 from the National Institute of Mental Health.

CHAPTER IV

VOICE AND ARTICULATION

JAMES L. FITCH

THE MODIFICATION of voice and articulation behaviors through the systematic application of principles of learning can provide the individual working with these disorders with an efficient, predictable method of treatment. Properly employed, behavior modification takes much of the guesswork out of the clinical setting and provides a reasonably objective evaluation of the efficiency of therapy procedures. While the approaches taken to the use of principles of behavior modification in voice and articulation are varied, they share much in common. It is from the commonalities of the work that has been done that the practitioner can derive those principles of behavior modification which are most effective.

There is presently enough literature available on the efficiency of operant techniques in the modification of verbal behavior to convince all but the most doubtful that behavior modification has a permanent place in disciplines related to treatment of disordered speech and language. In this chapter, a review will be made of studies pertaining to the manipulation of voice and articulation behaviors through use of materials and techniques adapted from current behavior modification principles.

The first section of the chapter will deal principally with four studies in the manipulation of vocal behavior through the use of electronic devices programmed to respond to specific acoustic events. The second section will discuss current materials and techniques designed for the treatment of articulation disorders.

MODIFICATION OF VOICE BEHAVIOR

The first study to be discussed was concerned with the manipulation of pitch, or vocal fundamental frequency* (Roll, 1968).

In this study, filters were used to isolate the desired behavior, vocal fundamental frequency (VFF). Three electronic filters* were connected in series to obtain a combined roll-off of approximately 72 dB per octave. Input to the filters was from a microphone located in a soundproof room, through a preamplifier. Output from the filters was to a set of relays which controlled a timing device (electric stop clock) for recording data and a bright white light situated in the soundproof roof room for reinforcement. In pilot studies it was noted that the filters did not function properly at high intensities. It was necessary, therefore, to include an overload circuit which overrode the filter output. When intensity reached the critical level, the output to the clock and reinforcing white light were deactivated and a time-out device (a red light situated in the soundproof booth) was activated.

Subjects were instructed to read a prose passage of approximately three minutes duration into the microphone. See Figure IV.1 for a schematic diagram of the experimental setting. Baseline was

* Asterisk indicates that term is defined in glossary at end of chapter.

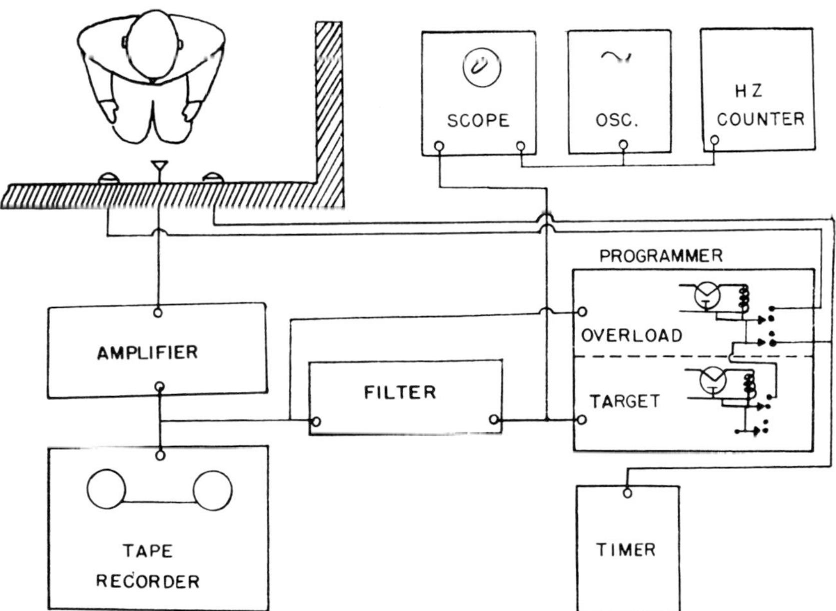

Figure IV.1. Schematic diagram of experimental setting. Roll, 1968, p. 10.

taken in the following manner: with the light in the soundproof room disconnected, subjects read the prose passage, of which a portion was recorded for analysis. Analysis was made by setting the filters (20 Hz* bandwidth*) at a setting below the vocal fundamental frequency (VFF) and at which no energy was recorded from the filters. The 20 Hz bandwidth was then raised in five Hz steps until sufficient energy passed through the filters to activate the relays.* The activated relay triggered an electric stop clock which provided data in hundredths of a second. As the filter band settings were raised, the duration first increased, then decreased (occasionally to zero time), then increased a second time. The second increase indicated the involvement of the first harmonic and thus data recording was stopped at that point. From the duration at each filter setting a profile of VFF was constructed. The midpoint of the filter band setting with the greatest accumulation of time was designated the modal VFF.

The bandpass frequency durations were plotted graphically. When over three days the plotted profiles were stable, a frequency band with a low probability of occurrence (less than 10% of the possible time) was selected for conditioning. Before the experimental condition was initiated, the filters were set for the low probability frequency band. Using trials four minutes in duration, the experimenter recorded the total time at the selected frequency. When the ninth trial was within the range of the previous eight trials, the baseline was considered stable. When this was achieved, the experimental condition was begun.

Subjects participated in the study a minimum of three days a week. On each day four, four minute trials were run. The reading material consisted of factual prose, a portion of which was the previously analyzed prose passage.

Subjects were asked to read the passages and to keep the bright white light on as much as possible. They were also told that the red light indicated that they were doing something wrong. The slow delay red light was activated by an overload which triggered when intensities great enough to distort filter functioning were present.

Trials under the experimental condition continued until the subject achieved a high stable rate of target behavior. In other words, when the low probability behavior was no longer a low probability behavior, the experimental condition was satisfied. The standard fifty-five-word passage was recorded and stored for analysis and extinction trials were begun.

During the extinction trials, the lights were disconnected. Data was taken as before. Extinction trials continued until a low rate

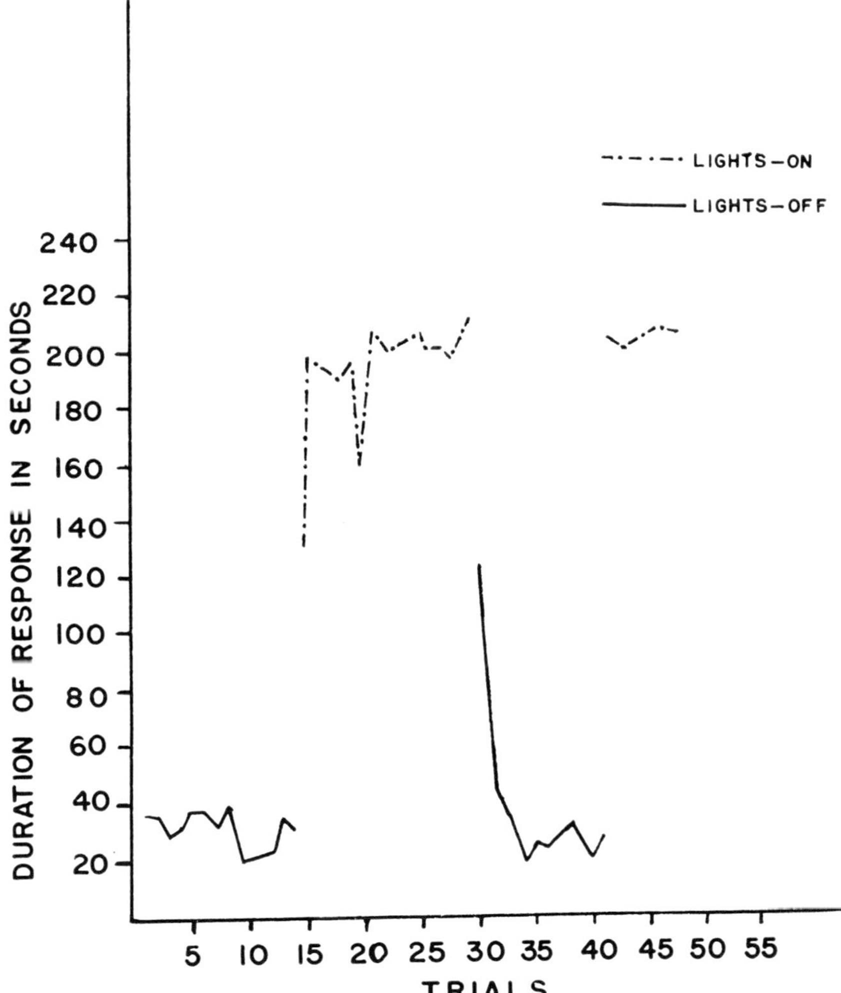

Figure IV.2. Response duration in seconds as a function of trials for subject 1. Roll, 1968, p. 19.

of target response was obtained at which time the lights were reconnected into the circuit and the behavior reinstated. Figures IV.2, IV.3, IV.4, IV.5 and IV.6 show the results of the experimental conditions. It is obvious that there was a marked increase in time recorded at the experimental frequency band during conditioning and reinstatement phases.

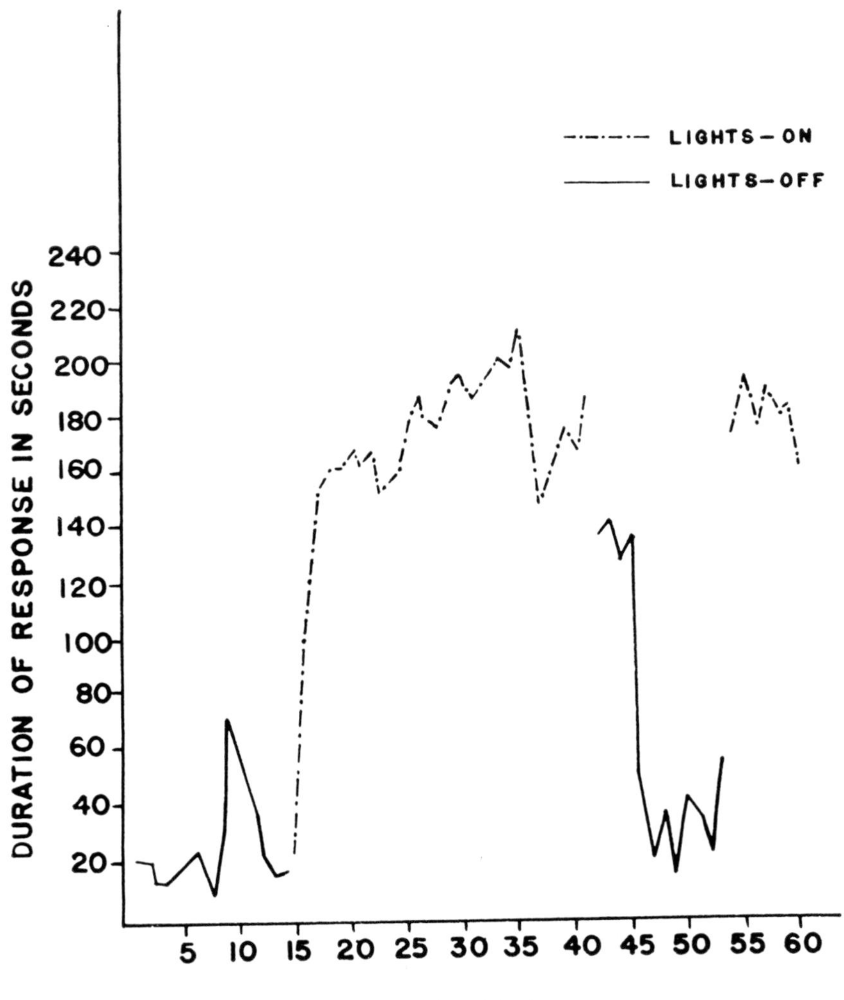

Figure IV.3. Response duration in seconds as a function of trials for subject 2. Roll, 1968, p. 20.

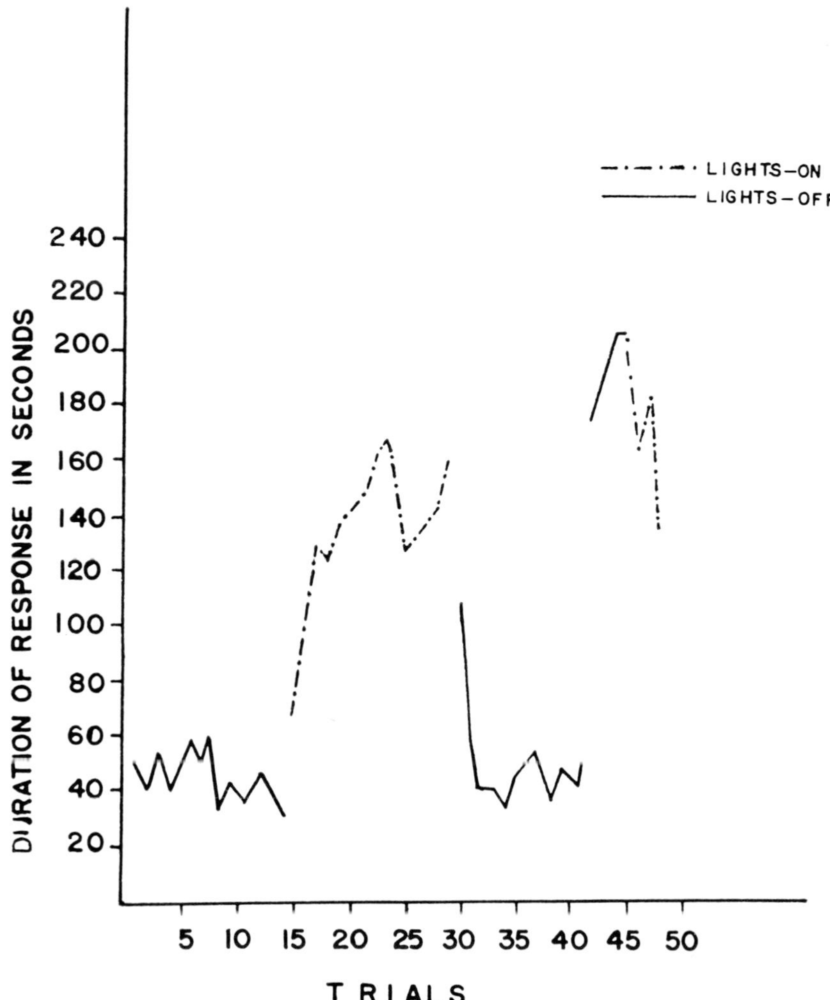

Figure IV.4. Response duration in seconds as a function of trials for subject 3. Roll, 1968, p. 21.

Analysis of the profiles of VFF range for the subjects, figures IV.7, IV.8, IV.9, IV.10 and IV.11, indicate the corresponding movement of the pitch range toward the target frequency. It can be noted that the profiles of the lights-on and lights-off condition vary somewhat in each subject, with the greatest variation being in the extinction profile of subject 5. At the conclusion of the study all sub-

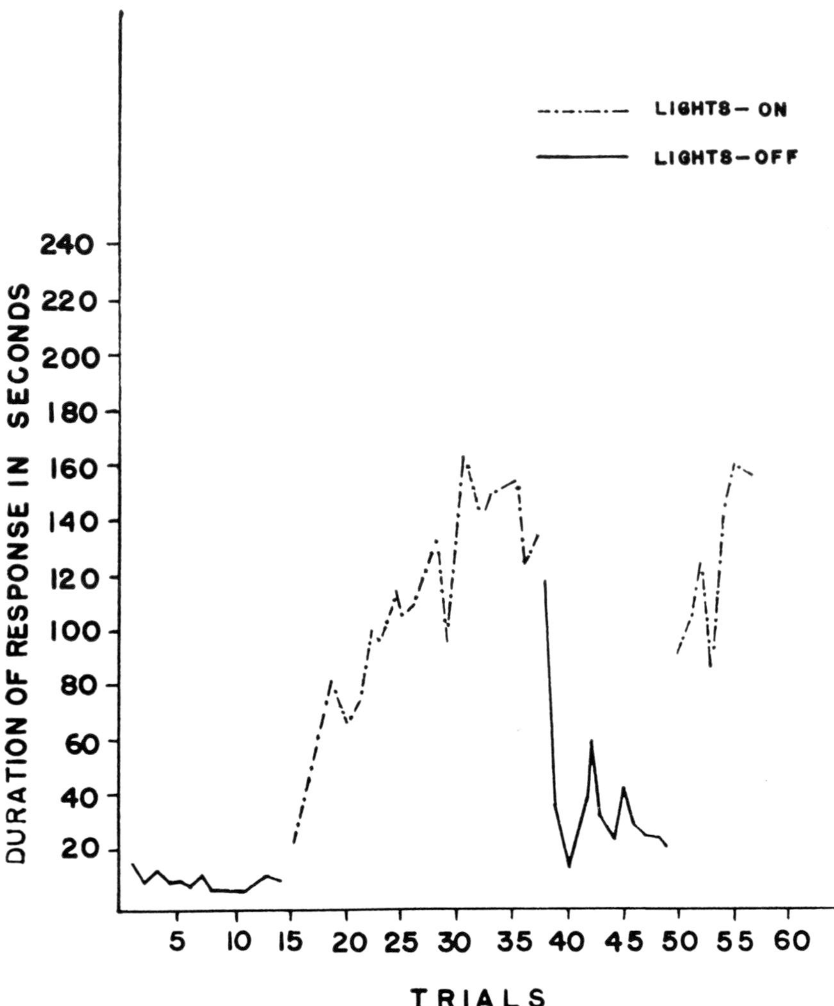

Figure IV.5. Response duration in seconds as a function of trials for subject 4. Roll, 1968, p. 22.

jects were able to verbalize the contingency of the white light and those who had encountered the red light were aware of its contingency.

Roll (1969) later applied the manipulation of vocal fundamental frequency to persons with functional pitch disorders. The same apparatus was used, and basically the same procedure. First VFF was measured using the techniques described in the previous study. Then an appropriate experimental target setting for the filters was determined. The determination was made in consideration of a number of factors. First of all, the new pitch level was to be within the range for the person's age and sex group. Secondly, consideration was given to vocal quality at different pitch levels. All subjects were seen by an otolaryngologist to eliminate cases of possible organic involvement.

The baseline was taken by setting the filters on the target VFF

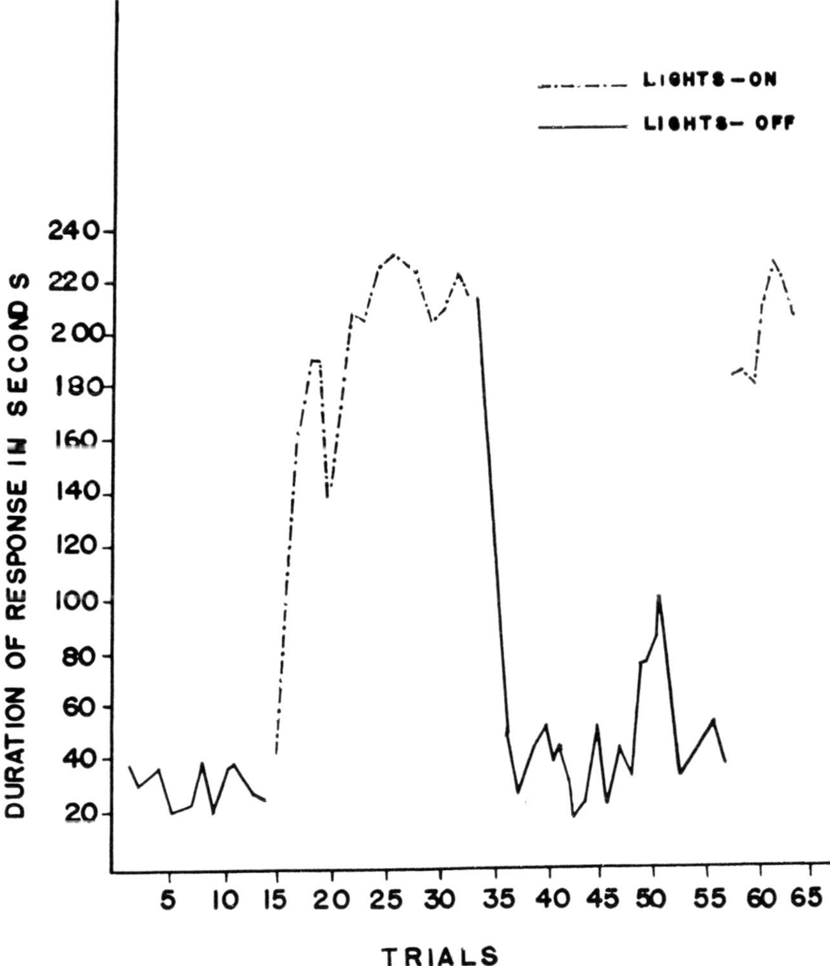

Figure IV.6. Response duration in seconds as a function of trials for subject 5. Roll, 1968, p. 23.

and recording the duration of energy passing through the filters in a three minute trial. Again the baseline was considered stable when the ninth trial was within the previous eight. When the baseline stabilized, the lights were connected to the system and feedback provided. In this study, the contingencies of the lights were explained to the subjects before the study was begun.

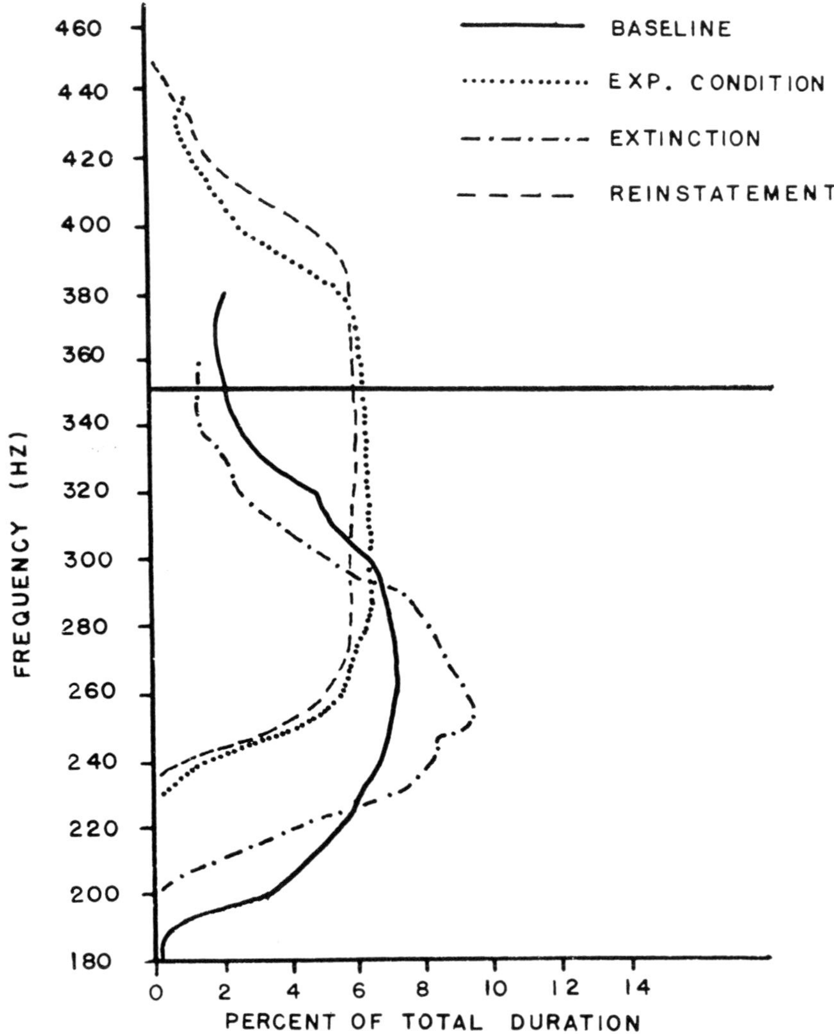

Figure IV.7. Percent of total duration as a function of frequency, subject 1. Roll, 1968, p. 25.

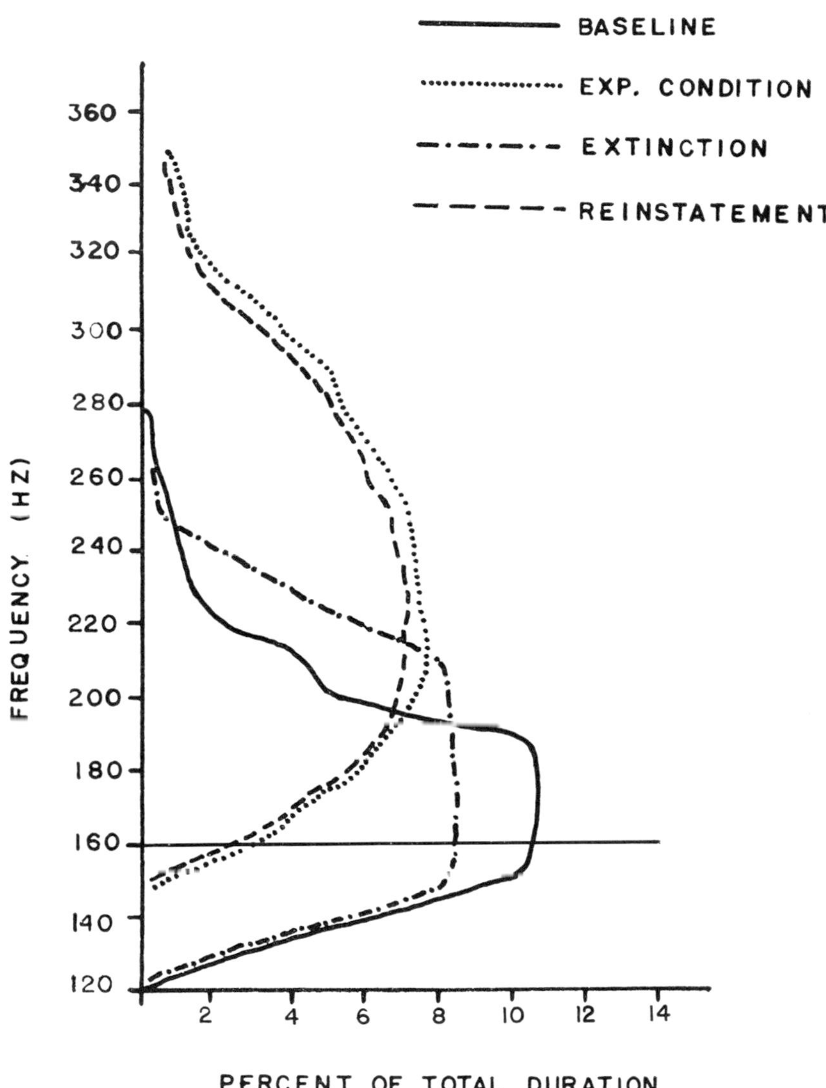

Figure IV.8. Percent of total duration as a function of frequency, subject 2. Roll, 1968, p. 26.

If the baseline rates were of zero duration, i.e., no energy recorded at the target VFF level, a shaping procedure was introduced. The shaping behavior was a frequency band between the habitual modal VFF and the target VFF which occurred with low probability. The shaping target was used in the experimental condition until it became a high probability behavior, at which time the shaping target was moved more closely to the target VFF

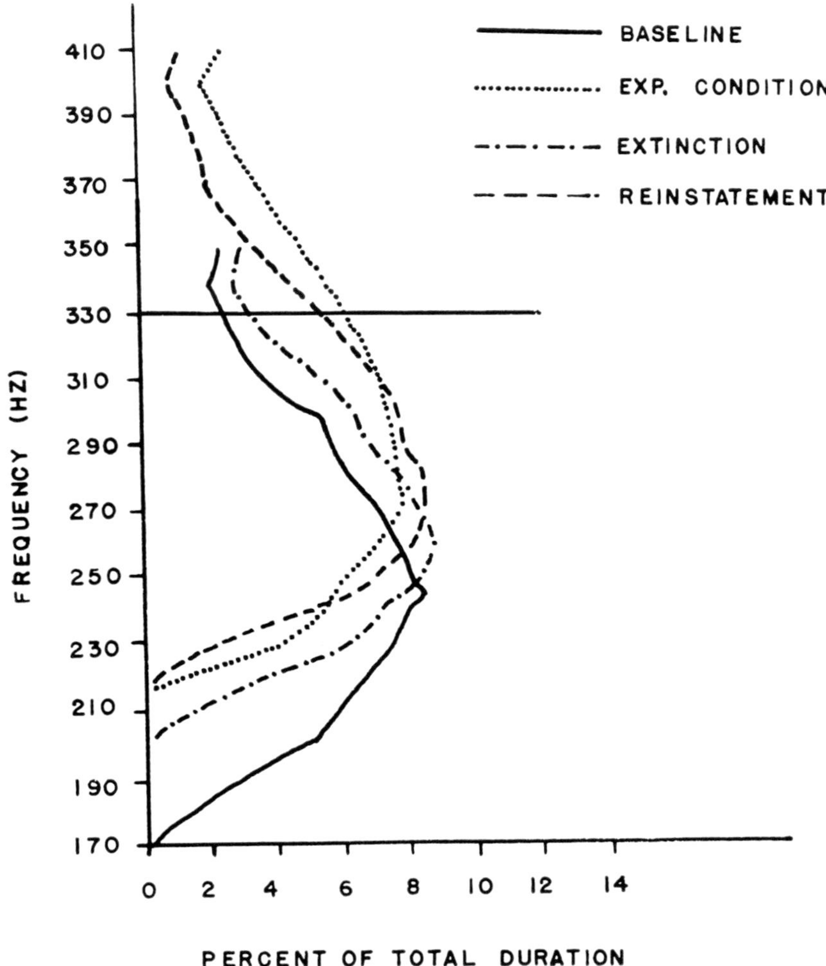

Figure IV.9. Percent of total duration as a function of frequency, subject 3. Roll, 1968, p. 27.

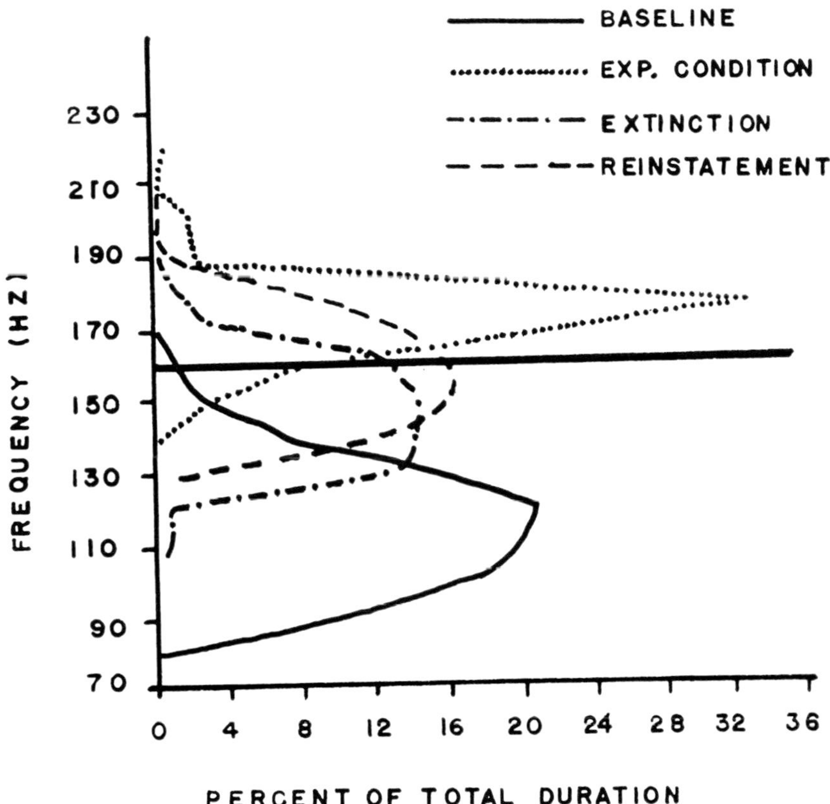

Figure IV.10. Percent of total duration as a function of frequency, subject 4. Roll, 1968, p. 28.

level. Shaping continued until the subject achieved the experimental target VFF level.

After each trial the subject was told how much time had accumulated on the clock compared to previous efforts. Verbal praise was contingent on trials of high duration. When the experimental VFF was being achieved at a high rate of response, a no-feedback condition was introduced. As this study was concerned with persons whose terminal behavior was to be stabilized, this phase deviated from a true extinction situation. During the no-feedback phase the subject was told that the lights were going to be disconnected, but that he should continue to use his new voice. The

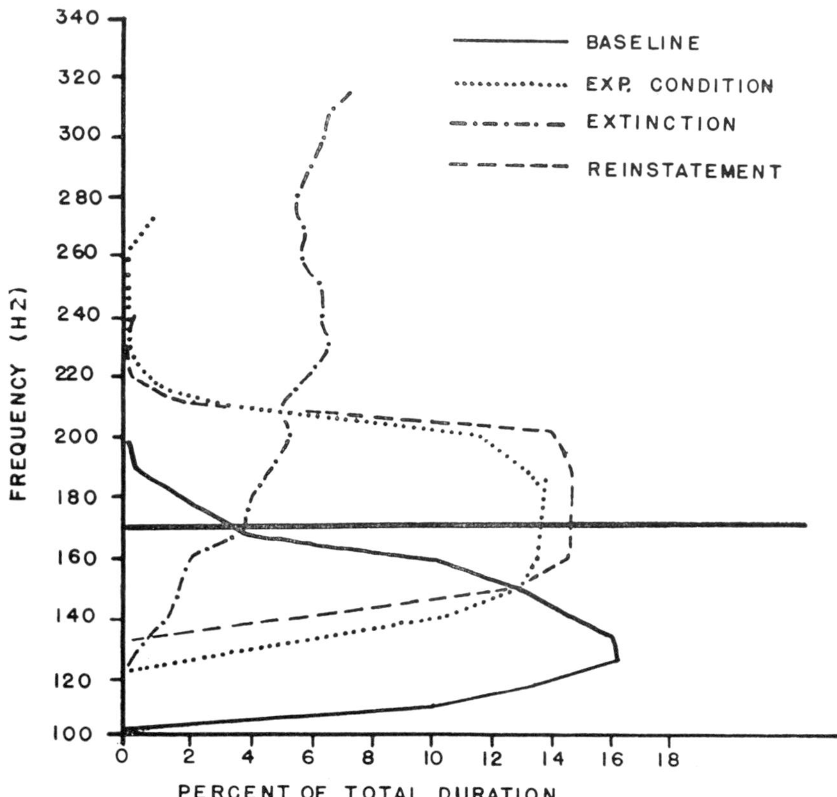

Figure IV.11. Percent of total duration as a function of frequency, subject 5. Roll, 1968, p. 29.

purpose of this phase was to determine if the experimental VFF could be maintained in the absence of the contingent light. If the high response rate at the experimental VFF continued through the no-feedback phase, generalization procedures were introduced. If the high response rate did not continue, the reinforcing light was connected and feedback was again presented to reinstate the behavior.

The purpose of the generalization procedures was to fade the experimental conditions while continuing a high response rate at the experimental VFF. This was done by having the person first read material other than the factual prose used in the first phase of the study. If the high response rate continued during reading, the subject was asked to speak on a list of topics provided him. The last of the generalization procedures consisted of having another person sit in the room with the subject and engage him in conversation. If during any of the generalization procedures the response rate decreased significantly, the previous condition at which a high response rate had been achieved was reintroduced. Profiles of the subjects were made at all stages.

Three of the five subjects who participated in the study will be discussed. Data were incomplete on two subjects who moved before the study could be completed.

Subject 1 was a male college student whose habitual modal VFF was 210 Hz, which is within the range of normal female VFF. He had, in fact, been mistaken for a female when talking on the telephone. The lowest tone he produced while humming was 156 Hz. It was not clear whether he was using a falsetto voice in the pre-study evaluation.

The experimental VFF was set for a band of 110 Hz to 130 Hz as this is within normal limits for his age-sex group. Each of the ten baseline trials were zero. A shaping target of 120-140 Hz was used initially as this band allowed some of his normally produced speech to activate the relays.

> During the second shaping trial, the subject's voice suddenly broke and continued to break from the high pitch to a very low pitch. The low pitch was found to be approximately 105 Hz. by Lissajous figure on an oscilloscope by comparison with a known frequency from a frequency generator. The filter band was changed to 100-120 Hz to allow feedback for the low frequency that he was using during his voice breaks. The vocal quality during these breaks was very poor, but the subject reported no vocal strain or pain connected with production of the low frequency. He reported that he could not voluntarily control the breaks, but total response duration per trial consistently increased. After shaping trials at the 100-120 filter band, the filters were adjusted to the experimental filter setting of 110-130 Hz.
>
> (Roll, 1969, p. 27-30)

The change was so obvious, and dramatic, that the author and another person working in the laboratory at the time did the traditional double-take.

> The subject's total response duration per trial steadily increased and stabilized during the conditioning phase of the investigation. The

> vocal quality and control of breaks also consistently improved. After 50 trials, the subject was reading for the entire three-minute trials without an upward break. (Roll, 1969, p. 30)

It became obvious that the subject had been using a falsetto voice and that rather than shaping downward from the habitual VFF it was actually easier for him to lower his VFF by an octave to his optimal VFF. This lower pitch had not been elicited in the pre-experimental clinical evaluation. The results of the entire experimental procedure are shown in figure IV.12.

It can be noted that the high response rate at the lower frequency remained stabilized through generalization procedures. An evaluation of range after completion of the experiment indicated lowest tone at 50 Hz and the highest before beginning falsetto at 160 Hz. At the end he also reported strain in using the falsetto voice. Figure IV.13 shows the pitch profile from beginning to speaking generalization. A follow-up after eight months found that he was using the new VFF and was pleased with it.

Subject 2 was a thirty-five-year-old female who reported hoarse-

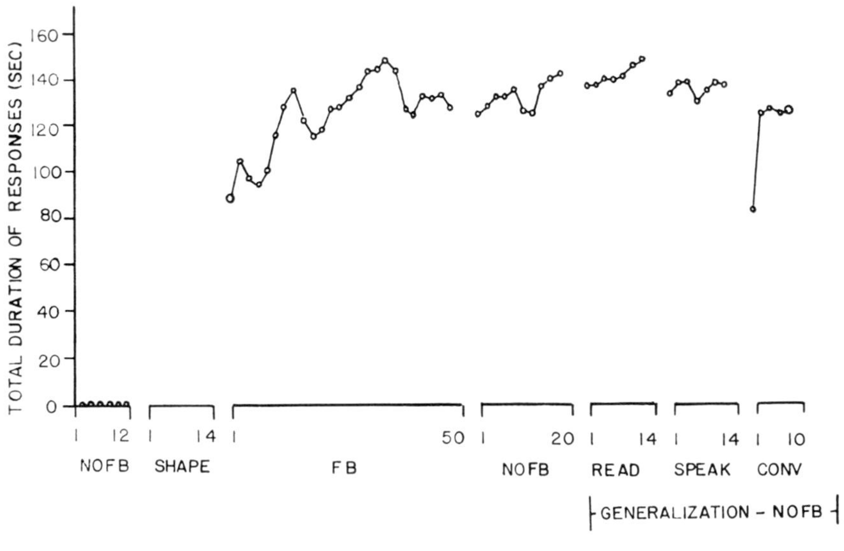

Figure IV.12. Total response duration as a function of trials. Each data point represents the average of the duration of two trials. (FB-Feedback present.) Roll, 1969, p. 29.

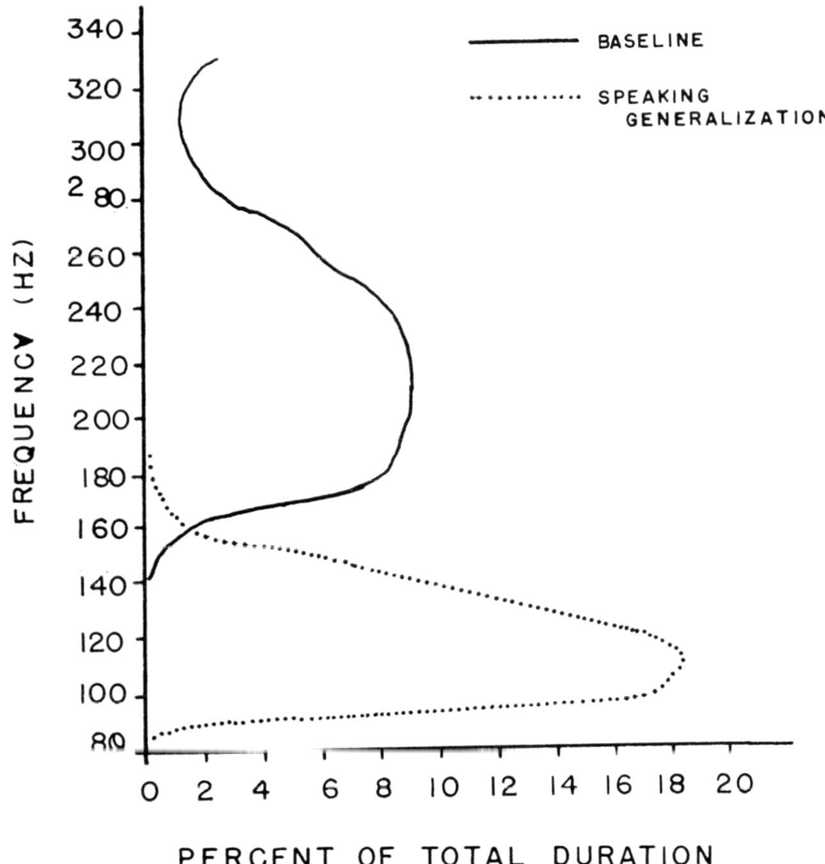

Figure IV.13. Modal fundamental frequency profiles for each phase of the investigation. Percentage of total duration as a function of frequency. Roll, 1969, p. 33.

ness and loss of voice when speaking publicly. As her profession required public speaking the vocal disorder was creating an uncomfortable situation. An evaluation of pitch yielded a VFF of 230 Hz, within normal limits for females of her age sex group. It was noted, however, that hoarseness accompanied tones produced about 200 Hz. An analysis of her pitch profile (figure IV.15) indicated that she was using a high percentage of frequencies near the top of her pitch range.

Using the experimental technique, her VFF was lowered to

180 Hz. Vocal quality remained good. Figure IV.14 indicates that the subject achieved a high rate of response during the light contingent condition. There was a decrease in rate during the initial phase of the no-feedback condition, but the rate rose and stabilized. It remained high throughout generalization procedures. Figure IV.15 shows the pitch profile from baseline to speaking generalization. A follow-up eight months later indicated that the lower VFF had been maintained and the subject reported pleasure with her voice.

Subject 3 was a nineteen-year-old male with a habitual modal VFF of 220 Hz, within normal limits for females, but well above the normal limits for males. After shaping to his experimental VFF there was variability in the response rate. To better stabilize the experimental level, the VFF was shaped to a frequency band below the experimental VFF. On figure IV.16 it can be noted that after shaping to the lower frequency, the rate of response at the experimental frequency stabilized at a high rate of response.

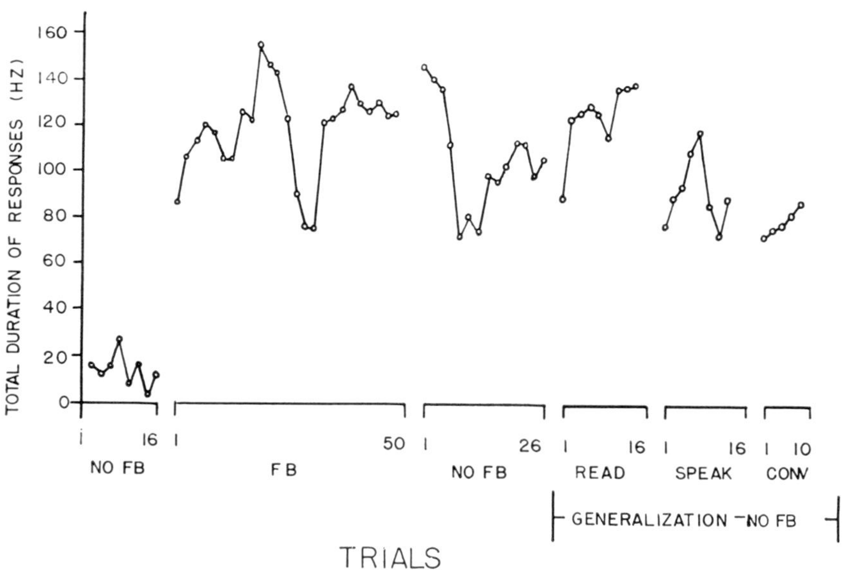

Figure IV.14. Total response duration as a function of trials. Each data point represents the average of the duration of two trials. (FB-feedback present.) Roll, 1969, p. 37.

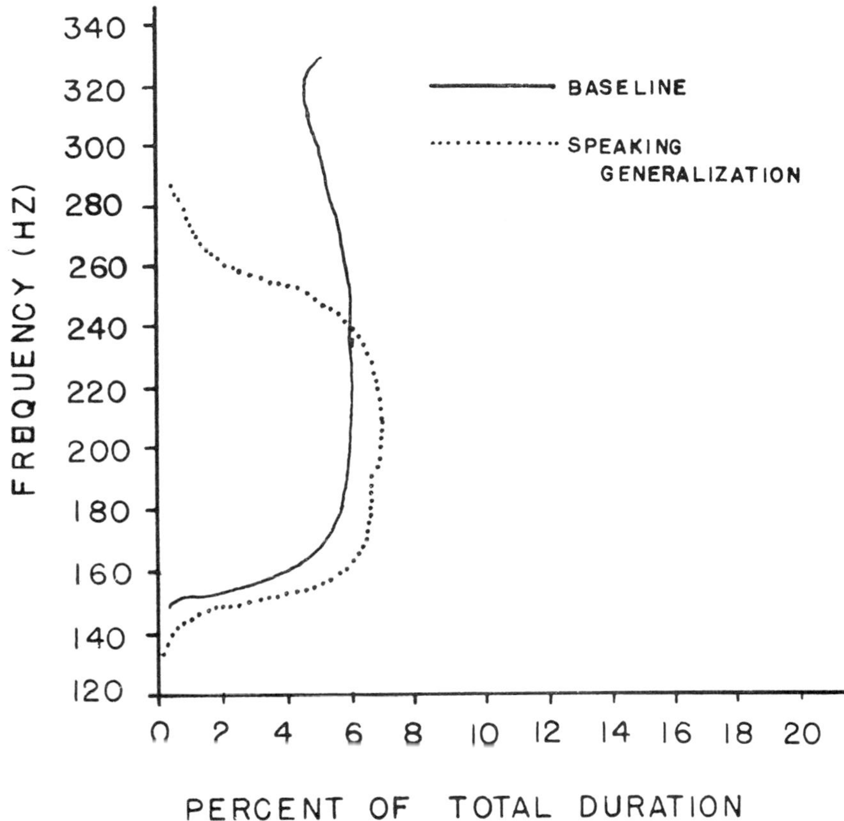

Figure IV.15. Modal fundamental frequency profiles for each phase of the investigation. Percentage of total duration as a function of frequency. Roll, 1969, p. 40.

During generalization in the reading phase with no-feedback, there was a decrease in response rate. A high rate of response at the experimental setting was reinstated and a variable interval reinforcement schedule used to fade the response contingent light. When the no-feedback condition was reintroduced, rate decreased slightly, but remained well above baseline levels. Figure IV.17 portrays the change from baseline profile to impromptu speaking with no feedback. The subject was not available for further measures.

Moore (1968), using the apparatus developed in the Roll study, applied various schedules of reinforcement to the modification of VFF in four normal speakers. After determining the experimental VFF level, conditioning began with reinforcement presented on a continuous schedule. Two of the four subjects were then presented with reinforcement on a fixed ratio followed by reinforcement on a fixed interval. The other two subjects were presented with reinforcement on a fixed interval, then a fixed ratio. All subjects were lastly placed on a series of variable ratios, with reinforcement presented progressively less often. When each schedule of reinforcement was terminated, the behavior was extinguished. Behavior was reinstated before beginning the next schedule of reinforcement by providing continous reinforcement.

The fixed interval was FI-twenty-two seconds consisting of ten seconds of opportunity for reinforcement after twenty-two seconds of response. The fixed ratio schedule, FR-fifteen seconds, consisted of the presentation of ten seconds of opportunity for reinforce-

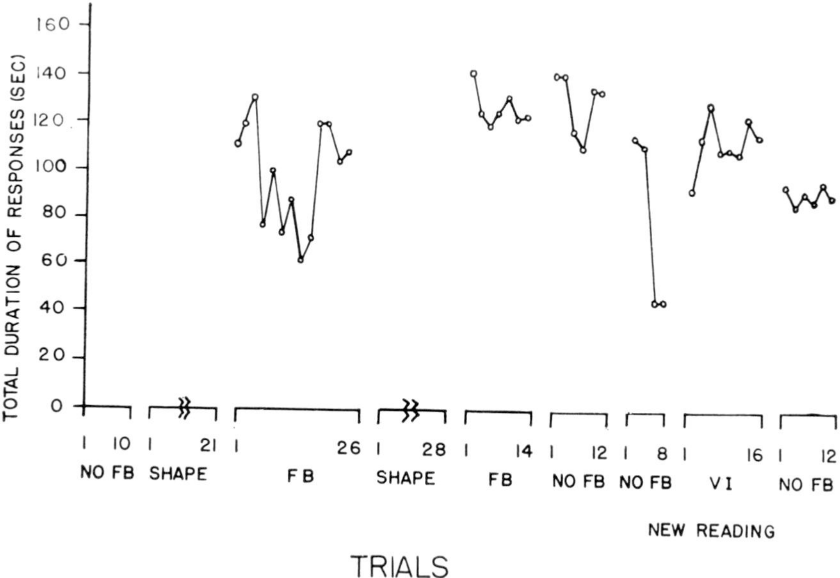

Figure IV.16. Total response duration as a function of trials. Each data point represents the average of the duration of two trials. (FB-feedback present). Roll, 1969, p. 43.

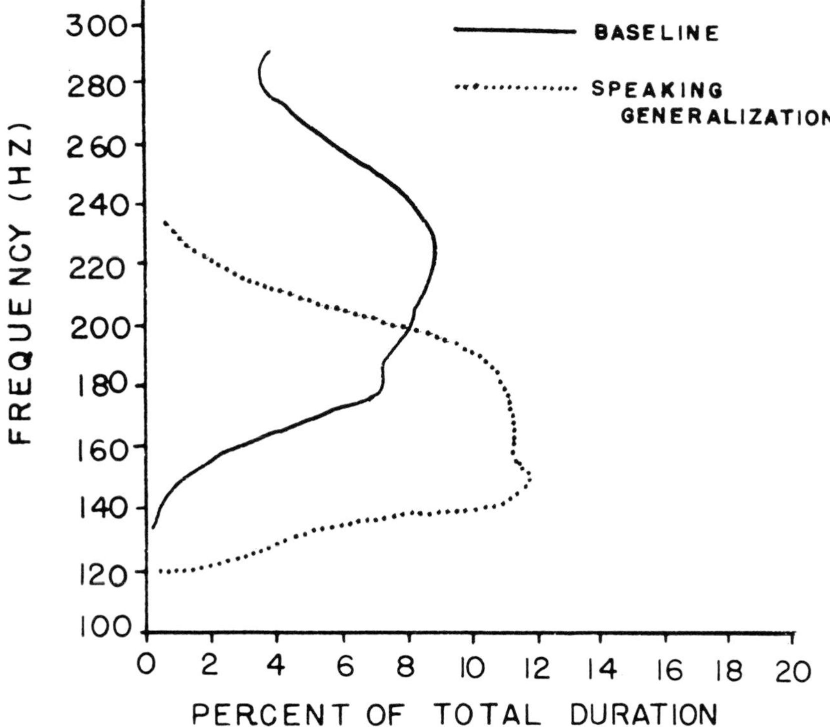

Figure IV.17. Modal fundamental frequency profiles for each phase of the investigation. Percentage of total duration as a function of frequency. Roll, 1969, p. 46.

ment after the subject achieved fifteen seconds of on-target behavior.

Graphic representation of the results can be seen in figures IV.18 through IV.21. It can be noted that in all experimental conditions there was a noticeable rise in rate of target response. Extinction after each phase was relatively rapid and reinstatement of experimental VFF was immediate by use of continuous reinforcement. The results of the effects of the various schedules of reinforcement were as follows:

> The fixed schedules tended to produce a pause or reduced rate of responding following a period of reinforcement. The responses in-

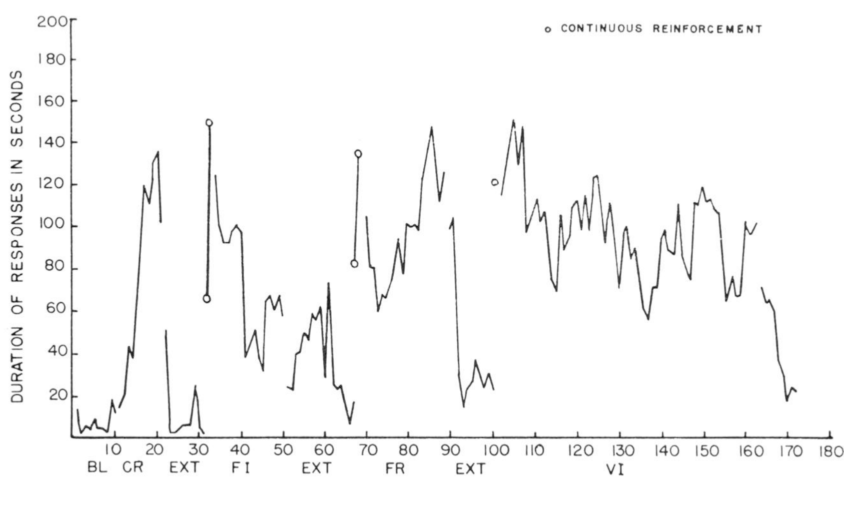

Figure IV.18. Response duration as a function of trials for subject 1 (female). Moore, 1968, pp. 25, 26.

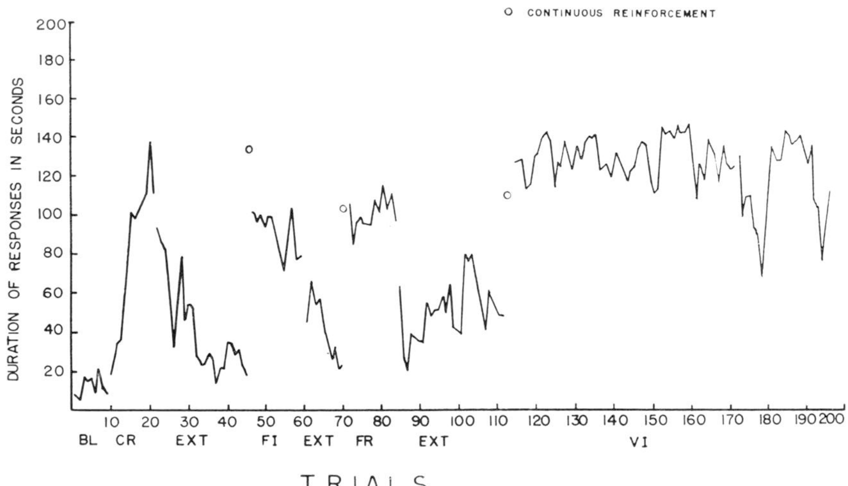

Figure IV.19. Response duration as a function of trials for subject 2 (female). Moore, 1968, pp. 33-34.

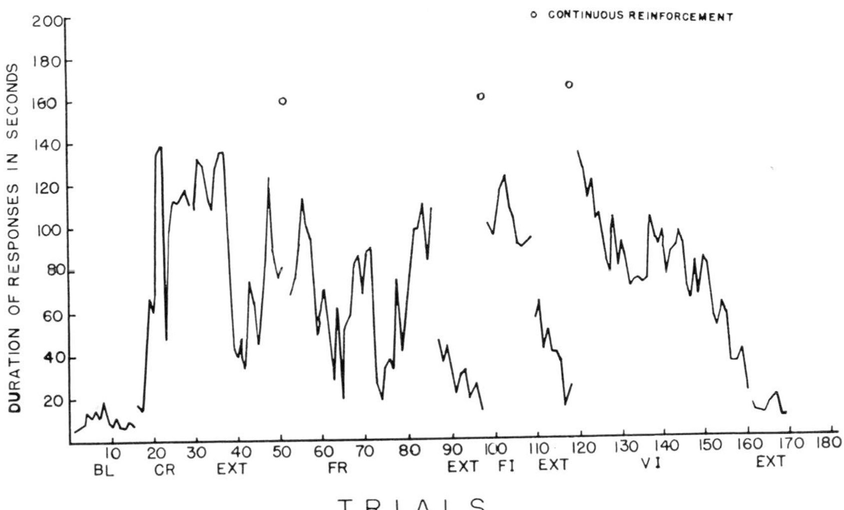

Figure IV.20. Response duration as a function of trials for subject 3 (female). Moore, 1968, pp. 40, 41.

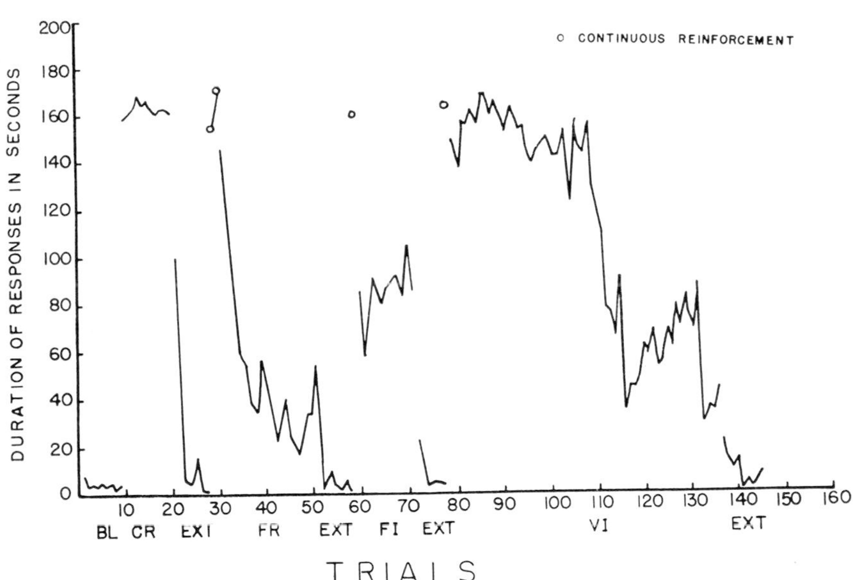

Figure IV.21. Response duration as a function of trials for subject 4 (male). Moore, 1968, pp. 46, 47.

> creased, however, as the approach of the next reinforcement period neared. The VI schedules, on the other hand, produced a steady rate of response in all *S*s. The VI schedules were also the most efficient schedules in that they produced high durations of response with a minimum of reinforcement. (Moore, 1968, p. 62)

A study of the graphs indicate rapid extinction in almost all cases.

> This investigation did not show that the VI schedules of reinforcement produced the greatest resistance to extinction as one might expect, based on previous research. Extinction from all schedules was fairly rapid for three of the four *S*s. The one *S* who developed great resistance to extinction following the VI schedules, tended to resist extinction from all conditioning phases of the study. The aversive nature of the required response probably accounts for the tendency of most of the *S*s to extinguish rapidly. (Moore, 1968, p. 63)

Aversive nature of the required response refers to the fact that all the speakers had normal VFF and the experimental condition was requiring use of a VFF not normal for the subjects.

Throughout the studies of pitch control it became obvious that vocal behaviors could be manipulated with exceptional efficiency through the use of electronic programming. In relation to behavior manipulation by a clinician, electronic programming has several advantages. First of all, the target behavior is maintained precisely from day to day. The clinician, in the judgment of pitch, cannot provide the constancy of expected response with nearly the accuracy of the machine. Secondly, the machine responds immediately with a consistent *yes-no* feedback. It takes longer for the clinician to do so and often the clinician gives ambiguity to feedback, i.e., "I'm not sure, try it again" or "I think that was better." While precision may be approached by an exceptional clinician on a good day, the machine responds the same at all times. The constancy of target behavior, immediacy of feedback, and consistency of performance evaluation contribute to a more efficient therapy procedure.

It was noted that intensity had to be controlled during the experiments because of the limitations of the equipment. The control of intensity added a new dimension to the research—two behaviors could be controlled simultaneously. In somewhat logical thought progression, it appeared that the same efficiency of behavior manipulation could be obtained for other parameters of speaking behavior if they could be defined precisely in acoustic description. If the control could be extended to articulatory behavior (a large portion of many speech clinician's case load) a major breakthrough in therapy could be achieved. The next study to be discussed, under the section in voice, was a step in that direction.

Through a series of pilot studies it was found that sounds could be defined acoustically in such a way that electronic identification was possible. [s] and [i], particularly, were amenable to this treatment, however, even these sounds varied greatly from individual to individual. In other words, the control of articulation would require a much more discrete type of electronic programming. Also, while pitch and intensity are *relatively* constant through speaking behavior, the acoustic spectrum for the sounds of speech have tremendous variety, overlap, and occur within very small time dimensions. Rather than attempt to program individual sounds, it was proposed that speech be programmed with attention to the distinctive features of the phonetic elements. The following study treats the modification of phoneme voicing through application of principles of reinforcement.

In this study (Fitch, 1971), the purpose was to determine the feasibility of modifying the production of a voiced sound, [z], to approximate its unvoiced cognate, [s]. The electronic equipment used in the previous studies was used with modifications. One set of filters, designated the target filters, passed a frequency band of 5000 Hz to 8000 Hz, a band in which there is considerable energy for the sounds [s] and [z], but little energy from other phonetic elements. A second set of filters, designated the reject filters, passed an energy band from 200 Hz to 4000 Tz. While [z] has considerable energy in this region, [s] has little. Energy passing through the target filters (5000 Hz to 8000 Hz) triggered the target relay which controlled the reinforcing light. Energy passing through the second set of filters triggered a *reject relay* which cancelled the target relay. An attenuator was connected to the reject input to allow for gradual shaping of decreasing voicing. To activate the reinforcing light the subject had to emit a high frequency with attenuated voicing. Thus, an [s] triggered the machine readily while [z] brought about no reinforcement.

Three subjects read lists of nonsense syllables beginning with the letter *z*. Shaping consisted of setting the reject attenuator so that only slight de-voicing of the [z] sound would activate the response contingent light. When the subject received three consecutive reinforcements, the attenuator to the reject relay was decreased so that in order to obtain further reinforcement the subject had to reduce the intensity of the voicing component. Shaping trials were continued until the attenuation to the reject

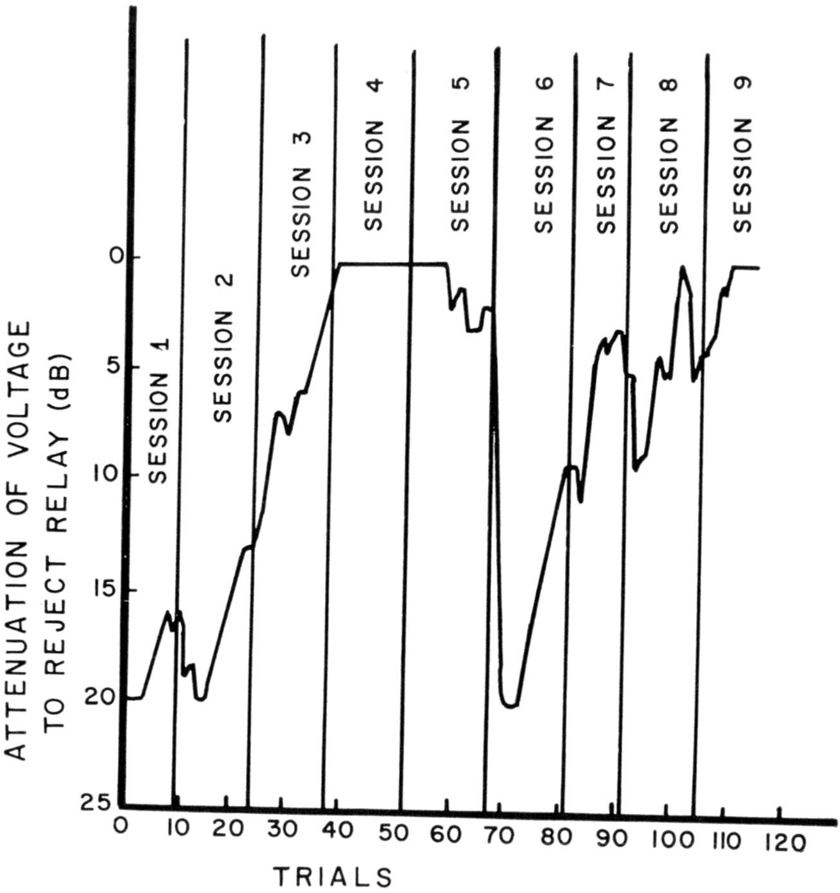

Figure IV.22. Shaping curve of subject 1. Fitch, 1971.

relay was zero, at which point the subject was unvoicing the initial sound of the syllable. Reinforcement was continuous and a program of reinforcement constructed that would allow the subjects to receive a maximum of reinforcement, thus keeping overall response rate high.

All subjects met the experimental criterion of reducing phoneme voicing to the point at which it would not activate the reject relay with zero attenuation. The manner in which they did so, however, varied considerably.

Perceptual and spectrographic analysis demonstrated that subject 1 learned to control the light by prefacing the syllables with high intensity target frequencies of short duration, but still voiced the initial sound through most of its duration. Subject 2 clearly unvoiced the sound during the conditioning and reinstatement phases of the study. While the responses of subject 3 during conditioning and reinstatement were perceptually identified as voiceless, spectrographic analysis found that there was still a small degree of voicing present.

Figures IV.22 and IV.23 show the shaping curve and the conditioning, extinction and reinstatement trials of subject 1. It can be noted in figure IV.22 that the subject met the conditioning criterion on the fortieth trial, but could not maintain it. A decrease in target response rate then occurred, followed by a more gradual climb to criterion behavior. In figure IV.23 it can be noted that extinction and reinstatement of the behavior was rapid. Subject 1 was in the experimental condition a total of two and three-fourths hours.

Figure IV.24 depicts the shaping curve of subject 2. After an initial climb there is again a decrease in response rate of the target behavior. It was followed by a steep climb to criterion behavior. In figure IV.25 it can be seen that the extinction and reinstatement phases are again rapid. Total time in the experimental setting for subject 2 was one and one-half hours.

Subject 3 achieved the target criterion behavior after a minimum of shaping trials (figure IV.26). In figure IV.27, it can be seen that the extinction phase was not successful. The wide range of response rates at target behavior indicate that subject 3 was

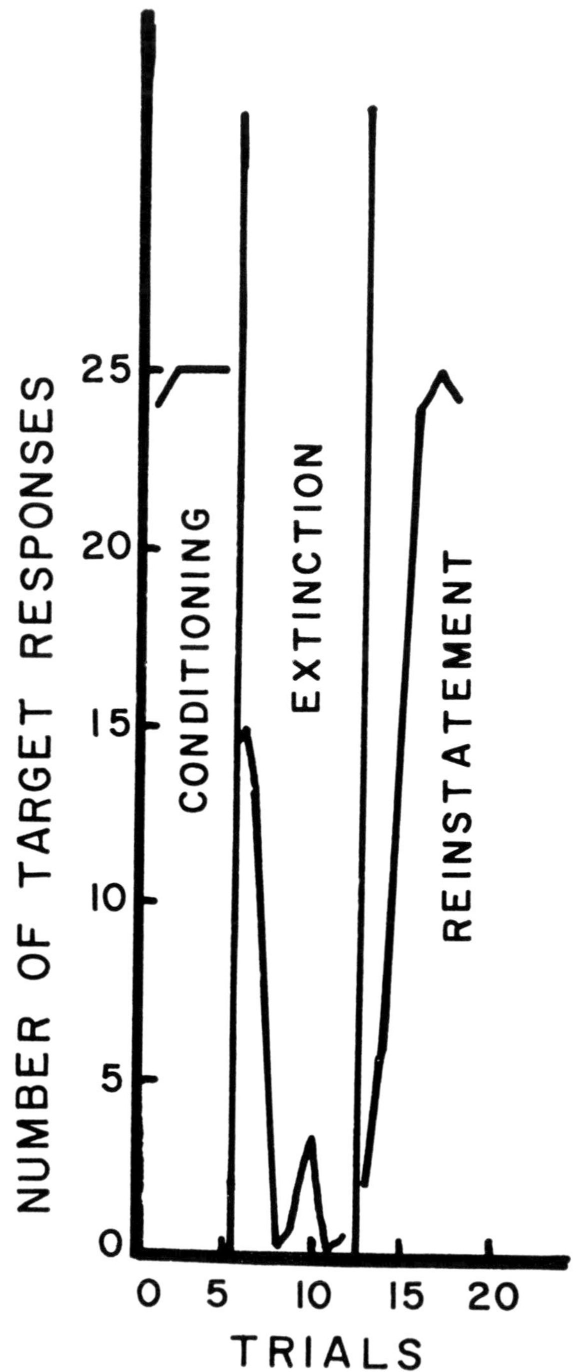

Figure IV.23. Conditioning, extinction and reinstatement trials of subject 1. Fitch, 1971.

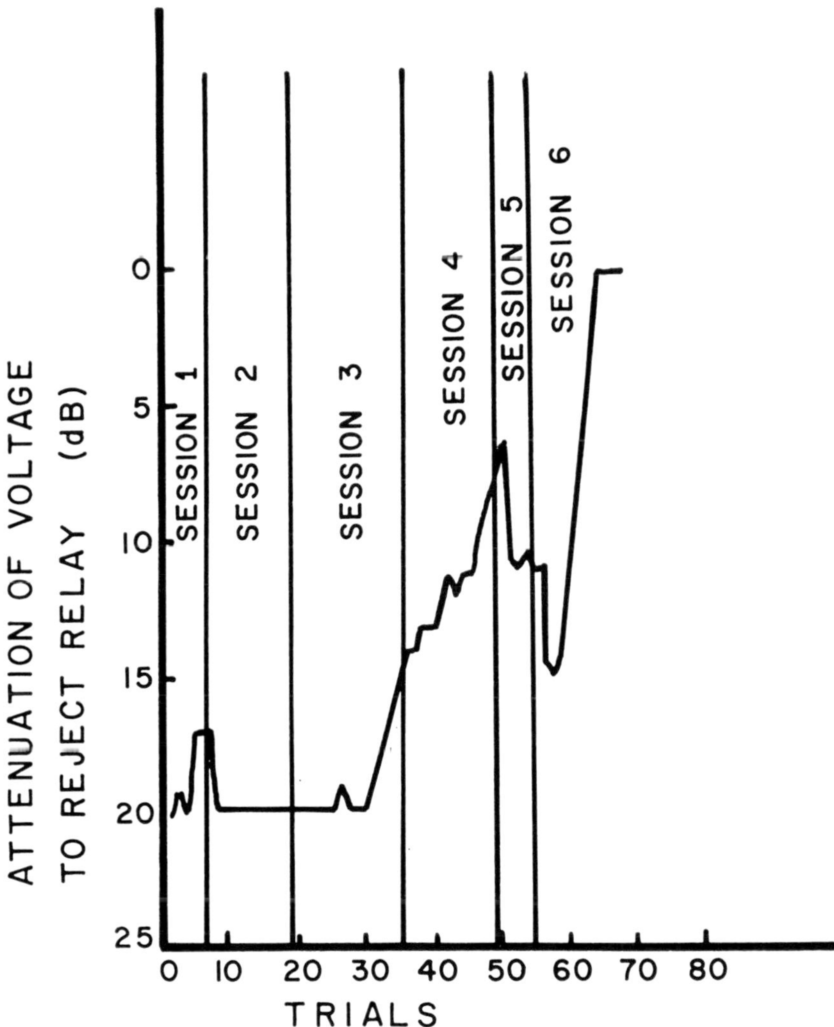

Figure IV.24. Shaping curve of subject 2. Fitch, 1971.

searching for a behavior that would be reinforced and that the searching behavior was becoming progressively more varied. As a low stable rate of behavior could not be stabilized, the extinction phase was terminated and reinstatement not included. Time in the experimental setting for subject 3 was one hour.

All of the subjects were given only the instructions that they

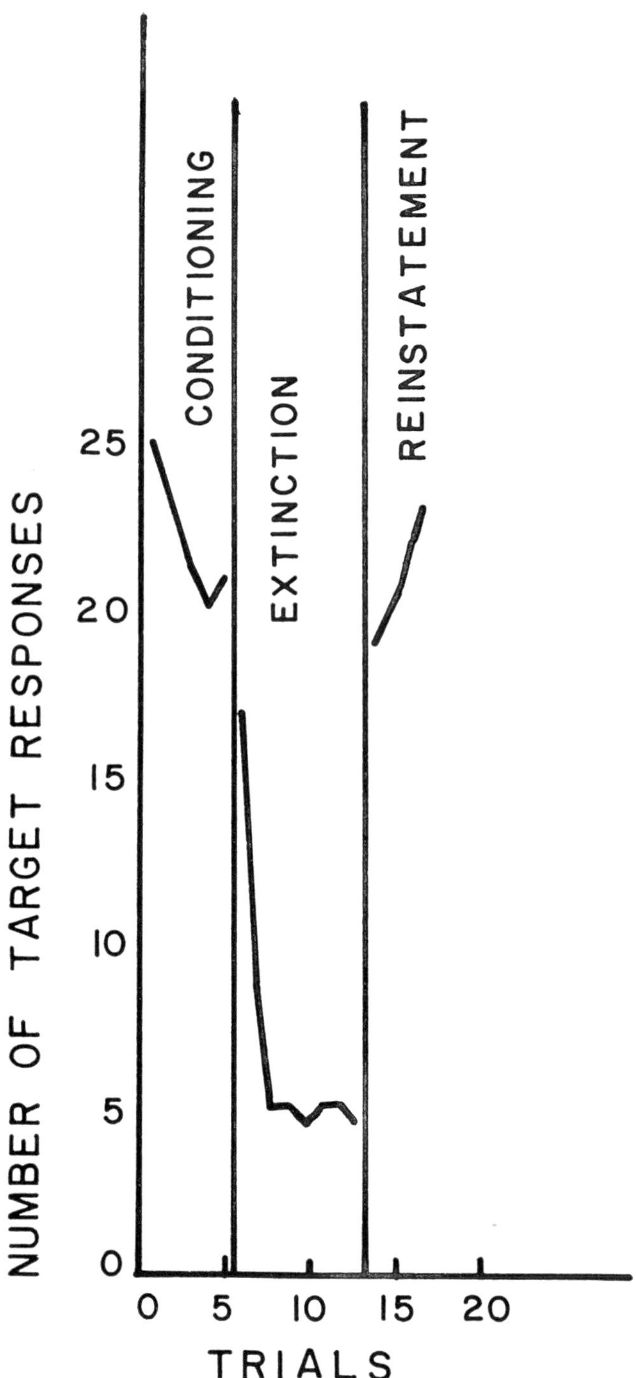

Figure IV.25. Conditioning, extinction and reinstatement trials of subject 2. Fitch, 1971.

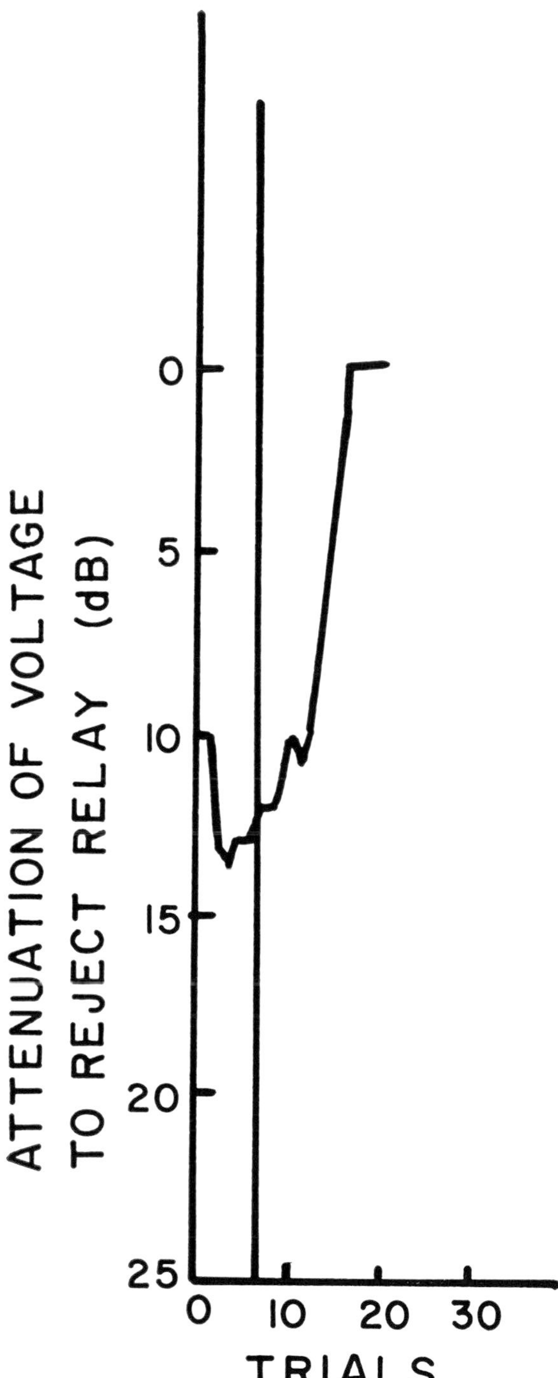

Figure IV.26. Shaping curve of subject 3. Fitch, 1971.

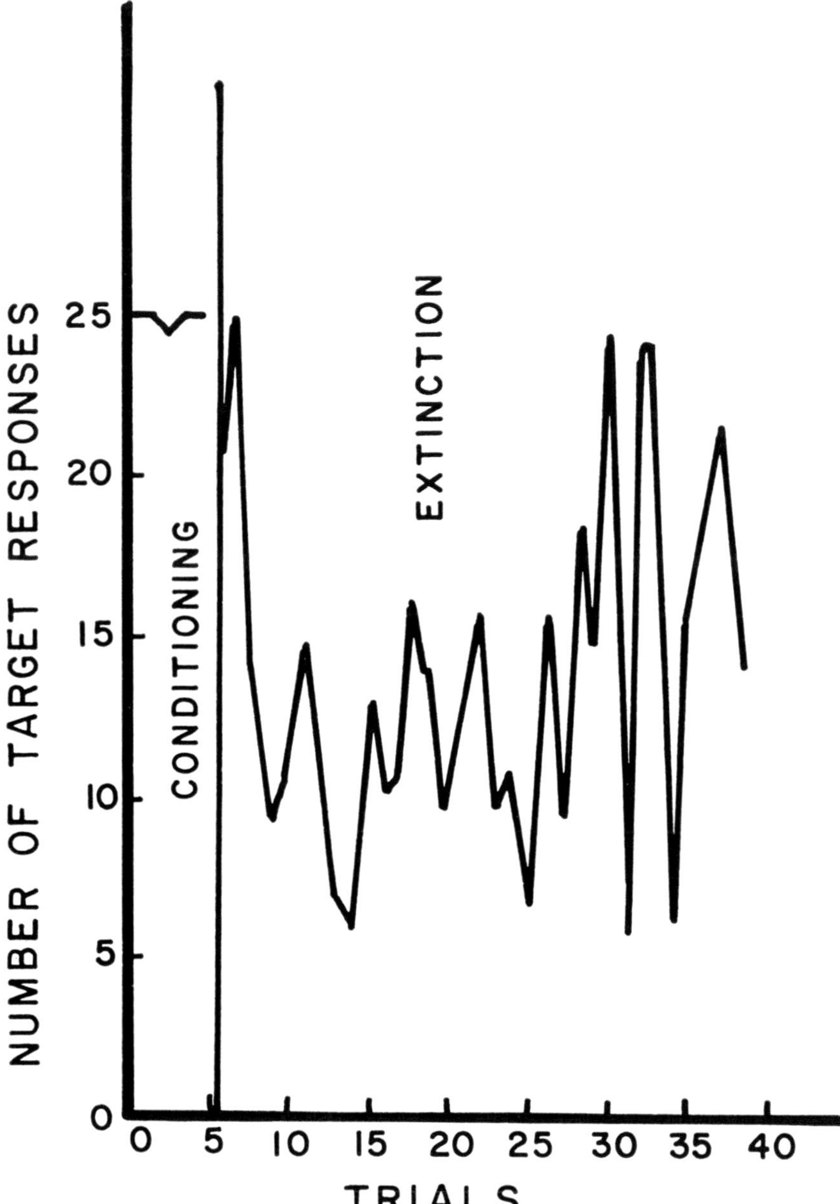

Figure IV.27. Conditioning and extinction trials of subject 3. Fitch, 1971.

were to read the syllables and try to make the white light flash. At the end of the study one subject, when asked to verbalize the contingency, stated "it's something you do with your mouth just before you say the syllable." Another said "it's the way you say the sound at the beginning of the word." Subject 1, who altered the stimulus sound considerably replied "you have to say it from the stomach." Considering her responses, this statement may have been the most accurate.

In summary, the study indicated that phoneme voicing is amenable to modification through use of a response contingent stimulus. As the subjects approached the task in a different manner, it is also obvious that programming of behavior must be done with great care to prevent the reinforcement of inappropriate responses. Currently there is not enough information available on the acoustic spectra of phonetic elements of speech to program their characteristics confidently. The advances in computer technology in relation to rapid waveform analysis and the possibility of programming the probability of phoneme occurrency may result in a system that would be conducive to electronic programming of speech through the identification of acoustic parameters.

MODIFICATION OF ARTICULATORY BEHAVIOR

While electronic programming of articulatory behaviors is still at the embryonic stage, programs to be administered by a clinician are gaining in number and degree of refinement. In the treatment of articulation disorders several systems of programmed therapy have been developed. Each have contributed something unique to the therapy situation and all have demonstrated efficiency in the use of therapy time.

Early attempts at programming articulation therapy were based on teaching sound discrimination. Holland and Matthews suggested that "the training of speech sound discrimination was chosen for programming, not only because it is recognizedly useful for the early phases of articulation therapy, but also because it appears especially suited to teaching machine programming" (1963). Holland and Matthews developed a program for teaching discrimination of the [s] phoneme. They concluded that "it seems clear from this study that techniques for improvement of [s] discrimination in children who misarticulate [s] are amenable to teaching machine programming." The average time per session was forty minutes and the average time of students to complete the program was approximately two hours and fifteen minutes.

Winitz (1969) reported that "for some children sound discrimination improves following sound discrimination training and that sound discrimination training effectively facilitates sound production." (p. 279) He also "takes the point of view that for some children intensive speech sound discrimination training between the error sound and the correct sound will facilitate the subsequent learning of the correct sound." (p. 276) MacDonald (1964) also suggested that "while some children definitely need to study the characteristics of the model which they are trying to duplicate, many children do not need to make such a detailed analysis of the externally produced model, but, instead, need help in becoming aware of and in interpreting sensations associated with their own articulatory efforts." (p. 183)

Garrett (in press), Leonard and Webb (1971), and others have also employed discrimination as an integral part of modifying articulatory behavior. In view of the ambiguity of the role discrimination plays in articulation disorders, it would appear that it has received an overemphasis in the development of therapy programs for disordered articulation. This may be accounted for by two obvious factors: 1) sound discrimination as proposed by Van Riper (1954) has been an accepted step in the treatment of articulation disorders, and 2) sound discrimination can easily be programmed so that the response of the client can be evaluated by a machine.

In the study by Leonard and Webb (1971), discrimination of the response by the client was paired with discrimination of the response by the clinician. Basically, the program consisted of tapes of the target sounds presented to the client and clinician through ear phones. The client imitated the sound and then moved a switch to indicate that he felt that his production of the sound was correct. If the sound was produced correctly, as determined by the clinician, the clinician moved a switch that allowed the client's sound production to be played back to him after a short delay. If the client's production of the sound was in error, the clinician did not move the switch and the client's production of the sound was not played back. Reinforcement, then, was derived from the client hearing his own sound production repeated. This, in effect, was teaching the client to produce the sound in the stimulus-response-contingency paradigm while also teaching the client to reinforce himself for correct productions of the target phoneme.

Garrett (in press), over a period of eight years, developed and tested several versions of a program for articulatory disorders. In a carefully documented presentation he indicated that on a cost-effectiveness basis the programmed materials were much more effective than traditional therapy. He also suggested that sound discrimination exercises, while effective in teaching sound discrimination, did not significantly affect the achievement of correct sound production.

Mowrer, Baker, and Schutz reported on studies of a behavioral approach to articulation which lead to the development of a program for the correction of the frontal lisp. This program dealt directly with the behavior, i.e., the retraction of the tongue so that protrusion through the lips was not visible. The program was administered in several ways. From these studies were made several conclusions. First, it was indicated that a highly structured program with detailed instructions could be extremely efficient in therapy beyond the experimental condition. Secondly, he suggested that reinforcers were "dramatically effective in facilitating the learning of correct articulation responses" (Mowrer, et al., 1968, p. 320). Thirdly, he suggested that group therapy may limit efficiency in therapy because only one child can actively participate in the learning task at one time. He also indicated that the presence of the therapist was not necessarily an important factor in achieving positive results. The suggestion was made that an aide could administer the program with results equal to that of a therapist, thus increasing the efficiency of the program further.

Carrier (1970) reported on a program for articulation therapy that could be administered by persons outside the school setting. Using poker chips as reinforcers, mothers of children with articulation disorders learned to reinforce the child's correct responses.

The poker chips could be traded for a prize at the end of the therapy session. After an hour of training at the clinic, the mother took the program home. Instructions were thoroughly explained. Before the program was given for home training, the clinician was to have achieved correct imitation of the sound in isolation at the clinic.

The home program consisted of six lessons progressing from sounds broken from the target words (such as s—aw), to natural pronunciation of the picture words, to saying the words without a model. After completing those steps, an object was then used to elicit the response. Finally the child moved about the house to the various natural locations of the objects. While significant improvement was found on sound testing, generalization of the sound to connected speech was not significant.

A program of articulation therapy is being developed by the author based on the research presented on voice modification earlier in the chapter. The approach places emphasis on the principles of reinforcement applied to articulation therapy. The rules used in the construction of the program, derived from the studies in voice manipulation, can be applied to language program in general. The rules are as follows:

1. *Economy through use of carefully planned target behaviors.* Although behavior modification has been shown to be efficient, it is only so through reinforcement of appropriate behaviors. As articulation disorders are labelled as such through the judgment of a client's *productive* speech, the target behaviors used in therapy should be only *productive* behaviors. Because sound discrimination is not a part of productive speech behavior, discrimination training was not a part of this program. Nonsense syllables, commonly used as a step in articulation therapy, were also not employed as they are not a part of the client's normal productive speech.

2. *To maintain a high response rate, the success-to-failure ratio of the client must be high on success and low on failure.* Mowrer (1970) treated this topic thoroughly. Through laboratory experiments the author programmed success into a treatment in such a way that the successes would always outweigh the failures to a satisfactory degree. The determinant of how great the success-to-

failure ratio must be to maintain a high rate of response should be an individual decision based on the performance of the child. It is suggested that children who have achieved a great deal of success in the classroom may maintain a high rate of response with a minimum ratio, while children who have received less reinforcement in the classroom may require a higher rate to assure them of their ability to achieve the target behaviors. That is, for the child who is not accustomed to receiving reinforcement for responding, it may take a higher success-to-failure ratio in the therapy situation to establish a high rate of response.

3. *The pace of therapy should be determined by the client's success-to-failure ratio.* As opposed to successfully completing a program, or a list of target behaviors, the client proceeds to the next higher step when he has the backlog of success to tolerate a possible failure. Also, as soon as the client has experienced a minimum number of unreinforced attempts, he is allowed to return to a step that will allow him to stockpile successful attempts.

4. *Intermediate steps between baseline and terminal behavior should not be allowed to stabilize.* If a child *masters* an intermediate step, it may impede his attainment of the next higher step. For instance, the child who masters the [s] in isolation may separate the [s] from the rest of the sounds when trying to learn to put it into a word, i.e., *sssss-top* as opposed to *stop*. He is doing so because an intermediate step between baseline behavior (error production of the sound in all occurrences in spontaneous speech) and terminal behavior (correct production of the sound in all occurrences in spontaneous speech) has been mastered. Therefore, intermediate steps should be incremented while the behavior is still viable.

5. *Linguistically meaningful material should be introduced immediately.* MacDonald (1964) and others have indicated nonsense syllables as an intermediate step in articulation therapy. It is logical that they should be easier to produce than words which the client uses meaningfully. Mowrer, et al. (1968) suggested that words which contain the error sound may serve as a discriminative stimulus for the incorrect production of the sound. The strong bond between the error sound and meaningful words thus becomes an obstacle to the generalization of the target sound

in spontaneous speech. The sooner the target sound is introduced into linguistically meaningful words, the greater the chances of generalization to spontaneous speech. In the program to be presented here, all material beyond the first step are commonly used linguistic occurrences.

In addition to the above stated rules, many more concepts (mostly borrowed) were incorporated into the construction of the programs. Factors such as readability and ease of manipulation of materials also played an important role. Even common sense occasionally played a part. Items were (and will be) added, modified, and deleted as the programs are tested further in the clinical setting. It is hoped that the reader will not view the programs as a finished product or an inviolate prescription. Rather it is desirable that the clinician draw from the program those principles which they may include in programs of their own construction.

Programmed Therapy for the [s] Phoneme

The program for the [s] phoneme follows the same pattern as the programs developed for other phonemes, [t, l, r, p, g, k, f, d, ʃ, tʃ] (Knott and Fitch, 1971). It is broken into ten steps, each with definite criterion for either progressing to the next step or returning to the previous step. Again, in clinical usage, it is suggested that the clinician might need to vary the criterion to maintain a high enough success-to-failure ratio to insure a continued high rate of response.

Each successive step contains targets that are progressively more complex either linguistically, phonetically, or both linguistically and phonetically. An explanation of the steps and justification for the steps will be given.

Each step identifies the linguistic event to be treated under the heading of *task*. In each step there is a suggested stimulus, or list of stimuli, under the heading of *target*. Criterion for either advancing to the next step or returning to the previous step is explained under the heading *if*. Each correct response by the client is reinforced.

The type of reinforcement used is at the discretion of the clinician. If verbal reinforcement (which is recommended as the first choice) does not elicit a high rate of response, the clinician should try other things, such as cereal, M&Ms, trinkets, tokens to be exchanged, etc., until a suitable reinforcer can be found.

Step 1: In the initial step the target behavior of the client is the correct production of the [s] in isolation. By isolating the desired behavior the most simple behavior related to the production of the sound is presented and the locus of therapy to follow is instated.

To achieve correct production of the sound in isolation several techniques are suggested, most of which are familiar to the practicing therapist. The criterion for advancement to step 2 is the production of five consecutive reinforced (correct) [s] sounds. The use of five consecutive reinforced productions is suggested, recognizing that more or less reinforcement may be warranted depending on the child. The level should be dictated by the response rate of the child. That is, if a child is responding at a high rate of behavior, the number of consecutive reinforced productions of [s] might be reduced so that the program may be presented more quickly.

Step 2: There are three phases to step 2; steps 2a, 2b, and 2c. In all three the target [s] is presented in a single word. In step 2a the [s] is presented in the initial syllabic position, in step 2b the [s] is presented in the final syllabic position, and the [s] is presented intervocalically in step 2c. Three phases are included as it is recognized that the production of the sound in different syllabic positions requires three allophones of [s]. Figure IV.28 is a sample of the program cards.

Beginning with 2a the same criterion for advancement is used as was used in step 1. If the client has two consecutive errors on step 2a, 2b or 2c he returns to step 1, and the particular phase on which he failed is placed at the end of the step. This is recognizing that the client may produce the sound more easily in one syllabic position than another. For example, if in step 2a the client makes two consecutive unreinforced responses, he returns to step 1, and step 2a is placed after steps 2b and 2c. After succeeding at step 1, he is then presented with step 2b. This continues until he has met criterion on all three phases of step 2.

Steps 3 through 8: In all of these steps the criterion for advancement from one step to the next is the same; five consecutive reinforced productions for advancement, two consecutive unreinforced responses for returning to the previous step. The steps differ in that they become progressively more complex linguistically and/or phonetically. In all steps the client repeats a model produced by the clinician.

Step 9: In step 9 the client is presented with a picture and read an accompanying story. The client is asked to repeat the story, which is loaded with the [s] phoneme. If there is hesitation, the story is repeated until the client is familiar with it. The clinician records the first ten productions of [s] as either correct or incorrect. If eight of the ten are correct, the client advances to step 10. If the criterion of eight of the first ten is not met, the client returns to step 8.

Step 10: While step 9 requires correct production of the sound in a structured occurrence, the task of step 10 is the correction production of the sound in free speech of the client's creation. If in spontaneous speech production the client produces eight of ten correct[s]'s, the program is terminated. At this point the client is asked to take the program with him for home administration twice a week and he is checked at the end of the first week. If the

STEP 4

TASK: ***Make the "s" sound correctly in 3-word phrases.***

IF: ***"s" sound correct in 5 phrases in a row, move to STEP 5.***

IF: ***"s" sound incorrect in 2 phrases in a row, return to STEP 3.***

TARGETS:

I like cats.
Three blind mice
Chase the ball
Good hot soup
Desk and chair
One blue spot
I saw Tom

Cold ice tea
Milk and toast
That's my coat.
Ask a question
A snow cone
Halloween mask
Cold gray snow
Sweep the floor

Figure IV.28. Sample of articulation therapy program card.

behavior is maintained, home administration is suggested for a period of one month to stabilize sound production. Therapy is terminated if the client maintains the behavior at the end of one month.

Home administration is recommended only after the client has demonstrated good success so that the home presentation is most likely to produce results that will please both the person presenting the program and the client, insuring a maximum of reinforcement. Four graphic records are presented and short case histories reported. The program for [s], and programs for other phonemes, have been tested on a larger group with equivalent results. It is presently being tested with different modes of presentation.

Subject 1 was an eight-year-old female who was referred to the speech clinic by her pediatrician for having a *short palate*. The inadequate velopharyngeal closure was mainfested only in the production of the [s] sound; she substituted a nasal snort for [s]. The velum was observed to be of normal length and had good mobility, but the nasopharynx was deep. In neither single word articulation tests or connected speech was the sound produced correctly. Stimulation was attempted with no success. As subject 1 produced the [t] correctly, she was told to "make a long t sound." The first session ended after the subject had produced several [s] sounds correctly in isolation, for which she was given strong reinforcement.

Subject 1 was seen for a second session a week later. She remembered how to produce her *long t sound* and could produce the [s] correctly through isolation. While a thorough analysis of connected speech was not made at the beginning of the session, it was observed that she was producing the [s] more correctly in connected speech, though inconsistently. The articulation program for [s] was presented. She completed the program with only two incorrect productions. For correct productions she was verbally reinforced. A tape made at the end of the second session revealed no incorrect productions of [s] in connected speech.

The mother of subject 1 was given the programmed cards and their use was demonstrated. She was asked to go through the program with her daughter daily and return to the clinic the

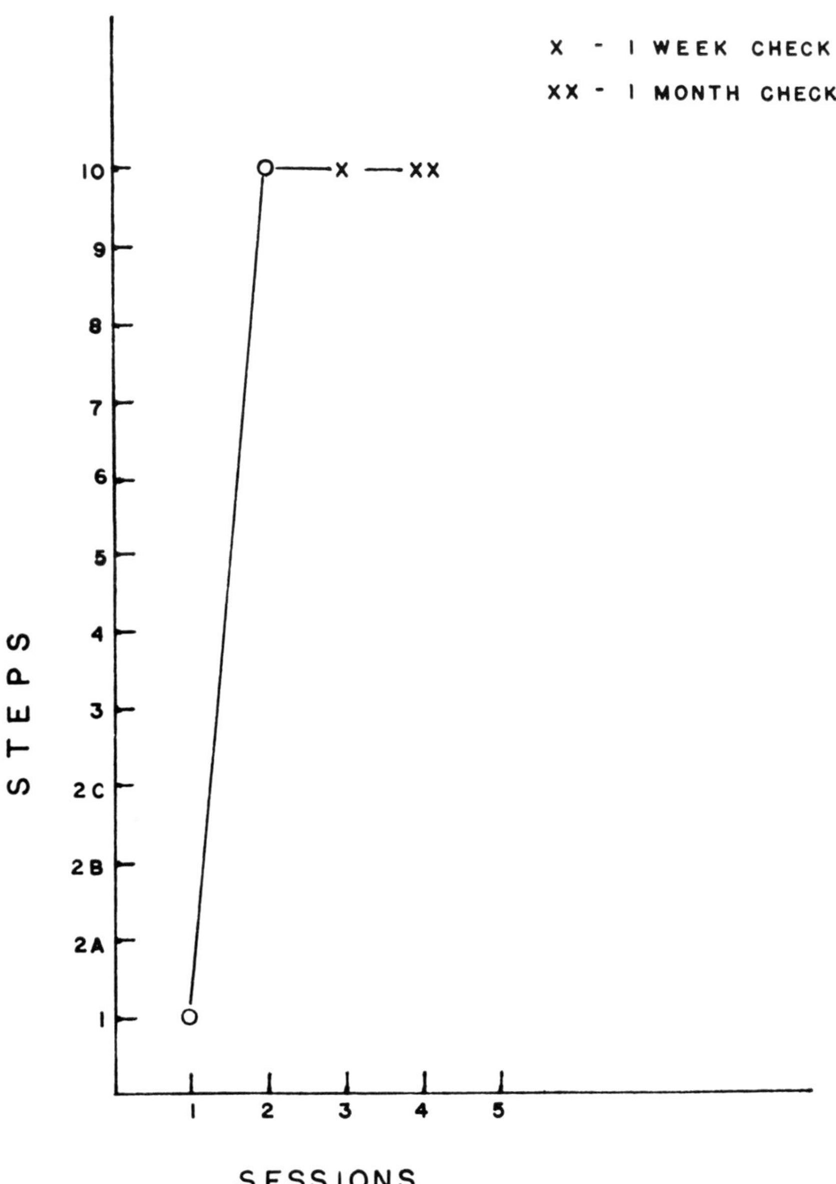

Figure IV.29. Program progress graph for subject 1.

following week. At the end of the week subject 1 returned. In free connected speech she produced the [s] sound correctly eight of the first ten attempts. The mother was asked to go through the program three times weekly. At the end of one month, all [s] sounds in free connected speech were produced correctly and the mother reported correct use of the sound in conversation at home. Total time in therapy was fifty minutes. Figure IV.29 plots the progress of subject 1 through the program.

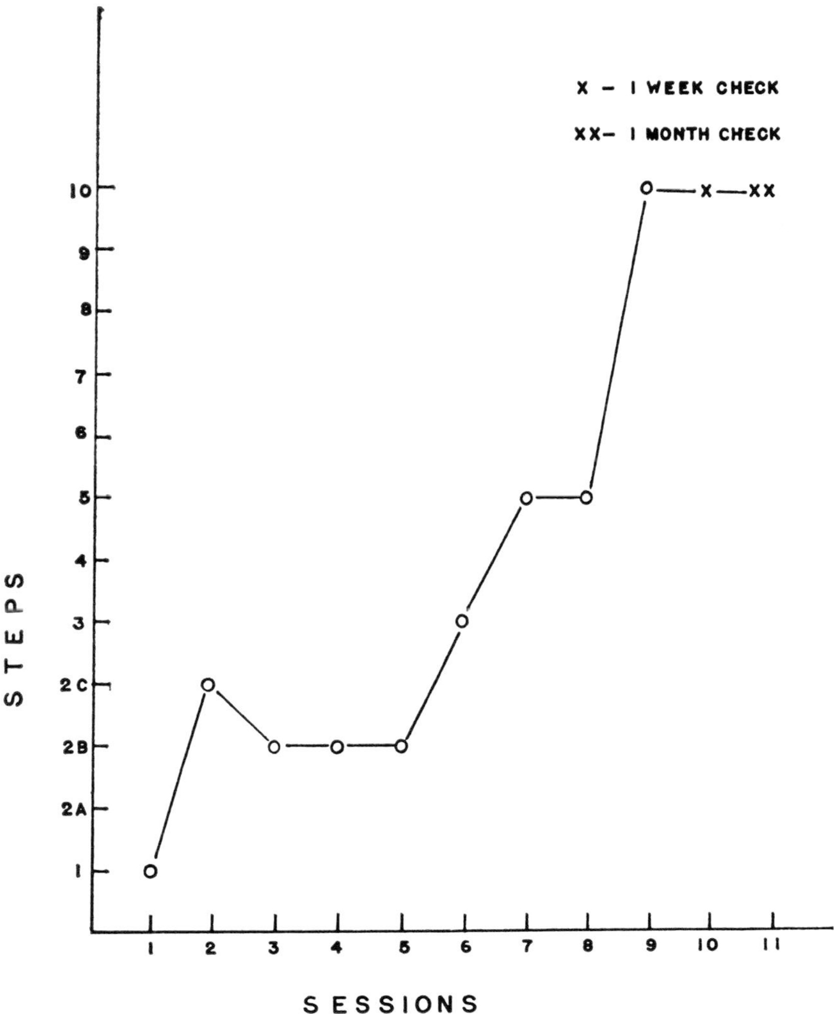

Figure IV.30. Program progress graph for subject 2.

Subject 2 was a five-year-old female who demonstrated multiple misarticulations, omissions, substitutions and distortions. She was stimulable on all sounds before entering the clinic. The child had had therapy for one year which included home exercises with poor progress reported. She is the youngest of five children, one of which is mentally retarded. The rest of the family history was unremarkable. Hearing was normal. For this child the phoneme selected was [k].

Subject 2 was administered the [k] program over a period of four weeks. Figure IV.30 shows the particular steps of the program that were the most difficult for the child to achieve. These were steps 2a, b, and c. They were presented at five sessions at which she did not achieve criterion on step 3. At that time she was not seen for two weeks (family vacation). When she returned she was able to progress to step 4. She again reached a plateau at step 6 for a week after which she progressed to step 10.

Upon achievement of criterion for step 10 the program was sent home. Subject 2 was seen at the end of one week at which time she demonstrated that the behavior was being maintained. She was checked at the end of one and two months; both checks indicated the behavior had stabilized.

The programs for other phonemes, [w], [g], [l], [ʃ], and [s] were presented to subject 2, all of which were completed with comparable efficiency.

Subject 3 was an eight-year, nine-month-old male with multiple articulation errors, omissions, substitutions, and distortions with a tendency toward nasality. Therapy was complicated by a severe neurological condition which was familial in nature. His initial behavior was listlessness and apathy. Subject 3 had received occupational and physical therapy for psychomotor and perceptual difficulties. He has a history of nephritic kidney and chronic kidney malfunction. He had been hospitalized on many occasions and kidney surgery has been performed several times since age two and one-half years. He had been seen for public school therapy for one year before coming to the clinic.

Subject 3 was administered the [f] program. It can be noted on figure IV.31 that progress through the program was consistent. Subject 3 achieved step 10 after six sessions at which time the program

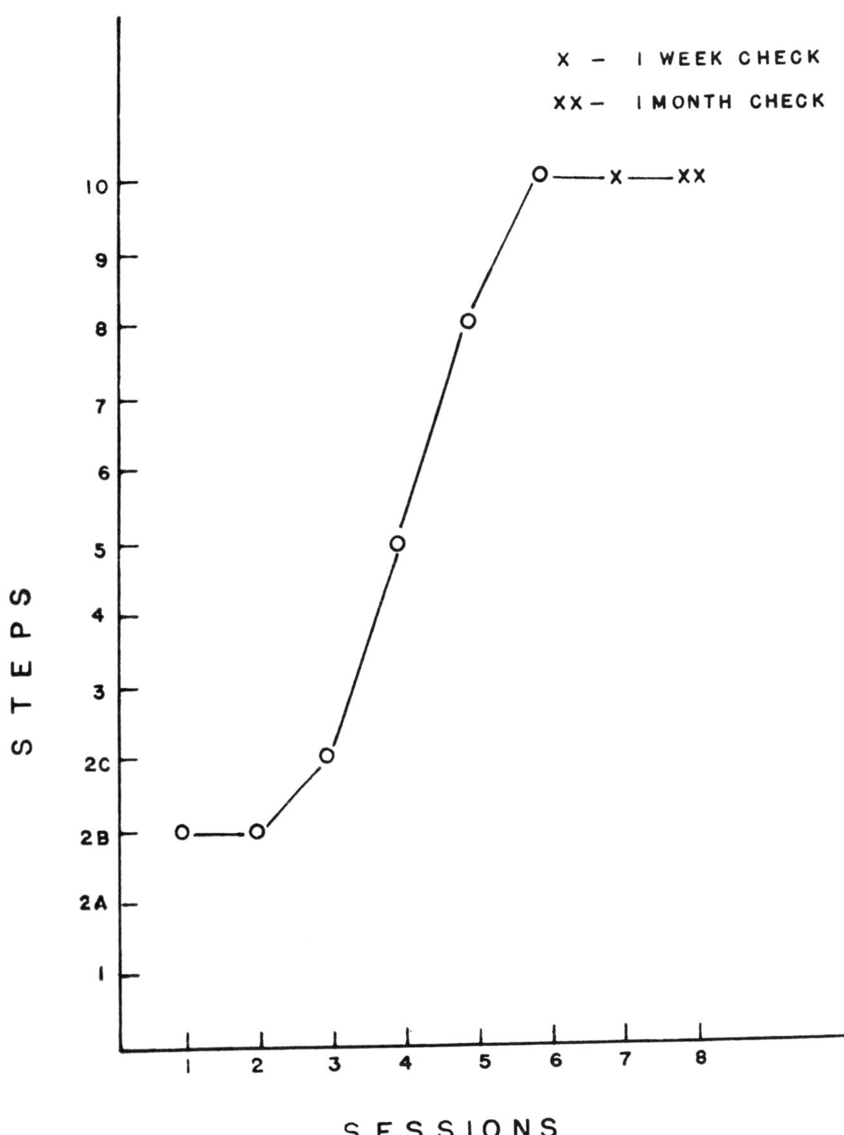

Figure IV.31. Program progress graph for subject 3.

was sent home. He was checked after one week and again after one month, at which times he demonstrated that the behavior was being maintained.

Subject 3 has been given programs for eight other phonemes with comparable results. Family cooperation was excellent throughout therapy. This appeared to be due in part to the fact that the child began communicating more, demonstrating more positive behavior, and exhibiting less listless and apathetic behavior; this the parents attributed to gains in speech.

Subject 4 was a six-year-old male who exhibited misarticulations of [s] and [z], with a frontal lisp in evidence. He had no previous therapy history and was not immediately stimulable to the sound. Subject 4's medical and social history were unremarkable. He was administered the [s] program on a once a week therapy schedule.

Figure IV.32 demonstrates the program progress for subject 4. He achieved step 10 after six sessions at which time the program was sent home. A check at one week and one month indicated that the behavior was being maintained.

Space does not permit the inclusion of many other cases who have been administered the programs with comparable success. Acceptance of the program has been positive by the clinicians involved in their use.

Discrepancies in the programs have become obvious through their use and should be noted. One problem which is now being studied is that of cycling, or vascillating back and forth between two steps, the more difficult of which is not achieved. While this is expectetd to a certain degree, on occasion it has become excessive. While no child has failed to achieve a higher step, a means of branching to subordinate steps is indicated.

Another problem now being corrected is the presence of only one level of the suggested story for each program. Above eight years of age story content must be varied to prevent *talking down* to the child. At older ages yet alternate stories should be used. The other steps have been accepted by all ages with no problems.

Problems in word content in the steps were noted, changed, and will probably be changed further. Also, the number of targets per step should be increased to prevent undue repetition.

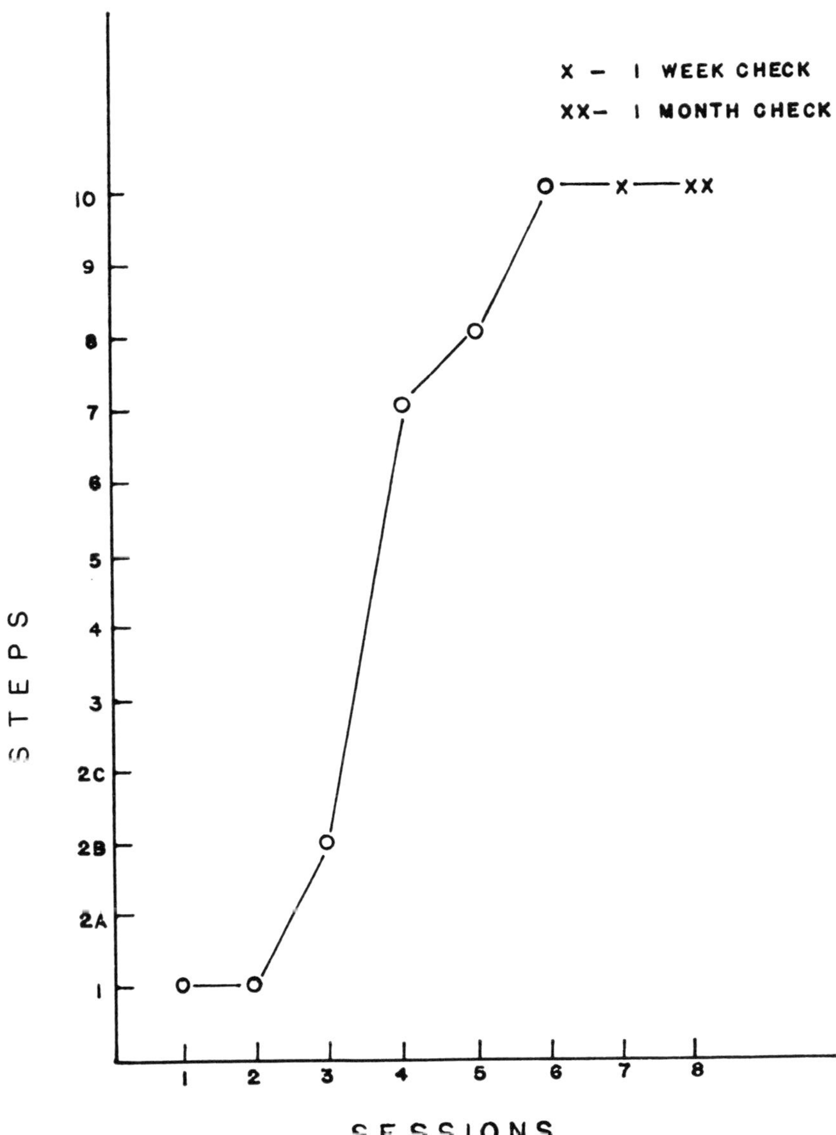

Figure IV.32. Program progress graph for subject 4.

While these problems have existed, their importance has been outweighed by the efficiency of the programs.

The articulation programs are being tested in other settings using different modes of presentation at the present time. A nationwide study using the programs will take place within the year that will further define the efficiency of their use in a greater variety of clinical settings.

CONCLUSION

It can be noted that the studies presented in this chapter have been applied clinically at an early stage of development. This is due in great measure to the growing need of persons working with speech and language disorders for clinical techniques that can quantifiably define habilitative procedures.

The surface has been broken in the use of behavior modification techniques with voice and articulation disorders, and the seeds sown. As the value of the systems developed becomes known and accepted by the field in general, a harvest of many more systems will be forthcoming. Persons who are in a clinical setting should first study the principles of behavior modification and set for themselves rules to follow in program construction. For the researcher there is abundant opportunity for investigation of the use of behavior modification with various kinds of cases; i.e., cerebral palsied, cleft palate, and others. It requires a minimum of cost and the results can be of much value to many people. In a period in which special services are being viewed with a critical eye, behavior modification can provide quantitative evidence of the efficiency being achieved in the clinical settings.

REFERENCES

Carrier, J.: A program of articulation therapy administered by mothers. *J. Speech Hearing Res., 35*:344-353, 1970.

Fitch, J.: Modification of phoneme voicing through application of reinforcement principles. *J. Comm. Dis., 4*:20-29, 1971.

Garrett, E.: Programmed articulation therapy. In Wolfe, W. D. (Ed.): Articulation and Learning. Springfield, Thomas, In press.

Holland, A., and Matthews, J.: Application of teaching machine concepts to speech pathology and audiology. *ASHA, 5*:474-482, 1963.

Knott, M., and Fitch, J.: Application of principles of reinforcement to articulation therapy in a clinical setting. Paper presented at *ASHA* convention, Chicago, 1971.

Leonard, L., and Webb, C.: An automated therapy program for articulatory correction. *J. Speech Hearing Res., 14*:338-344, 1971.

McDonald, E.: *Articulation Testing and Treatment: A Sensory-Motor Approach.* Pittsburgh, Stanwix, 1964.

Moore, J.: *The Effect of Certain Schedules of Reinforcement on the Experimental Manipulation of Fundamental Frequency.* Doctoral dissertation, Florida State University, Tallahassee, 1968.

Mowrer, D.: An analysis of motivational techniques used in speech therapy. *ASHA, 12*:491-493, 1970.

Mowrer, D.; Baker, R., and Schutz, R.: Operant procedures in the control of speech articulation. In Sloane, H., and MacAulay, B. (Ed.) : *Operant Procedures in Remedial Speech and Language Training.* New York, Houghton Mifflin, 1968.

Roll, J.: *Experimental Manipulation of Fundamental Frequency by Application of Reinforcement Principles.* Unpublished M.A. Thesis, Florida State University, Tallahassee, 1968.

Roll, J.: *Manipulation of Fundamental Frequency in Functional Voice Disorders by Application of Reinforcement Principles.* Doctoral dissertation, Florida State University, Tallahassee, 1969.

Van Riper, C.: *Speech Correction.* 3rd ed. Englewood Cliffs, Prentice-Hall, 1954.

Winitz, H.: *Articulation Acquisition and Behavior.* New York, Appleton-Century-Crofts, 1969.

GLOSSARY

Vocal Fundamental Frequency (VFF): The basic rate of vibration of the vocal folds. In young adult males the VFF is approximately 120 Hz and in young adult females VFF is approximately 220 Hz.

Hertz (Hz): A unit of measure of frequency; cycles per second.

Filters: Mechanical or electronic devices which serve to suppress selected frequencies while transmitting others.

Bandwidth: Bandwidth refers to the frequencies modified by a filter. May refer to either those frequencies transmitted or those frequencies suppressed.

Relay: Electromagnetic device which, when activated, acts as a switch to complete a circuit.

CHAPTER V

CLUTTERING

LAWRENCE SIMKINS

SEVERAL YEARS AGO the author worked with an emotionally disturbed child who had a speech defect. It was a type of deficiency that was difficult to describe except in a vague way such as *unintelligible*. She did not stutter but spoke rapidly and with such poor articulation that it was difficult to understand her. The author took a tape recording of her speech to a friend* who is the director of a well-known speech and hearing clinic in Kansas City. After listening to the tape he diagnosed her as a clutterer. This was the first time the author had heard of that classification of speech pathology, but after explaining his treatment strategy asked the friend what changes in treatment plan might prove to be most effective with a clutterer. His friend had no suggestions to make and explained that very little was known about cluttering or its treatment. A search of the literature on cluttering yielded little, if any, additional pertinent information concerning treatment. The brevity of this chapter, therefore, is a reflection of the paucity of literature in this area.

It might be added that the treatment plan for this child had been formulated prior to her diagnosis as a clutterer. Her subsequent diagnosis of cluttering did not provide any additional information with respect to treatment decisions. It was found that many of the basic modification principles that had been used with other forms of speech pathology (e.g. stuttering, articulation disorders) could be used effectively with a clutterer.

---

* The author would like to express his appreciation to Dr. Jack Katz who not only provided assistance at the time of the study but also for his critical reading of this manuscript and his suggestions. However, the author takes full responsibility for the views expressed in this final version.

It appears that the taxonomic system for classifying speech disorders may suffer one of the same limitations as the psychiatric taxonomy used for classifying behavioral disorders. Presumably, one of the major purposes of any diagnostic system would be to provide information upon which to base treatment decisions. As will be discussed later, the diagnostic category of cluttering meets this criterion only in a very limited way.

History and Definition of Cluttering

The literature on cluttering is sparse. Many texts on speech pathology make no mention of the disorder and other texts (e.g. Van Riper, 1963; West and Ansberry, 1968) limit their discussion to several paragraphs with an occasional mention of the disorder scattered throughout different segments of the books. The bulk of the literature on cluttering has originated from foreign countries, primarily Germany. Most of this work remains untranslated. However, the most comprehensive treatment of this topic written in English is by Deso Weiss (1964). A fairly recent translation of the second edition of a well-known German text on speech pathology (Luchsinger and Arnold, 1965) also contains an extensive section on cluttering. A recent issue of the journal, *Folia Phoniatrica* (22:241-384, 1970) is dedicated to Deso Weiss and its entire contents is devoted to cluttering. The majority of the literature is concerned with the etiology of cluttering and its differentiation from stuttering. There is very little information with respect to treatment, and speculation rather than data comprises most of the written material.

Weiss (1964) indicates that cluttering has been discussed in the literature of speech pathology for more than two thousand years; the first complete volume devoted to cluttering did not appear until 1963. This book was written by R. Luchsinger and published in German but has not been translated. According to Luchsinger and Arnold (1965) one of the earliest descriptions of cluttering to appear in the English literature was included in a text by Wyllie (1894), a British physician, who wrote a well-known medical text on speech pathology. In this book Wyllie described cluttering as a crowding of words so as to interfere with distinct articulation. Although the clutterer's articulation is normal when performed slowly, with an increase in speech rate, mental coordination is lost and there is an increase in poor articulation. Wyllie's observations seem to be consistent with the behavioral descriptions made by more contemporary authors.

Apparently, there has been much more concern about cluttering in countries other than the United States. The Luchsinger and Arnold text (1965), which was originally written in German, notes that "In fact no medical author of a general text in speech pathology would omit the presentation of his views on cluttering." According to Weiss (1964), in the United States there has been no incidence of cluttering reported in the White House Surveys simply because no category bearing that name has been included in the studies. It is difficult to estimate the incidence of cluttering. According to Powers (1957), the incidence of all functional articulation disorders of which cluttering is one class varies from 57% to 81% of all speech disorders. However, there is no information given as to the incidence of each of the specific articulation disorders.

From other countries, particularly Germany where cluttering is recognized as a specific form of speech pathology, it is possible to obtain some estimate of the frequency of cluttering. In a study conducted in Germany by Becker and Grundmann (1970) on school children ages seven and eight it was estimated that 1.8% of the children attending a normal school were clutterers. On the other hand it was found that 11.5% of the children attending special education classes were probable clutterers. These figures are relatively large if one takes into account the expected incidence of stuttering in a similar age group is 0.7%.

Some speech pathologists in the United States may not differentiate cluttering from other articulatory disorders or stuttering. It is possible that clutterers have been included within these categories. It is also generally agreed upon that cluttering is a less severe type of speech problem than stuttering, therefore, has not received the same amount of attention. Since cluttering is regarded as a relatively minor speech disorder, it is possible that many clutterers do not seek the attention of speech therapists. Because of these reasons it is difficult to estimate the actual incidence of cluttering but more than likely any incidence figures that have been reported represent underestimations.

Characteristics of Cluttering

Some of the confusion concerning cluttering may be due to the practice of assigning a different label to the same disorder. For example, the description that Anderson (1953) gives for *oral inactivity* fits the same description that other authors give for cluttering. On the other hand, Van Riper (1963) makes a differentiation between cluttering and oral inaccuracy; the latter referring to a wastebasket term for any mild articulatory defect.

One of the more basic descriptions of cluttering is given by Van Riper (1963, p. 26) as follows:

> Another disorder in which the time sequence is disturbed is called cluttering. It is frequently confused with stuttering because it, too, shows many repetitions. However, the major features of cluttering are first, the excessive speed of speaking; second, the disorganized sentence structure, and third, the slurred or omitted syllables and sounds. The clutterer can speak perfectly when he speaks very slowly, but it is almost impossible for him to do so except for short periods . . . The true clutterer has no seeming awareness of his excessive speed or garbled utterances. He is always surprised when others cannot understand him . . . Some clutterers become stutterers as well; most do not. Clutterers speak by spurts and their speech organs pile up like keys on a typewriter when a novice stenographer tries for more speed than her skill permits.

Berry and Eisenson (1942) describe a child that clutters as one who stumbles and repeats words and phrases, slurs and omits sounds and syllables while going at top speed. Powers (1957) notes that cluttering implies deviations in rate and rhythm as well as in articulation. She seems to indicate that cluttering represents a rather heterogenous class of speech defects in contrast to the more specific types of defects such as stuttering and the frontal lisp.

It would seem therefore, that cluttering refers not to a specific response deficit but rather to a heterogenous collection of speech anomalies. Thus, cluttering is characterized as involving an excessive speech rate (technically referred to as Tachylalia), faulty phonation, a faulty speech rhythm in which the speech is described as jerky or stumbling, a monotony in speech tone in which there is very little variation in pitch and stress, many articulation errors consisting of frequent transpositions, word or syllable substitutions, many of which are referred to as infantile (e.g. substitution or w for r as in wight for right), telescoping several syllables of a word (e.g. parlimentarian becomes pamerian) and spoonerisms (e.g. *many thinkle peep so* instead of *many people think so*).

One of the more frequent characteristics of cluttering is referred to by Weiss (1964) as a vowel stop which "consists of a stop before pronunciation of the initial vowel with the mouth opened as if frightened." Another common observation is that there are frequent interjections such as *ah, mn, ahem, well, you know.* There are also filled pauses which consist of a prolonged ah . . . ah, as well as the prolonging of vowels as if the person were groping for the next word. The clutterer may not necessarily demonstrate all of these characteristics but he usually displays a number of them so that collectively his speech can be most parsimoniously described as *unintelligible.*

Becker and Grundmann (1970) have performed one of the systematic investigations which compared normal speaking children with clutterers on a number of behavioral measures. Their results, however, are generally in agreement with most clinical observations. They found, for example, that clutterers had more omission of vowels, consonants, syllables and words than normal speakers. There were also significant differences in rate of word delivery and word additions. Transposition of letters as well as revisions and confusions were particularly frequent in the handwriting of clutterers.

Cluttering is also referred to by several authors as a syndrome rather than a specific speech disorder to the extent that deficiencies in other language abilities such as writing and reading are correlated with the defective speech patterns. The oral reading behavior of the clutterer quite often consists of running sentences together, omitting words, and substitution of words or syllables. In many instances the clutterer's handwriting is also of a poor quality. It is illegible, contains many misspellings, frequent transpositions, and frequent revisions. The cluttering syndrome extends not only to expressive language functions but seems to be a pervasive characteristic in social interactions and other behaviors.

Children who are clutterers tend to be hyperactive. Their excessive rate of speech seems to suggest a *compulsive* talkativeness, the content of which is poorly articulated and delivered in a monotonous whiny tone. As a consequence other people begin to avoid this individual or at least *tune out* the seemingly endless flow of *verbal drivel.* The restlessness and hyperactivity which is often noted is associated with poor concentration and an inability to focus on details or sustain attention for prolonged periods of time. For example, in a study referred to by Weiss (1964, p. 34), there were differences found between normal children and clutterers in their attention span as measured by the length of a series of nonsense syllables that could be recalled. As a result of their inattentiveness, many clutterers tend to be underachievers in school.

The lack of concentration or poor memory span reported by Weiss and others does not have unequivocal support in the experimental literature. For example, Langova and Moravek (1970) compared some parameters of memory for a verbal acoustic signal in clutterers and normal speaking subjects. They examined twenty-two normal speaking subjects and twenty-two clutterers who varied in age from sixteen to forty. The subjects first read two lists of words used in speech audiometry tests under normal or non-distracting conditions. After reading each list they were asked to repeat all the words they remembered. Subsequently, another list was read under conditions of delayed auditory feedback (referred to in the speech literature as the Lee effect) in which the delay was 0.145 seconds. The subjects then read another list under the influence of 80 db. white noise. In each condition they were asked to recall the words read. Under the no distraction condition, there were no significant differences in recall between normals and clutterers. During conditions of interference clutterers had significantly better recall than normals. This finding would be in opposition to that which would normally be predicted on the basis of clinical observation. Apparently, lack of concentration is not characteristic of clutterers that holds under all conditions.

Another part of the cluttering syndrome is the apparent inability to simulate rhythm and a general lack of musical talent. Weiss (1964) and Luchsinger and Arnold (1965) make repeated reference to the clutterer's inability to perform rhythmic exercises. Arnold (1970) goes so far as to suggest that certain brain structures which may affect both language ability and musical talent may be involved. Once again the data that is available is not wholly consistent with respect to these observations. Becker and Grundmann (1970) report a study in which they investigated the rhythmic ability of clutterers and normals. They had their subjects beat four-four time, three-four time and the rhythm of a song, as well as testing their ability to change from clapping hands to clapping on knees. Although the authors report that the clutterers had more errors than the normals, it is difficult to evaluate their results since the results of their statistical tests were not presented.

Langova and Moravek (1970) also conducted an investigation to determine some of the relationships between musical talent, impaired speech and some electrophysiological data. They examined a group of thirty-two clutterers who ranged in age from twelve to fifty-three. The tests included an evaluation of the ability to perceive and reproduce rhythm, perceive and differentiate between the pitch of sounds and melodies and to reproduce them. The patients were divided into groups according to their musical talent: (1) very good (2) average (3) poor and (4) complete amusia.

The results showed that musicality was preserved in twenty-three of the thirty-two subjects (72%). On the other hand impaired musicality was observed in nine subjects, 40% had very good musicality, 10% average musicality and 22% a poor or very poor musicality. In 12% of the subjects the expressive component was impaired. In about 6% of the subjects expressive and receptive musicality was preserved. About 10% had complete amusia. It is likewise difficult to interpret these results as the authors do not provide explicit criteria by which musical talent was categorized into good, average, poor, etc. They also do not provide any interjudge reliability estimates of their rating scale and consequently those results should be viewed with caution. Nevertheless, assuming the reliability of these data, the results would certainly bring into question the so-called *syndrome* nature of cluttering. That is, should cluttering be conceptualized as a disorder affecting many channels of communication as suggested by a number of authors or should it be more narrowly defined in terms of a language deficit?

The majority of the behaviors described above are relatively easy to describe and to denote. However, one inferred characteristic which appears in almost all of the material written on cluttering is that these individuals seem to be unaware that their speech is deficient. Despite the fact that clutterers may often be requested to repeat what they have said, these individuals are either unaware of their speech disorder or else are simply unwilling to acknowledge that they have a problem. Consequently, clutterers do not typically seek speech therapy and when coerced into therapy are poorly motivated clients. The present author takes the position while the *awareness* of the clutterer may be of some explanatory value, it is of little use in accounting for the deficient motivation. It is further contended that in all likelihood the cluttering behavior is maintained by the failure of the verbal community to attach differential consequences to the clutterer's behaviors. Despite the unintelligibility of speech, there are a sufficient number of intelligible elements and motor cues such as facial gestures and lip movements to which the listener is responding so that in effect the clutterer is able to communicate. Although perhaps annoyed, the listener does respond to the total context of speech including all of the paralinguistic indicators and thus is able to infer that which he does not understand and make an appropriate response to the clutterer. Since differential consequences are not attached to the intelligible and unintelligible components of the clutterer's speech, it is not difficult to understand why the clutterer's speech pattern remains unchanged. Thus, unless the ratio of unintelligible to intelligible speech is quite extreme, the clutterer is able to communicate, therefore, has no problem and hence no motivation to seek help for a problem that does not exist.

The problem of cluttering in this respect is somewhat analogous to the problem of alcoholism. One does not have a drinking problem unless his drinking behavior is correlated with some effect on his environment. Thus the definition of alcoholism is not dependent directly upon the amount nor frequency of alcohol that is imbibed, but rather upon the correlation of drinking behavior and other socially deviant behaviors. The wife of a heavy drinker may threaten to divorce her husband but does not execute this action. When he is so intoxicated that he cannot go to work, she protects him by calling his employer and saying that he is sick. If the man had held this job for a number of years his employer, upon finding out that he was an alcoholic, may even contribute further to this behavior by giving him *one more chance*. Since his wife and employer engage in similar loving and/or protective behaviors when the man is not drunk or when he has genuine physical ailments, why should the man admit to having an alcohol problem or be motivated to do anything about it? It is only when the wife divorces him and/or his employer terminates his job, that he may acknowledge he has a drinking problem. Although cluttering is by no means in the same category as alcoholism, nevertheless, both types of problem behaviors may be maintained by environmental consequences.

In the description of cluttering there is also a tendency on the part of some authors to make inferences to unobserved variables that they believe relate to the clutttering behavior. The result is a confusion of the description of the disorder with its assumed etiology. This is an issue that is basic not only to the treatment of cluttering but probably other speech disorders as well.

One characteristic that is often inferred to account for the clutterer's speech is that he has poorly integrated thought processes. There is an inferred discrepancy between his rate of thinking and the rate of word emission. On the basis of clinical evidence Weiss suggests that the clutterer thinks too slowly. According to Weiss (1964, p. 34-35);

> . . . If we interrupt a clutterer who has reached an articulatory dead end because of what appears to be an attempt to speak as quickly as he is thinking and ask him to state his thoughts slowly and clearly, we find that he is still unable to proceed with facility. Either he has no clear thoughts to express, or he has several indefinite and amorphous ideas. . . .

On the basis of this type of evidence Weiss concludes that a poorly integrated and incomplete thinking process rather than the rate of thinking *per se* is an important factor in cluttering.

In a similar vein Weiss talks about the *inner language,* a characteristic which is similar to thinking but which is also inferred from the speaker's behavior. Thus, Weiss characterizes normal speech as that which conveys to the listener the impression that the speaker knows what it is that he wants to express and is able to transform his thought into spoken words with facility. Apparently, the clutterer's speech lacks such inner harmony and thus again according to Weiss (1964, p. 36-37);

> One of the most basic characteristics of cluttering is a lack of clarity of inner formulation, and as a result, delivery is hackneyed, haphazard and studded with moments when the clutterer seems to lose the thread of thought completely, or to forget what he has said or the next word to be spoken. We can say, then that normal speech reflects inner order and cluttering is the mirror of inner disorder.

Whether or not Weiss's formulations are correct is impossible to say at this time since the factors postulated for the faulty speech have not been specified independently of the speech behavior. Such characteristics as *inner language* and *inner harmony* are inferred from the speech itself. That is, we do not have a set of measurement operations for defining *inner language* so that we are in a position to assess the extent to which changes in such events are associated with changes in speech clarity. The only observable event is the verbal behavior. In this instance, however, the verbal behavior is being used to both describe the speech defect and as an indicant of something else that is unknown but which is referred to as inner language or inner harmony which in turn is used to account for the speech defect. Such explanatory accounts put us in the position of running around in circles. If presumably the normal person speaks clearly because of inner language harmony and the clutterer speaks poorly because he lacks such harmony, we would be in good position to remedy the speech defect if we could change the inner language harmony. However, since the inner language is an unknown event which we have inferred from the verbal behavior, basically all we really know is that normal people speak clearly because they speak clearly whereas clutterers do not speak clearly because they do not speak clearly!

We have chosen to elaborate on this point because it is a basic issue relevant not only to cluttering but probably other speech disorders as well. There is a tendency among clinical investigators to infer the determinants of the disorder from the disorder itself. In the absence of any other information, there may be no other choice, but this procedure does have certain risks. If such events are hypothesized, they should at least be capable of definition and measurement and preferably capable of manipulation. Many of the variables that are believed to be associated with or responsible for cluttering do not meet this criterion. The postulated events are often hypothetical and inferred from the speech. When this is done the so-called etiology and the behavior defect become confounded. Thus, initially it may be hypothesized that some form of thinking deficit gives rise to cluttering. It is on the basis of the speech defect that the thinking defect has been inferred. The danger involved is going the additional step and concluding that cluttering is the result of a thinking deficit. By this time we have confused the verbal deficiency with the inferred characteristics believed to regulate it. Furthermore, the relationship between the speech defect and its controlling variables should be specified. Presumably, if a thinking deficit is the variable controlling the speech deficit, then the manipulation of the thinking deficit is necessary to attenuate the speech defect. However, if the thinking deficiency has not been measured independently of the speech deficiency, then we are neither in a position to assess the relationship between the thinking disorder and the speech disorder nor to remedy the speech disorder.

Etiology of Cluttering

Most of what is known regarding the etiology of cluttering is based more on speculation rather than upon data. Weiss and many other individuals believe that cluttering is determined by heredity. However, many investigators while implicating heredity as a primary determinant of cluttering also believe that organic changes involving the central nervous system particularly those cerebral functions concerned with expressive and receptive language functions are more directly responsible for cluttering behaviors. We will first review some of the data which is suggestive of organic deficits and then review Weiss's theory that cluttering is a central language imbalance.

Seeman (1970) suggests that cluttering may be the result of damage in motor areas of the brain. He notes that in children clutterers there is a striking motor restlessness of the entire body. This restlessness also occurs during sleep and is similar to the general motor hyperactivity seen in children with extrapyramidal disorders. He believes that the central disturbance is localized in the striopallidar system. The reason for this opinion is that many patients who have definite extrapyramidal disorders manifest some of the same symptoms as clutterers; that is, rapid acceleration of speech and deviations in general motor ability.

Deviations in sensory-motor coordination were also demonstrated in experiments conducted by Seeman. In one study clutterers and normals were asked to repeat the nonsense syllable *tah*. Initially the articulation is precise but after awhile acceleration begins, precision is lost, and the verbalization changes into unarticulated muttering. In one study he found that clutterers pronounced this syllable at a rate ranging from 100-180 responses per minute faster than the normal controls. Seeman suggests that his results indicate there is no inability of the articulatory musculature but that there is a *pathological propulsion of speech* caused by some central mechanism. He also indicates that whereas some authors assume that cluttering is caused by the discrepancy in the rate of thinking and the motor ability of the speech organs, his data suggests the acceleration appears even repeating the same syllable when articulation is not controlled by thinking as in the case of forming sentences.

Seeman also found deficiencies in visual motor coordination. There were no differences between clutterers and normals on a simple reaction time experiment which involved depression of a switch when a light came on. But in a multiple discrimination reaction experiment which involved the depression of one of two keys dependent upon which of two colored lights were presented, the number of errors made by clutterers was almost double that recorded for normal subjects.

The accelerated motor behaviors of the clutterer were also the concern of Langova and Moravek (1970). They were also interested in examining some electrophysiological concomitants of cluttering. In a group of fifty-seven clutterers they noted the frequent occurrence of electroencephalographic abnormalities (50% abnormal findings and 11% atypical findings). The electrophysiological activity was characterized by a relatively low incidence of alpha rhythm. These electroencephalographic abnormalities were not uniform nor was the extent of the abnormality related to the severity of the speech defect. It is interesting to note the reactions of these authors in reviewing their own results (Langova and Moravek, 1970, p. 332):

> The anomaly of the electroencephalographic findings is striking. This very remarkable fact must be, however, evaluated with regard to another remarkable fact, that is, that clutterers are able to improve their speech by volitional effort. If the electrical abnormality we found on EEG examination were the expression of an organic disorder, the patient would hardly be able to eliminate this disorder by his will.

Langova and Moravek are certainly not representative of the majority of investigators in this area who in their attempt to account for cluttering in terms of a genetic or organic component overlook the common observation that the clutterer is able to control his own behavior. Therefore, an important locus of control may be found in terms of environmental consequences.

Since Weiss's theory of the etiology of cluttering is frequently cited, it is desirable that a critical review of his theory be presented. As in any field where little information is known, any book written on the subject tends to be considered authoritative in the field and cited quite often. To the author's knowledge Weiss's book is the only book in English that is devoted entirely to cluttering and there are a number of secondary sources that refer to his work in a noncritical fashion.

At the beginning of his book Weiss indicates his theoretical bias by defining cluttering in terms of what he assumes to be its etiology. According to Weiss (1964, p. 1);

> It (cluttering) is a disorder of the thought processes preparatory to speech and based on a hereditary disposition. Cluttering is the verbal manifestation of Central Language Imbalance, which affects all

> channels of communication (e.g. reading, writing, rhythm and musicality) and behavior in general.

Weiss goes on to elaborate his position to indicate that many disorders in communication such as delayed speech, dyslalias, cluttering, stuttering etc. are all interrelated and symptomatic of a central language imbalance, the prime characteristics of which are a lack of concentration, short attention span and lack of awareness of the function of communication. He uses an iceberg analogy to demonstrate his theoretical conception. This is shown in Figure V.1. The picture indicates that many seemingly diverse communication disorders are all symptomatic of an underlying central language imbalance. Weiss's use of the iceberg analogy is reminiscent of a similar analogy typically used to represent Freud's constructs of consciousness and unconsciousness. Thus, the psyche of the individual is represented by an iceberg of which only a small portion appears above the surface of the water. This portion represents consciousness or awareness. The much larger mass that lies submerged represented the storehouse of unconscious motivation. Disturbances at the conscious level were viewed as symptomatic of an underlying intrapsychic or unconscious conflict.

In a similar vein Weiss sees all disorders of communication which include cluttering as symptomatic of a central language imbalance. The disorder is central in the sense of bearing on a num-

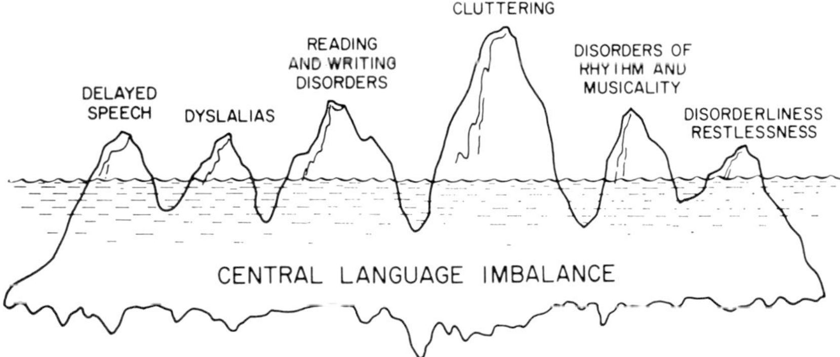

Figure V.1. Iceberg Analogy showing a Central Language Imbalance as an Underlying Determinant of Diverse Communication Disorders. (After, Weiss, D., 1964.)

ber of functions presumably originating in the brain and a central language imbalance affects the channels of communication. This central language imbalance is a hypothetical construct which, in addition, seems to have as its referents the hereditary or constitutional characteristics of the individual. Although Weiss never makes this relationship explicit, the central language imbalance is presumably the result of a faulty genetic endowment which manifests itself in the form of language and communication defects. At this point the similarity between Freud's and Weiss's iceberg analogy ends. Although there is considerable disagreement about Freud's theoretical constructs, at least there was a logical consistency between etiology and treatment. The goal of psychoanalytic treatment was to release the repressed *submerged* material and bring it into conscious awareness. As far as the present author can determine, there seems to be very little, if any, relationship between Weiss's etiological model which is presented in the first part of his text and the therapeutic procedures that are presented in the latter part of the book.

Presumably this central language imbalance may affect the central nervous system in the form of neurological disease or some structural dysfunction. Weiss does not make this point very explicit. However, his genetic orientation is so strong that he concludes that when neurological involvement is definitely present or associated with cluttering, that this does not represent *true* cluttering. Only when there are symptoms of cluttering present and lack of neurological involvement, can it be said that *true* cluttering is present.

Weiss goes on to indicate that although the central language imbalance may be responsible for a retardation of neurological development and some specific anatomical defects, the major effect is on the feedback function of the central nervous system. This feedback principle is based on the assumption that during every controlled bodily movement proprioceptive information on the position of the moving organs is fed back to the central nervous system. Awareness of the movement makes control possible and it also enables us to correct erroneous movement. According to Weiss there is some disturbance in the feedback system of the clutterer and he, therefore, is completely unaware of his errors. As a rule he tends to be an inattentive listener and reader and even less attentive to his own speaking.

The evidence presented by Weiss for the role of genetics in the development of cluttering is very sketchy and is mainly based upon clinical case histories in which there is a history of speech defects in the family of the clutterer. Weiss presents neither actuarial data on the number of such families that have been surveyed, nor for that matter is there data presented on the actual number of clutterers that he has treated.

Luchsinger and Arnold (1965) do not take as strong a position with respect to a genetic determination as does Weiss, but they do present some information that seems to be supportive of a genetic etiology. They conceive of cluttering as a congenital language disability that always begins with severely delayed language development. It is typically diagnosed about the tenth year of life. In common with other types of language disorders cluttering occurs about four times more often in the male sex of all ages than among females. Although Luchsinger and Arnold do not present any actuarial data, they do report that such information may be available from the world's largest collection of case histories at the National Hospital for Speech Disorders in New York. According to Luchsinger and Arnold the anlysis of such histories strongly suggest an hereditary influence. Seeman (1970) reports a family pedigree where cluttering appeared in four generations. From eighteen family members, sixteen were clutterers pointing to the strong possibility of an hereditary predisposition.

Luchsinger and Arnold (1965) differentiate between two types of hereditary influence; specific and nonspecific inheritance. Specific inheritance brings about the transmission of the cluttering syndrome in families containing clutterers or stutterers. Nonspecific inheritance manifests itself in the transmission of a general language disability. Thus, delayed speech, dyslalia, dyslexia and dysgraphia are often associated with other signs of delayed neural maturation. The classification of nonspecific inheritance seems similar to Weiss's central langauge imbalance. However, unlike Weiss, Luchsinger and Arnold seem willing to attach more importance to neurological deficits as a determinant of the disorder. Arnold (1970), like Weiss tends to view cluttering as a genetic syndrome which probably has some organic components. Although Arnold acknowledges the possibility of some environmental influence, he takes the position that the initiation of cluttering is determined by heredity and that the environment may influence the further course of the disorder.

By ruling out definitive neurological involvement as contraindicative of *true* cluttering, Weiss is able to pull a tour de force. If *true* cluttering is defined in terms of its etiology (i.e. a genetic defect) then there is no need to search for the controlling variables since they are already known. This position may be almost unassailable except for the fact that it would be impossible to diagnose *true* cluttering without first demonstrating that there was an hereditary determinant. Weiss suggests that cluttering is a symptom of a central language imbalance and that this imbalance is under hereditary influence. The only evidence for such hereditary influence is the presence of a family history of speech deficiency. However, in the absence of actuarial data, the reliability of clinical observation can be questioned. Furthermore, even if there was a high degree of congruences between the presence of cluttering and family history of speech disorders, this alone would hardly constitute a strong case for genetic determination since many other concomitant events could play an important role. As a matter of fact, it is generally acknowledged that imitation plays a major role in the acquisition of speech skills particularly during the early developmental phases. A number of faulty environmental events could be as much responsible for the development of speech pathology as can faulty genes.

Once again the definition of the behavior in terms of its etiology is responsible for some of the confusion. If the definition of cluttering can be restricted to a description of the verbal behaviors involved, this may serve to alleviate some of the confusion. It is quite possible that the acquisition of such behavior is under the control of hereditary, neurological-physiological, and/or environmental variables. It is also quite possible that the variables that were primarily responsible for the initial acquisition of the behavior are different than the variables responsible for the further development and maintenance of the behavior.

It is conceivable, for instance, that a faulty genetic endowment is responsible for delayed speech development but when verbal behavior does appear whatever deficiencies are emitted are then regulated by environmental influences. Whether this is indeed what happens is really unknown at the present time. It is quite clear that research is needed to substantiate this notion. We can only conclude at this time that the etiology of cluttering is for the most part unknown.

Cluttering Vs. Stuttering

As was mentioned earlier, since cluttering is a diagnostic category that has not received much attention in this country, it is possible that a number of clutterers have been included within the stuttering category. Weiss (1964) and Luchsinger and Arnold (1965) devote considerable attention to differentiating between these two types of speech anomalies. A table summarizing the major differences between stuttering and cluttering as reported by Luchsinger and Arnold (1965, p. 601) has been reprinted on following page.

In general stuttering is a more constricted range of behavior than is cluttering. Although there are some clutterers that may stutter, typically the clutterer represents a much more heterogenous collection of speech deficiencies. One of the key differences is that the true stutterer is most unhappy about his nonfluencies while the clutterer seems to be unaware of any speech abnormality. However, when the clutterer does concentrate on his speech, he is temporarily able to overcome his defects whereas the stutterer experiences increasing difficulty the more his attention is directed to his oral performance. Another difference as reported by Weiss is that under stress the stutterer tends to increase his nonfluencies but there is a decrease in their occurrence as he becomes more relaxed. The reverse is characteristic of the clutterer who is on his guard under stress conditions and speaks relatively fluently, but as he becomes more relaxed exhibits more nonfluencies. Because of these differences, Weiss suggests that there should be differences in therapy for clutterers and stutterers. In general he advocates that the therapist focus attention on the articulation problems in treating cluttering whereas in the treatment of stuttering less stress should be placed directly upon the speech

TABLE V.I

DIFFERENCES BETWEEN GENUINE (IDIOPATHIC) STUTTERING AND CLUTTERING (OR TACHYPHEMIC CLUTTER-STUTTERING) (AFTER, LUCHSINGER AND ARNOLD, 1965)

	Stuttering	*Cluttering*
Interpretation	Acquired social neurosis	Inherited language deficit
Heredity	Neurotic predisposition	Familial language disability
Onset	Usually sudden, in childhood, or after traumatic events	Always gradual, following developmental language disorders
Language development	Normal or early	Severely delayed
Intelligence	Normal to bright, verbal-social	Normal to bright, practical
Aptitudes	Good to superior in most areas	Superior in sciences and mathematics but poor in languages
Psychomotor ability	Emotionally inhibited	General dysrhythmia
Musical talent	Average to superior	Usually very poor, and tone deaf
Singing	Average, not disturbed	Usually melody-mute and monotonous
Underlying predisposition	Neurovegetative dyscrasia	Congenital language disability
Course	Spontaneous remissions or relapses, eventual compensation	Persisting if untreated, worse in puberty
Physical findings	Normal, or vegetative dystonia, allergic tendencies	Congenital dyspraxia
EEG	Preponderantly normal	Diffuse dysrhythmia
Spontaneous speech	Clonic or tonic blocks, grimaces, parakinesias	Rapid, jerky, truncated, repetitive, stumbling
Silent reading	Not disturbed	Often dyslectic or slow
Reading aloud	Often less disturbed	Rapid, jerky, cluttered
Graphologic findings	Difficulties in beginning, carrying out, and maintaining the sequence of motions	Disintegrated and incoordinated handwriting
Handedness	Normal distribution	Familial laterality disorders
Combination with other speech disorders	Not typical	Residual dyslalia, dysgrammatism, dyslexia, dysgraphia
Consciousness of defect	Greatly concerned	Unconcerned and disinterested
Speaking to superiors	Worse	Better
Speaking to familiar persons	Better	Worse
Short answers	Difficult	Easy
Calling attention to speech	Aggravates	Improves
Having to repeat	Aggravates	Improves
Phonophobic concerns	Stereotyped sounds or words	Any difficult blends and long words
Treatment	Psychotherapy and specific techniques	Instruction in all language functions
Prognosis depends on	Emotional adjustment	Diligent learning

defect since to do so seems to enhance the amount of stuttering. Weiss has observed a number of stutterers who also clutter. He feels that there is a developmental progression from cluttering to stuttering. In treating stuttering problems he has noted that as the stuttering problems begin to decrease, there is an increase in cluttering. It is as though the original stuttering was masking underlying cluttering behavior.

In terms of differences in the etiology of the two disorders, there has not been agreement on the variables that are involved. For the most part there has been speculation and not data concerning the events that contribute to cluttering. Weiss has speculated that both cluttering and stuttering result from constitutional differences which give rise to a delay in the development of speech. The clutterer is usually late in speaking and quite often has a family history of cluttering, stuttering and/or retarded speech development. Weiss has observed that cluttering usually occurs before stuttering develops. Cluttering also persists in the early stages of stuttering until suppressed by the patient's efforts. In the treatment of stuttering, Weiss has reported that he has never observed a case in which cluttering symptoms have not appeared after there has been a reduction in the stuttering behavior.

Despite these clinical observations, the evidence thus far has not substantiated the notion that a history of cluttering is a necessary condition for the development of stuttering, although the two conditions often coexist. Freund (1953) has reported for instance, that approximately 50% of children whose stuttering first appeared at puberty had a history of cluttering. In addition Freund seems to disagree with Weiss that all cluttering is the result of a constitutional defect and tends to take the position that many forms of cluttering are symptomatic of basic neurotic or intrapsychic conflicts. Van Riper (1963) has observed that whereas some clutterers become stutterers, in the majority of instances cluttering does not progress to stuttering. It is Van Riper's position that it is only when a pattern of cluttering coexists with stuttering either in the presenting symptomatology or in the past history of the individual is the presence of a constitutional predisposition suspected. However, Van Riper seems to allow for the possibility of a multideterminant etiology to the extent that cluttering could result from minor brain damage, environmental conditions as well as genetic defects or any combination of these events. It would appear insofar as etiology is concerned, the relationship between cluttering and stuttering is ambiguous. There seems to be discrepancies in the number of cases in which cluttering and stuttering coexist and presently there is no definitive evidence that stuttering develops from cluttering.

Cluttering Therapy

In our discussion of the etiology of cluttering the suggestion was made that the definition of cluttering be restricted to a description of the types of behaviors which are considered to be deficient. The etiology of the behavior (s) could then be determined by investigating those variables which are believed to be associated with the acquisition and maintenance of cluttering behavior. It has also been postulated that three large categories of variables (genetic, physiological or neurological and environmental events) may be possible determinants of cluttering. It is of interest to note that the least attention has been paid to the role of environmental events. A factor to be considered if only for pragmatic reasons is that even if genetic and/or neurological events were known to relate to cluttering in a systematic fashion, that most speech therapists and psychologists do not have the tools at their disposal to manipulate such events. It would seem more reasonable, given our present state of knowledge and level of technology, to search for the controlling events of cluttering in the environment. If such relationships are found, then it may be possible to systematically alter such events in order to bring about a reduction in cluttering.

The failure to take into account more fully the role of environmental control is rather striking in that one common observation is that the clutterer is able to speak fluently when he wants to or when he is concentrating on his speech. This would certainly seem to suggest that motivational variables in terms of the types of consequences that are made contingent upon cluttering may be playing a major role on the maintenance if not the acquisition of cluttering behavior.

Another clue that the environment is a contributing factor to cluttering is implied in the clinical observations that clutterers speak well under stressful conditions. Also when given instructions to speak clearly or to repeat what they have said there is a decrease in the amount of nonfluent speech. If the rate of nonfluencies vary in such a systematic fashion, it would seem more plausible to search for the controlling variables in the environment than to postulate determinants which are relatively inaccessible to measurement and manipulation. It is suspected that there may be certain environmental conditions setting the occasion for high rates of cluttering while other environmental conditions set the occasion for low cluttering rates. If that were the case, it would be conjectured that cluttering may be under stimulus control. It would then be possible to modify cluttering rates by systematically manipulating certain stimulus conditions.

This type of strategy would be used by those who advocate a behavior modification approach to speech pathology problems. Unfortunately, whereas cluttering has been paid but scant attention by investigators in the field of speech pathology, it has attracted even less attention by investigators who make use of behavior modification techniques. On a recent bibliography of the behavior modification literature which had over 1,100 references there was not one citation made to the treatment of cluttering. In a recently edited text (Sloane and MacAuley, 1968) which dealt specifically with operant procedures in remedial speech and language training, there was again no reference made to treatment of cluttering. In fact the only behavior modification study with cluttering that could be found was the one conducted by the present author (Simkins, Kingery and Bradley, 1970). Even in this instance the investigation was more of a case study than a systematic research effort.

Since research on cluttering that makes use of behavior modification techniques is virtually nonexistent and since there is but minimal data reported by investigators using techniques which have originated from other than a behavior modification approach, it is obviously impossible to evaluate which technique or set of techniques would be most effective in the remediation of cluttered speech. We will therefore, review some of the therapeutic procedures used by earlier investigators and go into some of the procedural details and results of the study conducted by Simkins. It is contended that despite the lack of studies with cluttering, that many of the behavior modification procedures used in the treatment of stuttering and articulation defects would probably be effective with clutterers. Since these procedures are discussed in detail in other chapters of this text, we will make brief mention of some of these procedures and how they might be applied to cluttering behavior. Finally some of our discussion will be devoted to outlining the types of research that seem to be needed and how such problems could be conceptualized within a behavior modification framework.

Traditional Therapy Techniques

The majority of treatment techniques used by speech pathologists have a common sense rationale underlying them. Some of these techniques involve an attempt to achieve stimulus control over the clutterers' behavior and therefore, are compatible and in some instances bear a great deal of similarity to the behavior modification procedures that have been used with other types of speech problems. Other techniques such as group singing, poetry reading, mental concentration exercises have a great deal of appeal in terms of their logical validity but the actual effects produced on cluttering have not been clearly demonstrated. At this point we will briefly review some of the more traditional speech therapy techniques.

In order to reduce the excessive speaking rate, the client is simply instructed to speak more slowly. Weiss has found that this procedure is effective in producing a temporary reduction in speech rate. In many instances it has been found that the clutterer's oral reading rates are as excessive as their conversational speech rates. In order to reduce oral reading speed, Froeschels (as reported in Luchsinger and Arnold, 1965) used a window reading technique. A paper shield in which there was a hole large enough to expose only a single letter or a short word is placed upon the printed text. Later the size of the hole is gradually expanded to reveal words. Moving the paper over the line forces the eye to look long enough at each word. By moving the shield faster the therapist allows the clutterer to increase his reading rate as his ability improves. Froeschels' technique is very similar to a procedure developed by Goldiamond (1962) in which a page is projected on the screen and the subject is required to read aloud or silently. Through the same optical system an opaque loop is presented that masks the projection and a transparent slit on the opaque loop exposes part of a line of type. With each frame, the slit moves lineally and sequentially exposing successive reading material. Unlike Froeschels' technique in which the therapist controls the stimulus presentation, in Goldiamond's procedure the subject controls the loop by pressing a microswitch to advance the frame. The pressing of the microswitch can also be used to define a monitoring response during silent reading.

Since clutterers typically make frequent articulation errors and also have dysrhythmic speech, a variety of procedures for ameliorating these effects have been attempted. For example, Weiss has made use of a syllabization technique which consists of requiring the patient to speak in slowly pronounced syllables, giving each syllable an equal time allotment. Another technique consists of exaggerated stress on every accentuated syllable, e.g. YESterday I MET a VERy GOOD FRIEND.

The disordered rhythm of the clutterer's speech is frequently described as being jerky, stumbling and full of temporal abnormalities. In order to produce a normal speech rhythm, a combination of a rhythmical tapping technique and the syllabization technique have been tried. This consists of tapping on the desk with every pronounced syllable. It is a reinforcement of the syllabization exercise allowing the patient greater control over his speed of delivery. Weiss reports in using this technique that the clutterer initially experiences difficulty in integrating the two activities. He might speak in syllables and tap haphazardly or tap regularly and speak irregularly.

In order to improve the rhythmical sense a metronome has been used to control the rate of syllable emission. This frees the clutterer from having to execute a hand movement response as well as a verbal response. One of the difficulties with this technique is that quite often there is very little transfer to situations once the metronome has been removed. However, a recent study by Brady (1971) which involved the use of a miniaturized electric metronome which is worn behind the ear like a hearing aid demonstrated a marked increase in the speech fluency of stutterers. More than likely this procedure could also be employed with clutterers. Presumably techniques such as practice in discrimination of pitch, training the patient to recognize and identify different rhythmical patterns, and singing exercises are designed to alleviate the temporal abnormalities in the clutterer's speech. There is, however, very little information pertaining to the extent to which such exercises carry over to the clutterer's conversational speech.

Another procedure reported by Weiss is to have the therapist and patient read a text simultaneously. The therapist imposes a slow speed, permitting variation and rhythmical accentuation of syllables. The therapist then makes use of a fading technique to ascertain whether the patient has begun to spontaneously follow the therapist's lead. The therapist begins to lower his voice slowly and imperceptibly until he is no longer emitting any sound. Weiss has found, however, that while this technique produces a decisive improvement in articulation and rhythm while reading, the quality of the clutterer's spontaneous conversational speech often remains unchanged. A similar effect was noted by Simkins, Kingery and Bradley (1970).

Since inattentiveness or lack of concentration is a frequent characteristic of the clutterer, a variety of procedures have been employed in an attempt to remedy this defect. One frequent observation has been that there is a decrease in the rate of nonfluencies when the clutterer encounters unfamiliar materials. Therefore, one technique that has been used is to have the clutterer read aloud materials printed in a foreign language. His unfamiliarity with the material forces him to concentrate on each word. The effect is not only a reduction in the rate of nonfluencies but also a reduction in his total rate of oral activity.

Another technique recommended by Weiss to increase concentration is to have the clutterer count backwards by threes starting from one hundred. A technique to improve concentration reported by Beebe (1944) makes use to material from a syllabic memory test. This material consists of meaningless syllable sounds in which there is a gradual increase in the number of syllables that are to be memorized and repeated. Although there are undoubtedly a number of other techniques available to improve concentration, again there is no data available to indicate whether or not improvement on such tasks is related to either improvement in the clutterer's conversational speech or on his reading habits. Until such data are available, it is difficult to estimate the extent to which such concentration exercises are of benefit in terms of decelerating the rate of cluttering.

Behavior Therapy Techniques

Thus far we have been discussing some of the traditional techniques that have been employed by pathologists in treating cluttering. While some of these techniques bear some similarity to the stimulus control procedures used in behavior therapy, contingency control and reinforcement procedures are notably lacking. Although Weiss and others make frequent reference to the recalcitrant nature of the clutterer, there are only some vague hints as to how the motivation problem is handled. Thus, the patient may be encouraged, he may be told of the benefits of therapy, or he may be coerced into attempting to improve his speech. Since lack of motivation seems to be of major importance in cluttering patients, it would seem that reinforcement principles could be used to alleviate this problem. Another major advantage of behavior therapy procedures over more conventional techniques is that specific behaviors are defined and measured. The continuous recording of the specific behaviors provides the therapist with a more sensitive measure of the behavior and allows him to assess fairly rapidly the extent to which his procedures are producing the desired effect.

At this time we will consider in some detail the study conducted by the present author (Simkins, et al., 1970). Although the results of that study are by no means conclusive, some desired effects were achieved and the study does provide an illustration of how behavior modification procedures could be used in the treatment of cluttering.

The subject (C) in this study was a nine-year-old girl who had been diagnosed as a childhood schizophrenic. She was in residence at a parochial school for emotionally disturbed children. C engaged in a number of deviant behaviors, such as excessive masturbation and withdrawal from social contact.

We noted that in ordinary conversation C spoke very rapidly, and that many of her words were cluttered. Nevertheless, in conversation or oral reading, one was able to understand, with some difficulty, what she was saying. However, when her speech was recorded, it was estimated that only approximately 20% of her words were intelligible. The reason for this apparent difference in intelligibility was that the listener did not have the benefit of lip movement cues or the printed text.

As a point of departure, we decided to work on C's oral reading. If we were successful in modifying this behavior, we planned to proceed to work on her conversational speech. We used several different procedures in working with her oral reading.

During the first few sessions, or what is referred to as the baseline phase, we requested her to read passages from one of her fifth grade reading books. A count of words per minute was made. As can be seen in the upper graph of Figure V.2 her word rate was fairly high, averaging about 145 words per minute. She ran sentences together, did not pause for commas or periods, mispronounced words, omitted some words, and occasionally substituted words. Since it was fairly evident that periods and commas exerted on control over her vocal behavior, our first goal was to reinforce pausing at these grammatical junctions. We also felt that pausing would slow her word rate, and this in turn might help her speech clarity.

We used stars as reinforcement. These stars were made contingent on the behavior we desired. C would paste the stars on a chart and whenever she obtained 100 of them, she would be allowed to go on a field trip to the library, the zoo, a children's movie, etc.

In the procedure in which pausing was reinforced, we had a face of Yogi Bear with two lights for eyes. Attached to Yogi was a counter and clicker. Each time C paused at a comma or period, the clicker would sound. Whenever she accumulated ten clicks, the experimenter (E) would say "Yogi Bear," C would push a button, Yogi's eyes would light, and a point would register on the counter. At the end of the session, C would receive one star for each point on the counter. As can be seen in Figure V.2 there was a definite reduction in word rate.

However, the intelligibility of her speech was not affected.

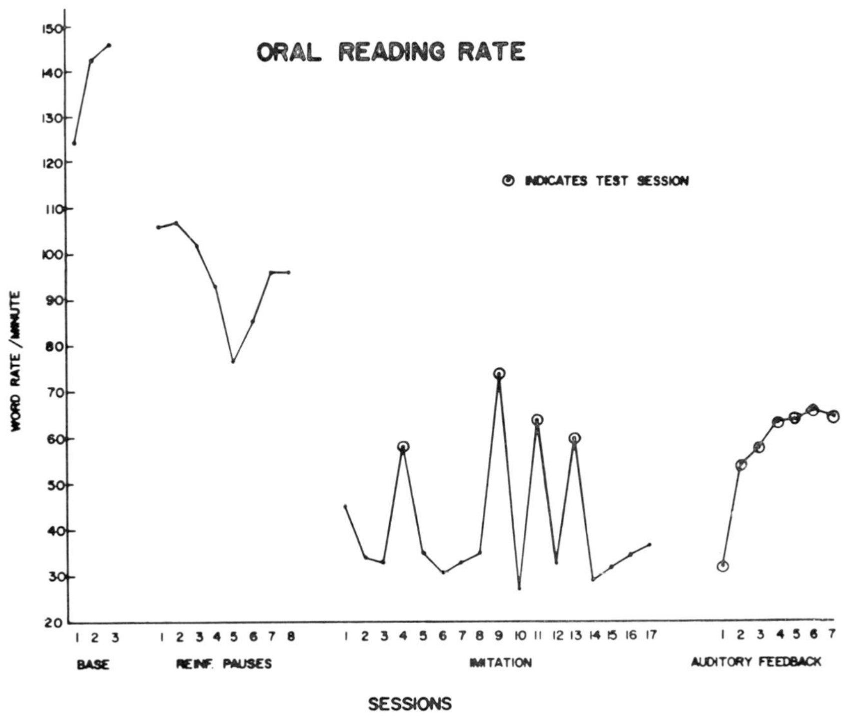

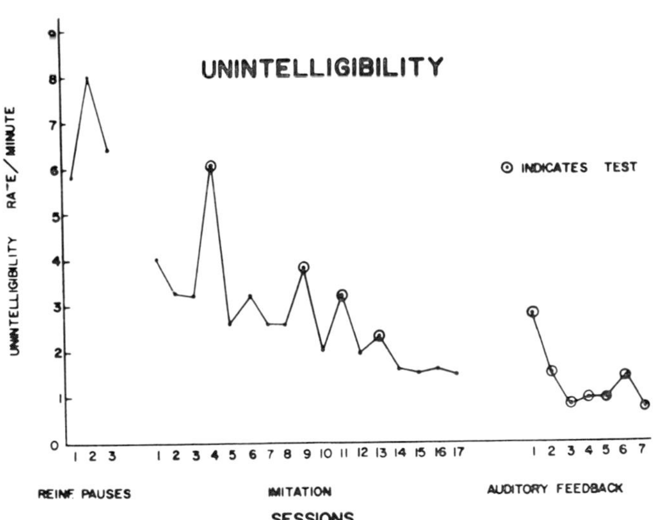

Figure V.2. Word Rate and Unintelligibility Rate as a Function of Manipulation of Oral Reading Behavior. (After, Simkins, Kingery, and Bradly, 1970.)

She still rambled words together, dropped the endings off words, and had pronounced difficulty articulating words having *th* and *sh* sounds. Toward the end of the first procedure, we began taking a count of unintelligibility. One of the investigators who did not have the book in front of her would tally each time she did not understand what C had read or when C did not properly articulate a word. A second investigator made a similar tally from the tape recording of C's oral reading. Several estimates were taken in this fashion. The inter-observer reliability of unintelligible responses averaged 0.89.

Despite the crudeness of our definition of unintelligibility, it was felt that the amount of agreement between the observers was sufficiently high to warrant using it as a response unit of measurement. Measures of C's unintelligibility rate were made on the last three sessions of the reinforcement of pause procedure. These data are presented as the first series of points on the lower graph in Figure V.2.

In order to increase intelligibility, we started a training procedure using imitation. E first read a few words from the text in which each of the words was carefully articulated. C was instructed to focus upon E's tongue and lip movements. She was then reinforced for each successful repetition. During this phase, tests were occasionally made, during which C would read by herself orally and the same procedure was followed as during the reinforcement of pause stage. That is, during the test sessions, there was no imitation training and C was only reinforced for pausing at the appropriate grammatical junctions. These test sessions are indicated by the dots enclosed in circles on the two graphs in Figure V.2. During the test sessions, word rate and unintelligibility seem to be high, relative to the days on which there was training on imitation. Nevertheless, as can be seen in Figure V.2, there was a progressive decrease in rate of unintelligibility across sessions.

Despite the improvement shown in the second procedure, we felt that the quality of C's speech could be further improved. Until this time, C's speech was in large measure under the imitative control of E. We wanted to use a procedure where the sound of her own voice would serve to control and modify her verbal behavior.

A passage of one hundred words was marked off in her book. She was told that she would receive one star for each 10 intelligible words. If she read the passage perfectly, she would receive ten stars. C read the passage into the tape recorder and we immediately replayed the tape. C was given a pencil and paper and told to tally each error made. When she made an error, the tape recorder was stopped, the error was replayed, E corrected the error, and C was requested to imitate E. Social approval was usually made contingent upon correct pronunciation. As the sessions progressed, C began to recognize her own errors and to tally them. Also, during the actual recording, she began to correct her speech spontaneously. In subsequent sessions, the passage length was gradually increased from one hundred to five hundred words. The reinforcement ratio was also increased from Fr:10 to Fr:50, i.e., one star for each fifty intelligible words.

Test sessions were inserted in which the procedure used was identical to that employed in the reinforcement of pause procedure. That is, C was reinforced only for pauses at grammatical junctions. Measures of her word rate and unintelligibility appear in the two graphs in Figure V.2. It is interesting to note that despite the increase in word rate, her rate of unintelligibility continued to decrease.

The proportion of errors to words spoken during the training sessions appears in the first series of points on the upper graph in Figure V.3. By the end of this procedure, her oral reading had reached a satisfactory level of clarity. However, this improvement did not generalize to her conversational speech. In fact, the differences in verbal behavior between speech and reading were quite dramatic. On several occasions, C would stop reading and pause to tell E something about the story. As soon as she would look away from the book, there would be an immediate deterioration in her intelligibility. It was evident that clear speech was under the stimulus control of the printed text. This stimulus specificity has also been observed by Weiss (1969) who found that improvement in an oral reading task did not generalize to conversational speech.

In the next phase of the study, an attempt was made to modify C's conversational speech. E would engage her in conversation

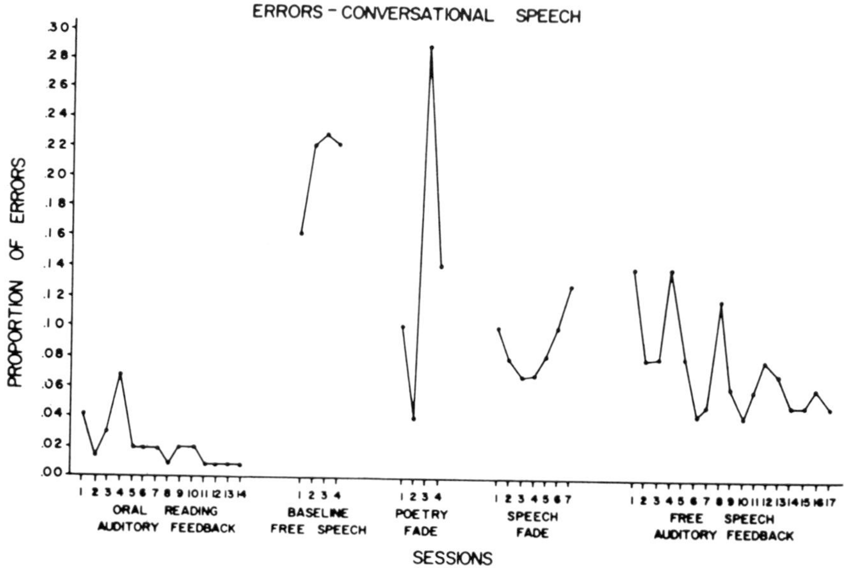

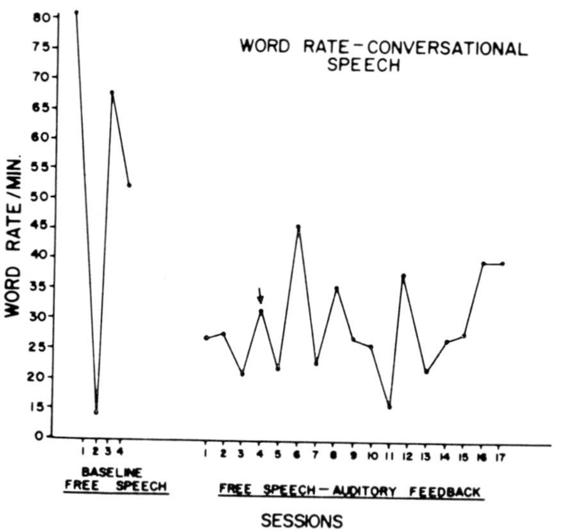

Figure V.3. Word Rate and Proportion of Errors as a Function of Manipulation of Conversational Speech. (After, Simkins, Kingery and Bradly, 1970.)

for approximately five minutes. This conversation was recorded. After the session, a count was made of C's word rate and errors (rate of unintelligible words). There were four such estimates made. These measures constituted the baseline of free speech. The proportion of errors to words spoken and word rate during the baseline of free speech are presented in Figure V.3. During this baseline period, her word rate was quite variable, while the proportion of errors remained fairly stable and was considerably higher in magnitude than the proportion of errors made during the auditory feedback phase of the reading procedure.

The first speech modification procedure will be referred to as the poetry-fade technique. C was given a series of 3 x 5 index cards. On each card was a nursery rhyme which had four lines. C was instructed to read the poem, but when she came to the last word on each line she was to turn the card over, look at E's eyes, and then say the word. If the word was spoken clearly, C received one point. For each ten points, she received a star creditable toward a field trip. This procedure was followed for three poems. The poems were then reread, but this time the last word on each line was blanked out with masking tape and the same procedure followed. The poems were read again, with the last two words on each line blanked out, so that C had to look at E while saying these words. More words on each line were faded until C was reciting the entire poem while looking at E. At each session C was given a new set of poems. We used this poetry-fade procedure for four sessions.

The next procedure used was referred to as a speech fade. In this procedure, C was also provided with index cards, the content of which related to *chit chat* conversations. Each card had a partially completed sentence, for example, "The color of my hair is ...." C would have to look at E and complete the sentence. Then E would say, "What is the color of your hair?" C would be required to answer with a complete sentence, such as, "The color of my hair is brown." Again C was reinforced at the rate of one point for each intelligible word spoken while looking at E. This procedure was used for seven sessions. The reasons for the poetry and speech-fade techniques were: (1) to provide a transition from oral reading to conversational speech, and (2) to reinforce intelligible speech while looking at another person, rather than having a printed text control this behavior.

As can be seen in Figure V.3, there was considerable variability in the proportion of errors during the poetry and speech-fade procedures. Nevertheless, there was a reduction in errors relative to her baseline conversational speech.

The final procedure used will be referred to as free speech-auditory feedback. During this procedure, E would bring to the school a box containing an assortment of different objects, for example, old keys, pictures, toy statues, and a medallion. C was instructed to select one object at a time from the box and describe the object while looking at E. The reason for the use of the box was to provide a fairly standard conversation topic. Each day the content of the box was varied, in order to sustain C's interest.

Tape recordings were made of the conversation and immediately played back. If an error was made, the tape was immediately stopped, E provided the correct pronunciation, and then had C repeat the word (s). This procedure was basically the same as had been used in the oral reading-auditory feedback stage. The proportion of errors for this procedure is presented in the upper graph of Figure V.3 and the word rate in the lower graph of Figure V.3.

The word rate was very low and during the fourth session (indicated by arrows on the graphs), a minor modification in the procedure was made. Until the fourth session, C's word rate had averaged twenty-five words per minute. The trials were five minutes in length. C was told that if she spoke 125 words or more, she was entitled to extra bonus points which she could exchange at the end of a session for a gift or an extra privilege in the dorm, such as watching TV for an additional hour. These points were in addition to those accumulated for the field trips. On the first day of the procedure, there was an increase in both word rate and proportion of errors. After that session, there was considerable variability in her word rate. We had planned to gradually increase the word rate requirement without also producing an increase in errors. However, because of the variability in her word rate, we retained the requirement of twenty-five words per minute. Also, since the school year ended, we were unable to collect any more data. On the last five days, there appeared to be an acceleration in word rate and the proportion of errors remained fairly low.

This case has demonstrated the effectiveness of a series of techniques in improving the intelligibility of speech. Whether or not all the procedures that were employed are necessary to achieve the same effect will not be known until investigations are performed which impose more controls than were feasible in our particular situation. Certainly, the efficiency of this procedure can be questioned when one takes into consideration the fact that this study spanned a nine-month period, in which C was visited for thirty-minute sessions three times a week. It must also be noted that C was an emotionally disturbed, highly withdrawn child. There was considerable variability in her behavior from day to day. We observed that sessions of low word rate seemed to be correlated with the display of atavistic behaviors in the dorm and/or the occurrence of some aversive environmental event. It is therefore quite possible that our procedures may be more effective with normal children, whose mood changes do not vacillate as unpredictably.

Another limitation of this study was that the changes in C's verbal behavior that were produced under restricted conditions did not generalize to more natural surroundings and with other people. The one exception may have been her oral reading behavior. This may have been a function of her teachers and her peers, who praised her for her improved reading performances. On the other hand, although no formal measures were taken, her conversational speech outside the experimental room showed only minimal improvement. Perhaps one of the reasons for the resistance to generalization was that differential consequences were not made contingent upon conversational speech. That is, other people in her natural environment continued to respond to her requests in much the same manner as they always had.

How to produce generalization of newly acquired verbal behavior patterns is a persistent problem in speech pathology. It would appear that in order to increase the probability of such generalization effects, it may be necessary to enlist the cooperation of all personnel who interact with the child.

The problem of generalization with the clutterer may be especially acute inasmuch as there is a tendency for these individuals to emit their usual speech patterns when they return to familiar surroundings or under conditions when they are relaxed. Therefore, in order to produce stable improvements in their speech behavior, it may even be necessary to initiate the speech therapy program in some of the clutterer's natural habitats. The development of radio telemetric devices (e.g., Hoshiko and Holloway, 1968, Stumphauzer, 1971, Brady, 1971) as well as other technological innovations for monitoring verbal behavior, may also enable us to extend our measurement and control procedures into the more natural environment.

The study by Simkins made use of a number of standard behavior modification procedures. Since cluttering does seem to bear some relationship to stuttering, procedures used in the treatment of stuttering could possibly be adapted to treat cluttering. For example, the delayed auditory feedback procedures used by Goldiamond (1965) to attenuate stuttering rates might also reduce cluttering behavior. Such a procedure might be desirable to the extent that it would force the clutterer to attend or listen to his own speech. Goldiamond's finding that one of the effects produced by delayed feedback was the emergence of speech prolongation may also be desirable with clutterers as this would tend to produce a reduction in the excessive speech rate. On the other hand there is some experimental data available which is somewhat puzzling with respect to the effects of delayed feedback on cluttered speech. Langova and Moravek (1970) report that delayed auditory feedback produced a striking deterioration of speech in 85% of the clutterers who were tested but produced improved articulation in 82% of the stutterers that were tested, Langova and Moravek found, however, in another study that when chlorpromazine was given in combination with delayed auditory feedback, the speech of the clutterers became slower and there was a systematic decline in the number of articulation errors in successive observation intervals. However, since they did not have a control in which only chlorpromazine was introduced, it is not known whether it was the chlorpromazine in conjunction with delayed auditory feedback or the chloropromazine itself that was responsible for the decrement in articulation errors.

Since articulation errors are a frequent characteristic of the clutterer's speech behavior, some of the procedures used by behavior therapists to treat specific articulation problems may be of some benefit for some of the more pervasive articulation problems of the clutterer. In working with a clutterer in which there are a number of articulation errors, it may be desirable to first teach sound recognition of correctly articulated sounds. Such sound discriminations could be taught through successive problems of delicately graded difficulty. Once such sound discriminations can be made without error, it may then be easier to verbally produce these sounds. Programmed instruction for the remediation of specific types of articulation errors have been developed by Mower, Baker and Schutz (1968) and by McDearborn (1968). Various steps of these programs could easily be adapted in treating the types of articulation errors made by clutterers.

Although the clutterer makes a number of articulation errors, clinical observers have frequently noted that such misarticulations are not as frequent when the clutterer is under stress or when he is admonished to speak clearly. This would suggest that some type of contingency control could be used to modify the clutterer's behavior. Although the use of response contingent punishment has not produced unequivocal results in terms of altering speech errors, nevertheless, some investigators do report effective suppression of errors. Marshall (1970) reports that the application of a mild shock contingent on misarticulation of the [s] and [z] phoneme produced a rapid decline in such errors by a twenty-year-old subject who had an inconsistent interdental lisp. A six month follow-up of this procedure indicated that such misarticulation errors remained at a low rate.

Siegel, Lenske, and Brown (1969) used a response cost procedure to modify the dysfluencies of normal college students. The dysfluencies consisted of interjections and/or repetitions of a word, sound, or syllable. The subjects in the experiment were paid $2.00 for participation in the experiment but it was possible to earn additional money in the experiment. The subjects sat in an experimental room facing a television monitor. On the screen of the monitor was a picture of a counter having the number *200*. The subjects were told that each point was worth one cent and that at the end of the session they would be credited with $2.00 plus one cent for every remaining point on the counter.

The experimenter sat in an adjacent room and monitored the subject's verbal behavior. A switch was activated each time a dysfluency occurred. During the first or baseline phase of the experiment dysfluencies were recorded but no points were subtracted. During the second or treatment phase, a point was subtracted for each dysfluency. During the third or recovery phase points were no longer subtracted. Although there were individual differences between subjects, the results generally indicated a systematic reduction of dysfluencies during the treatment phase. During the final phase in which points were no longer subtracted, the frequency of dysfluencies increased but remained at a level lower than the baseline. Although the subjects in this study were not classified as clutterers, the types of dysfluencies they emitted are frequently found in the speech characteristics of clutterers. The results of such studies would seem to suggest that some type of contingency control may be an important component of any rehabilitation work with clutterers.

Concluding Comments

Perhaps one major difficulty with the diagnostic classification of cluttering is that the term subsumes a variety of behaviors, many of which overlap with other classes of speech disorders. As a behavioral description the term cluttering conveys very little information. Although there are certain similarities between one clutterer and another, to communicate the differences it is necessary to specify the behaviors involved. Van Riper (1970) has also indicated the need for more precise behavioral discriminations. For example, a frequently reported characteristic of the clutterer is his short attention span. Weiss (1964, p. 34) has produced some data that would corroborate this observation. Yet Langova and Moravek (1970) were unable to find any differences between clutterers and normal speaking subjects. Whether or not clutterers have short attention spans may very well depend on the operations used to define attention span, the criterion employed for *short,* and the procedures and conditions under which such observations have been obtained.

If more attention were paid to the operations for measurement of the specific deficits, this would enable us to differentiate more clearly between cluttering and related disorders such as stuttering. Again Van Riper (1970) suggests the need for a standard list of behaviors to be used for differential diagnosis. Research is needed to derive empirical cut-off scores as a method for reliably differentiating cluttering and stuttering.

Perhaps one of the major differences between those investigators who make use of behavior modification procedures and those who use more traditional methods is in terms of the a priori assumptions made with respect to the etiology of cluttering. A frequent view expressed in the literature is that cluttering is a *syndrome* for which there is an underlying common denominator which is usually some postulated hypothetical construct. These constructs have vaguely defined referents such as *genetic predispositions* or *sub-clinical neurological defects.* While such constructs provide a plausible rationale for accounting for the disorder, their utility is limited with respect to specifying procedures for rehabilitating the clutterer.

The behavior therapist would take the position that the behaviors are neither symptomatic of some underlying state nor that it is likely that the entire collection of behaviors are regulated by the same variable or sets of variables. Furthermore, while it is quite conceivable that at least some of the behaviors described as cluttering may have originated as a function of certain genetic and/or neurological abnormalities, it is highly doubtful that these variables play a major role in the continued maintenance and regulation of all of these behaviors. The role of environmental events has not received much attention and it would be the strategy of the behavior therapist to search for the maintenance variables in the environment. Since the major types of therapeutic intervention used both by traditional investigators as well as behavior therapists involves environmental manipulation, the virtue of this strategy would be to provide a more direct relationship between the assessment of the variables that regulate cluttering and the development of procedures necessary to produce therapeutic changes. Given our limited technology and knowledge concerning the role of genetics and neurological events as they relate to cluttering, it would at this time seem more reasonable to search for the controlling variables in the environment(s) of the clutterer than to speculate about variables which are not immediately accessible to therapeutic manipulation.

At the present time there is very little systematic data available which would enable us to assess which of the assortment of available techniques would be most beneficial to the treatment of cluttering. However, since cluttering does refer to such a diverse collection of behaviors, it may be desirable to assess the effects of certain procedures and specific types of response measures such as word rate, articulation errors, pitch variation and tempo. In all likelihood we will find some modification procedures are highly effective with certain dimensions of cluttering but relatively ineffective with others. Our ability to produce an effective treatment of cluttering is dependent on obtaining some systematic data and the establishment of some reliable functional relationships. Obviously much research is needed.

REFERENCES

Anderson, V. A.: *Improving the Child's Speech.* New York, Oxford Univ. Press, 1953.

Arnold, G. E.: An attempt to explain the causes of cluttering with the LLMM theory. *Folia Phoniatrica, 22*:247-260, 1970.

Becker, K. P. and Grundmann, K.: Investigations on incidence and symptomology of cluttering. *Folia Phoniatrica, 22*:261-271, 1970.

Beebe, H. A.: Auditory memory span for meaningless syllables. *Journal of Speech Disorders, 9*: 59-65, 1944.

Berry, M. F. and Eisenson, J.: *The Defective in Speech.* New York, Appleton-Century-Crofts, 1942.

Brady, John: Metronome-Conditioned speech retraining for stuttering. *Behavior Therapy, 2*:129-150, 1971.

Freund, H.: Psychopathological aspects of stuttering. *American Journal of Psychotherapy, 7*:689-705, 1953.

Goldiamond, I.: Machine definition of ongoing silent and oral reading rate. *Journal Experimental Analysis of Behavior, 5*:363-367, 1962.

Goldiamond, I.: Stuttering and fluency as manipulatable operant response classes. In Krasner, L. and Ullman, L. (Eds.): *Research in Behavior Modification.* New York, Holt, Rinehart and Winston, 1965.

Hoshiko, M. and Holloway, G.: Radio telemetry for the monitoring of verbal behavior. *Journal of Speech and Hearing Disorders, 33*:48-50, 1968.

Langova, Jirina and Moravek, M.: Some problems of cluttering. *Folia Phoniatrica, 22*:325-336, 1970.

Luchsinger, Richard and Arnold, Godfrey: *Voice-Speech-Language: Clinical Communicology: Its Physiology and Pathology* (2nd Ed.). Belmont, Wadsworth, 1965.

Marshall, R. C.: The effect of response contingent punishment upon a defective articulation response, *Journal of Speech and Hearing Disorders, 35*:236-240, 1970.

McDearborn, J.: Programmed learning instruction in phonics. In Sloane, H. and MacAulay, B. (Eds.): *Operant Procedures in Remedial Speech and Language Training*. Boston, Houghton Mifflin Co., 1968.

Mowrer, D., Baker, L., and Schutz, R.: Operant procedures in the control of speech articulation. In Sloane, H. and MacAulay, B. (Eds.): *Operant Procedures in Remedial Speech and Language Training*. Boston, Houghton Mifflin Co., 1968.

Powers, Margaret: Functional Disorders of Articulation; Symptomology and Etiology. In Travis, Lee (Ed.): *Handbook of Speech Pathology*. New York, Appleton-Century-Crofts, Inc., 1957.

Seeman, M.: Relations between motorics of speech and general motor abilities in clutterers. *Folia Phoniatrica, 22*:376-380, 1970.

Siegal, G. M., Lenske, J., and Brown, P.: Suppression of normal speech dysfluencies through response cost. *Journal of Applied Behavior Analysis, 2*:265-276, 1969.

Simkins, Lawrence, Kingery, Martha, and Bradly, Patricia: Modification of cluttered speech in an emotionally disturbed child. *Journal of Special Education, 4*:81-88, 1970.

Sloane, Howard and MacAulay, Barbara: *Operant Procedures in Remedial Speech and Language Training*. Boston, Houghton Mifflin, 1968.

Stumphauzer, Jerome: A low-cost *bug-in-the-ear* sound system for modification of therapist, parent, and patient behavior. *Behavior Therapy, 2*:249-250, 1971.

Van Riper, C.: *Speech Correction: Principles and Methods,* 4th ed. Englewood Cliffs, Prentice-Hall, 1963.

Van Riper, C.: Stuttering and cluttering: The differential diagnosis. *Folia Phoniatrica, 22*:347-353, 1970.

Weiss, D.: *Cluttering,* In Van Riper (Ed.): The Foundations of Speech Pathology Series. Englewood Cliffs, Prentice-Hall, 1964.

West, W. Robert and Ansberry, Merle: *The Rehabilitation of Speech,* 4th ed. New York, Harper and Row, 1968.

Wyllie, J.: *The Disorders of Speech*. Edinborough, Oliver and Boyd, 1894.

CHAPTER VI

TRAINING SPOUSES TO IMPROVE THE FUNCTIONAL SPEECH OF APHASIC PATIENTS

Robert Goodkin, Leonard Diller and Nandini Shah

I. INTRODUCTION

APHASIA IS A PROBLEM central to rehabilitation. Although much work has been done in this area, there has been little agreement on ways of measuring specific aphasic deficits. There has been still less agreement on means of treatment. The goals of treatment and whether it works are still matters of speculation. In this study we attempt to develop a way to advance toward these goals. Standard speech therapy generally focuses on improving linguistic components of an asphasic's speech. This study aimed to improve the patient's talking behavior and train the patient's spouse to be an effective trainer of her husband's interpersonal talking behavior.

Although behavior modification has been applied in many different clinical situations, little work has been done in the area of effecting changes in the talking behavior of aphasics.

The purposes of this study were to: 1) apply a system for categorizing the functional talking behavior of aphasic patients and the responses of their wives in a controlled situation; 2) apply a measure for evaluating verbal interactions between aphasic patients and their wives in a naturalistic home setting; 3) determine if a spouse's proficiency as a trainer is related to several personal characteristics; and 4) apply a technology for teaching spouses of aphasics (or their surrogates) to train patients to improve their functional speech.

The first problem to be overcome in the controlled application of operant techniques is how to classify responses so that the behavior being observed can be quantified and the effectiveness of the intervention can be assessed. Ferster and Skinner (1957) and Skinner (1957) have indicated that responses may be classified if the operational nature of the responses are defined *a priori*. Alterations in the frequency of occurrence of each behavior may then be determined. Greenspoon (1956) was the first to apply specific response classes to quantify the effect which reinforcement had on verbal behavior. The literature on verbal conditioning was reviewed by Salzinger (1959), Krasner (1958) and Greenspoon (1961). Catania (1965) has discussed the techniques and application of simultaneous measurement of concurrent response classes. In the present study, concurrent response classes of aphasics and their spouses are recorded while a variety of verbal conditioning procedures are being employed.

There has been previous research involving the use of behavioral procedures in training individuals with language difficulties (Goldiamond, 1965; Holland, 1968; Kerr and Meyerson, 1965). Again specific response classes were used to indicate the gain which occurs in several dimensions of verbal behavior. These changes in verbal output were the result of various treatment procedures which involve verbal and token reinforcement and punishment.

The technique of eliciting speech in aphasics by asking open-ended questions was used in previous research by Vignolo (1964).

The means of altering the verbal behavior of the subjects in this study have been selected from the many procedures appearing in the operant conditioning (Honig, 1965) and behavior modification (Ullmann and Krasner, 1965) literature. The methods employed include the following: 1) positive and negative feedback (Lindsley, 1963; Ullmann and Krasner, 1965; Sidman, 1961); 2) token reinforcement and punishment (Staats, 1964); 3) additional questions and structuring of stimuli (Goldiamond, 1966; Terrace, 1965); 4) modeling (Bandura, 1965); 5) fading (Terrace, 1965); 6) filling in (Taylor, 1958; Goodkin, 1966). Holland (1968) has utilized programmed instruction in working with aphasics.

Mowrer (1970) has discussed the question of measurement in speech therapy. He indicated the importance of empirically identifying independent variables that produce changes in speech, and the value of specifying the effects of these variables on such performance variables as rate and ratio of particular responses. In this study the frequency of responses in key categories are concurrently evaluated in aphasics and their spouses. This enables one to quantify simultaneously several independent variables and the effects of these treatment variables on specific parameters of speech.

The response classes employed to classify the speech of the aphasics used in this study were selected on the basis of the observation of characteristic errors which aphasics make when speaking (Goldstein, 1958; Granick, 1947; Head, 1926; Schuell, 1964; Travis, 1931; Wepman, 1953; Jones and Wepman, 1961). There are many schemes for classifying the language disturbance in aphasics. However, in order to delineate the response classes to be modified some of these schemes are not relevant because they are designed to classify responses to specific test stimuli rather than to extended samples of talking in an interpersonal situation (Goodglass, Quadfassel, and Timberlake, 1964). The work of Halpern (1965) and Tikofsky (1962) on perseveration errors appear to be particularly appropriate for this type of study.

In order to classify speech in a way that would best fit our research aims, several pilot studies were undertaken. Prior to the onset of the present study, the basic procedure in dealing with the initial pilot subjects (Goodkin, 1966A; 1966B) was to employ two response classes: 1) clear words and phrases, and 2) unclear and perseverative utterances. Following the structure of a functional research design, after baserates were taken, various treatment procedures were introduced and their effects were assessed. Once it became clear that words and phrases could be increased and unclear and perseverative utterances decreased using this approach, other classical aphasic deficits were studied (Goodkin, 1969). The new target response categories included increasing frequency of sentences, length of utterances, relevant utterances, and self-corrections; and decreasing dysfluencies; irrelevant and self-critical utterances.

In the early stages of the present study, concurrent measures were taken (Goodkin, 1968) of sentences, words and phrases, unclear utterances, dysfluencies, perseverations, relevant responses and self-corrections. The aphasic subjects' responses to a variety of questions were recorded on tape and these tapes were scored independently by two raters. The raters counted the frequency of responses in each response category. Correlation coefficients of .95 were obtained between raters. This suggested considerable reliability in scoring. Several response classes were then studied and trained simultaneously.

II. METHOD

A. Population

Twenty-three aphasic patients and their spouses or spouse-surrogates were the subjects of this study. Seventeen aphasic-spouse pairs comprised the experimental group and 6 pairs made up the control group. In addition to subjects drawn from the patient population at the Institute of Rehabilitation Medicine, because of the difficulty in obtaining a sufficient number of subjects, several subjects were obtained from other institutions. Seven aphasic-spouse pairs were from the Kessler Institute of Rehabilitation, three pairs from the DeWitt Nursing Home, and one pair from the Burke Rehabilitation Foundation. The basic demographic data on the subjects is presented in Table VI.I.

Difficulties in obtaining subjects were encountered due to the demanding requirement of the experimental design: a) subjects had to be married; b) outpatients who were willing to attend regular sessions for at least a fifteen week period; c) many potential subjects could not participate because they lived too far away from the Institute to attend regular sessions; d) most of these patients were elderly, therefore, many spouses were deceased; e) other patients were too disabled to attend sessions; f) all of the patients must have plateaued in terms of gain in speech therapy as measured by the Functional Communication Profile (Taylor, 1964). Most patients were seen at least two years following the onset of their CVA, a period after which physiological gains are also considered to have plateaued.

For the experimental group, reinforcement and other procedures were contingent on target behaviors; whereas for the control group a comparable amount of reinforcement was randomly

TABLE VI.I

DEMOGRAPHIC DATA ON PATIENTS IN APHASIC-SPOUSE STUDY

Patient No.	*Sex*	*Age*	*Education*
Experimental:			
1	Male	63	Post Graduate
2	Male	64	High School
3	Male	61	High School
4	Male	53	Post Graduate
5	Female	32	College Graduate
6	Male	42	College Graduate
7	Male	69	High School
8	Male	70	College Graduate
9	Male	68	College Graduate
10	Female	66	High School
11	Male	50	College Graduate
12	Male	56	High School
13	Male	75	College Graduate
14*	Male	70	High School
15	Male	47	Some College
16	Female	43	High School
17	Male	44	College Graduate
Control:			
1*	Male	65	High School
2	Male	72	High School
3	Male	53	College Graduate
4	Male	58	High School
5	Female	38	High School
6	Male	66	High School
Discontinued:			
1	Male	53	High-School
2	Male	53	Post Graduate
3	Male	68	High School
4*	Female	47	Some College
5	Male	66	High School
6	Male	40	Post Graduate

* Patient worked with daughter rather than spouse. In each case the spouse was not available during the session.

presented and not contingent on any particular class of behaviors. This type of control allowed us to partial out the effects of any change due to the possibility that the experimenter's interest or spouse's involvement in treatment might be responsible for the gains.

The overall plan consisted of: a) obtaining a full day's sample of talking behavior between a husband and his spouse at home both before and after training; b) obtaining samples of talking behavior in a controlled setting; c) developing a system for analyzing the talking behavior of both aphasic subjects and their spouses; d) obtaining indices of the wife's personal characteristics which might influence her being an effective trainer (Buxbaum, 1967); e) teaching the wife principles and techniques of behavior modification; f) evaluating the effects of techniques introduced during the course of the study.

B. Measures Used

1. *Naturalistic speech.* A home tape recording, triggered off only when the patient or someone in the same room was speaking. This apparatus stops recording after a five second interval of silence. This device was specially designed after techniques of Suskin and John (1963), and has yielded running accounts of talking for periods up to twelve hours. The apparatus consists of a wireless transmitter which is about the size of a package of cigarettes and can be comfortably worn in the patient's shirt pocket. These samples of talking were obtained before and after treatment, and were analyzed according to the response categories listed in another part of this section.

2. *Samples of speech in controlled setting.* In working with aphasics it is often difficult to elicit speech. Vignolo (1964) found that asking open-ended questions facilitated their talking. Each spouse asked the patient to answer each of the following ten questions for two minutes (Vignolo, 1964; Goodkin, 1966):

a. What are some of the things you see in this room?
b. Name and describe the clothes you are wearing.
c. Describe some of the classes that patients have at the Institute.
d. What kinds of things do you do outside of your classes?
e. Tell me about your home and neighborhood.
f. Tell me about some of the people in your family.
g. Name as many animals as you can.
h. Name as many cities and towns as you can.
i. Tell me a little about New York City.
j. Tell me about the kind of work you did.

This part of the study took place at the Institute of Rehabilita-

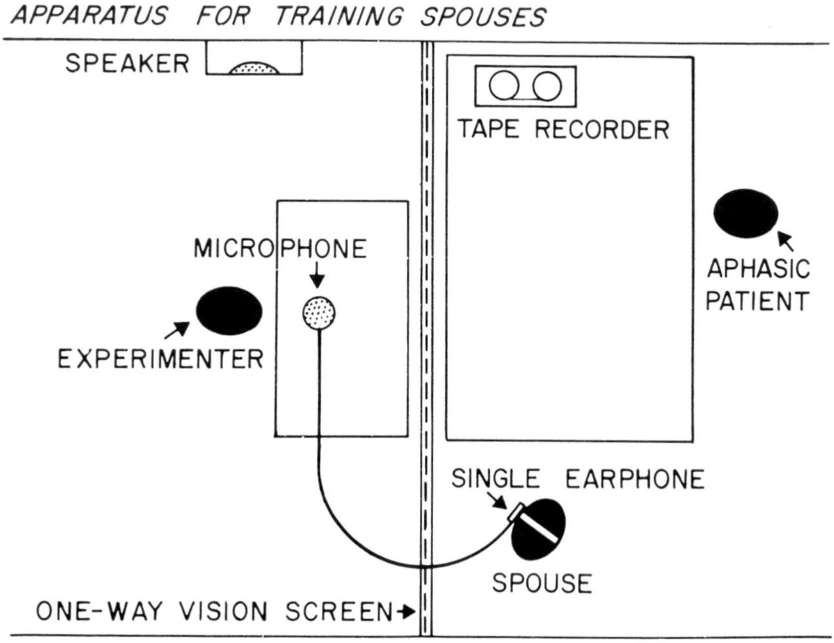

Figure VI.1

tion Medicine, where the experimenter observed through a one-way mirror. All verbal interactions were recorded on tape. The spouse wore a single earphone so that she was able to hear the experimenter but the patient could not (Figure VI.1).

3. *Scoring system.*
   A. *Patient categories*
      1. *Sentence*—Each group of words containing all of the grammatical elements of a sentence, even if minor grammatical errors, such as wrong verb tense or omission of a preposition, are made. Sentences containing perseveration are also scored in this category.
      2. *Words and phrases*—Words and phrases emitted that are not in the context of a sentence.
      3. *Unclear*—Utterances which are not understood as recognizable words.
      4. *Dysfluency*—When the beginning of a word is drawn

also repetition & blockage.

out (e.g., sssstore) or sounds such as *uhh* occur between words.

5. *Perseveration*—Any word or words repeated that do not express new material in response to a question (e.g., "a *bookcase* over here, a *bookcase* up there, a *bookcase* down there.").
6. *Direct answer*—Any word or words emitted which specifically relate to the questions asked.
7. *Self-correction*—Any response in which the patient states that what he has just said was in error, or in which he begins his utterances again and revises it.

B. *Spouse categories*

1. *Positive Feedback*—Words that objectively or subjectively convey that the patient's response was clear or correct (e.g., "That's right," "Correct," "Mm-hmm," "Very good.")
2. *Negative Feedback*— (objective)—Task-oriented negative feedback (e.g., "I didn't understand that," "You have already said that," "That was not a sentence.").
3. *Negative Feedback*— (subjective)—Person-oriented negative feedback (e.g., "Is that all you can say about it?" "No good," "You should do better than that.").
4. *Additional Questions*—Questions asked during the two minute response period after the initial stimulus question was asked.
5. *Modeling*—Examples of appropriate answers that might be given in response to a question.
6. *Starts Word*—Filling in the first letter or syllable of a word the patient is apparently searching for and allowing time for him to state the whole word.
7. *Supplies Word*— (immediately)—Filling in a word the patient is apparently searching for within five seconds after the patient uttered his last word.
8. *Supplies Word*— (after waiting)—Filling in a word the patient is apparently searching for after waiting more than five seconds after the patient uttered his last word.

This scoring system has proven highly reliable. Two raters independently scoring patient and spouse responses showed Pearson r's of .95 or better in each session scored (Goodkin, 1968).

4. *Functional Communication Profiles.* This scale designed by Taylor (1964), is a widely used instrument to assess the functional speech of aphasics. Results are reported as percentages of the patient's current speech in relation to his functional speech prior to his aphasia. Qualified speech therapists administered this test prior to speech therapy, following speech therapy, and following the experimental treatment. Spouses completed this form prior to the experimental treatment.

5. *Katz' adaptation of the Edwards Personal Preference Schedule.* This scale was completed by each spouse prior to the onset of the experimental treatment. One measure yielded by this scale is a nurturance score. In an associated study (Buxbaum, 1967) it was found that wives who were more nurturant rated their husbands as less severely aphasic than speech therapists. This finding suggests that less nurturant wives are less critical of their husbands. It raised the question posed for study: Will a nurturant wife make a more effective trainer than a nonnurturant wife? It also permits validation of the concept of nurturance defined by a paper and pencil inventory with the kind of criticism which the wife shows in an actual verbal interaction.

C. Procedure

Baserates were regarded as three consecutive sessions in which neither the responses of the patient nor those of the spouse deviated by more than five in any category for three consecutive sessions. The baserate material was used to select the categories to be modified in the study. The categories of talking behavior to be modified for both patient and spouse were determined from these baserates and were also based on the speech therapists' recommendations and clinical judgment.

1. *Training sessions with spouse alone.* After baserates had been obtained, each spouse was given a brief individual course on principles and techniques of behavior modification. These principles were related to how she was responding to the patient and how she might respond differently to improve the patient's speech. Such

topics as shaping, reinforcement, punishment, extinction, modeling and fading were discussed. Tapes of baserate sessions were reviewed with the spouse, relating the principles to how she was responding to the patient and what she might do differently in her effort to improve the patient's speech. Goals were discussed with the spouse both in terms of the target response categories to be increased and decreased in the patient, and the target categories to be modified in the spouse.

2. *Shaping the spouse's response.* This training involved both patient and spouse, utilizing the observation room. The same apparatus was used that was employed in obtaining baserates and various sets of stimulus questions were asked by the spouse and answered by the patient for the same period of time. The experimenter then gave feedback and suggestions to the spouse as to how she was responding with regard to the goals set for her and the patient. For example, if the goal was to have the spouse give more positive feedback, she was reinforced for reinforcing specified target responses. It was also suggested that she reinforce target responses more frequently after she had let some go by unnoticed.

Prior to the onset of this study, working individually with aphasic subjects, many variations of verbal operant conditioning procedures were employed (Goodkin, 1966). The procedures that were found to be most effective in producing favorable changes in speech during this pilot research period were taught to the spouse by instructing her in their use and by verbally reinforcing when she used them appropriately. These procedures include the following: (1) verbal reinforcement (complimenting a response, repeating a response, stating when a response was correct). The reinforcement to be employed was determined on the basis of its empirical effect on the patient's target behaviors; (2) tokens (using blue tokens in addition to verbal (social) reinforcement and red tokens in addition to verbal punishment to provide more tangible consequences for low level patients); (3) modeling (the spouse gave examples of good responses and reinforced her own responses); (4) self-reinforcement and self-punishment (after allowing the patient to take a blue token following responses he judged to be correct or a red token after responses he judged to be incorrect, the spouse took the appropriate token to indicate to the patient whether his self-judgment was correct or incorrect). This was one of the most effective procedures in eliminating errors; (5) patient reinforces spouse (the spouse intentionally gives appropriate and inappropriate responses, depending upon the patient's specific errors, and the patient verbally reinforces).

Each treatment in this phase of the study was continued until the responses of each patient and spouse category stabilized (i.e., did not deviate by more than five responses for each of three consecutive sessions).

After a minimum of fifteen sessions, new baserates were obtained in the laboratory and home settings, and these data were then compared with the pre-training baserate data. Pre- and post-experimental treatment Functional Communication Profiles were administered by qualified speech therapists in order that changes in the patient's functional speech could be assessed by an outside, widely used criterion measure. Prior to the experimental sessions, spouses completed: 1) Functional Communication Profile forms, and 2) Katz' adaptation of Edwards Personal Preference Schedules. A deviation score was obtained between spouses' FCP's and Speech Therapists' FCP's, to assess the degree to which spouses over-estimated or under-estimated their husbands' functional speech (e.g., if speech therapists' FCP score was 60% and spouses' FCP score was 68%, the deviation score was +8). These scores and the nurturance scores derived from the Katz adaptation of the Edwards schedule, were obtained to determine whether spouses who were good trainers could be differentiated from spouses who were poor trainers. These two measures were obtained from spouses in less than one hour.

In addition to the general data collection of responses resulting from the standardized procedures, each aphasic-spouse pair was also regarded as an individual case study. Several individualized specific procedures (independent variables) were employed to determine their effects on modifying target responses in the desired direction. In addition to presenting the general group findings in the results section, the individualized procedures used with five representative aphasic-spouse pairs and outcome data is presented as a series of case studies.

The questions discussed and the duration of the response periods remained consistent during baserate sessions. Methods of eliciting speech and the selected topics to be discussed during treatment sessions were individually determined. The topics, frequency of changing topics, and the treatment methods employed depended upon the level of the subjects' functional speech and the subjects' interests.

While treating patients at a low functional level (FCP below 40%), two or three series of questions were employed for many sessions. These subjects did not indicate any objection to the repeated use of the same content.

While treating patients at a higher functional level (FCP above 40%), topics were changed more frequently and the topics were drawn from the patient's general and daily interests. Focus was on: (1) the aphasic's specific deficit (e.g., building clear words and phrases or sentences, decreasing unclear or perseverative utterances); and (2) the content of the patient's speech. The spouse and the experimenter attempted to be responsive to both.

Several patients brought their own topics to be discussed during the sessions (in the form of outlines, letters, essays, etc.). Role playing was employed with several patients who wanted to develop specific skills (e.g., talking on the phone to clients; giving a cab driver directions or an address; ordering lunch in a restaurant). Some patients read a newspaper article and discussed it. Some patients, who were unable to read, listened to recorded articles from the *Reader's Digest* magazine (on records produced for the blind) and discussed them. With several patients, ongoing daily problems (e.g., feeling legs were getting worse, boredom at home, son being called into military service) supplied the subject matter for sessions.

In addition to the general treatment procedures described above, several individualized procedures were employed. An additional dependent variable employed with several aphasic subjects pertained to building awareness of the adequacy of their responses. For example, if the target category was to build clear words and phrases, after each utterance the patient indicated whether his response was clear or unclear. Then, contingent upon this self-judgment, the spouse verbally reinforced or punished. The aim of this procedure was to build the aphasic's awareness of his speech, thereby increasing his ability to monitor his responses.

A second procedure called for magnification of the stimuli presented and of the aphasic's own voice by means of an amplifier and a set of headphones. Gradually the cue of loudness was faded out until the headphones were no longer used. This procedure was employed with subjects who had particular difficulty in the area of repeating specific sounds.

A third procedure used with twelve subjects involved showing the patient and spouse their verbal behavior with one another by playing portions of their taped sessions back. In addition to hearing themselves and the effects of their interactions on one another, specific responses were commented upon and reinforced by the experimenter.

With several subjects, the experimenter modeled treatment sessions while the spouse observed the effects of the experimenter's procedures by means of a one-way vision screen (e.g., spouse observed the effects of allowing considerable time for the aphasic to respond before filling in a word, contingent reinforcement, cuing).

Wolpe's (1970) desensitization procedure, a means of training relaxation by classical conditioning procedures, was employed with three subjects who were functioning at a relatively high functional level. In this procedure, situations which produce high anxiety levels, and as a result interfere with the subject's speech, are repeatedly paired with induced relaxation in an effort to decrease anxiety in these situations. In order for subjects to profit from this procedure, it is necessary that they be able to follow simple verbal instructions and visualize themselves in various settings.

Fading, or errorless-learning, was employed in several ways. With some subjects, at a low functional level, visual presentation of the objects they were naming were introduced (e.g., items around the room, clothes). Then, the presentation of the visual cues were faded out, and the subjects were asked to name the items. Another approach concerned the fading of auditory cues. In these cases, the spouse modeled whole words during several (four or five) sessions and the patient repeated the words. Then, during the next four or five sessions the spouse gave the sound of the first syllable or letter of the word, and the patient stated the whole word. Finally, the spouse simply asked a general question concerning the practiced words with no auditory cues (e.g., "Name the items in the room." "Tell me about the clothes you are wearing.").

III. RESULTS

The results are presented in two ways. First, the general effects on the seventeen subjects in the Experimental Group and the six Control subjects are presented. Then, five representative aphasic-spouse pairs are discussed in the form of case studies.

Tables VI.II and VI.III summarize the basic data obtained in this study. Table VI.II indicates the speech therapist's clinical diagnosis of the speech disorder following speech therapy and shows the spouse's nurturance score and the Functional Communication Profile (FCP) scores obtained. FCP scores obtained from the spouse and changes produced in FCP scores following speech therapy and following the experimental procedures are shown in this table. Table VI.III indicates changes produced in target behaviors of patients and spouses in the laboratory and at home. Both frequency of occurrence and percentage of target responses (percent of total output in all response categories) are shown.

Table VI.IV is a summary of mean changes produced in patient and spouse target behaviors in the laboratory and at home. The number of subjects involved in each target category is indicated. Total Target refers to every target behavior of all subjects in the given group. Whereas some subjects had only one specified target behavior, others had two or three targets. Average changes in frequency and average percentage changes in target responses are indicated for experimental and control subjects. While the mean change in experimental patient target behavior was 14.9% in the laboratory, control patients changed -4.4%. At home experimental patients changed 12.5% and control patients changed 5.4%. Spouses in the experimental group made mean target changes of 11.6% in the laboratory and control spouses made mean changes of -3.01%. At home, experimental spouses made mean target changes of 3.0%, and control spouses made average changes of -2.4%. Because of the great differences existing

TABLE VI.II

DIAGNOSIS, FCP, AND NURTURANCE DATA

Patient No.	*Diagnosis R=Receptive E=Expressive*	*FCP1 Speech Therapy Pre-Sp. Ther.*	*FCP2 Speech Therapy Post-Sp. Ther.*	*FCP3 Speech Therapy Post-Ex. Trea*	*FCP4 Spouse Post-Sp. Ther.*	*Nurturance Score*
Experimental Subjects:						
1	R:Mod E:Sev	13.5	15.5	28.6	37.1	16
2	R:Mod E:Sev	50.8	54.0	59.1	46.8	11
3	R.Mod E:Sev	33.2	44.2	53.6	25.3	12
4	R:Mil E:Mil	76.2	76.2	79.8	96.3	10
5	R:Mil E:Mod	60.1	63.2	68.5	95.2	14
6	R:Mil E:Mod	34.1	43.6	68.7	75.2	15
7	R:Sev E:Sev	10.8	20.7	25.5	68.4	09
8	R:Mod E:Sev	52.1	65.0	81.3	77.1	14
9	R:Mod E:Sev	45.1	48.1	55.0	54.0	08
10	R:Sev E:Sev	43.6	42.5	37.0	70.3	13
11	R:Mil E:Sev	49.5	65.8	80.6	70.8	12
12	R:Mil E:Mod	63.2	64.7	81.3	97.3	15
13	R:Mod E.Mod	38.0	38.2	54.1	59.0	15
14	R:Sev E:Sev	—	—	—	58.5	12
15	R:Mod E:Mod	—	50.7	52.4	55.0	13
16	R:Mil E:Mod	—	65.8	70.0	78.0	14
17	R:Mil E:Mod	43.7	63.5	77:2	71.8	07
Control Subjects:						
1	R:Mod E:Sev	—	21.6	45.2	43.8	—
2	R:Sev E:Sev	—	21.5	20.0	67.2	15
3	R:Mod E:Sev	—	35.4	36.7	49.3	16
4	R:Mod E:Mod	—	52.3	52.8	55.7	16
5	R:Mod E:Mod	—	63.8	63.0	79.2	08
6	R:Mod E:Sev	—	34.7	35.2	39.4	04
Discontinued Subjects:						
1	R:Mod E:Sev	22.8	23.0	—	34.4	09
2	R:Mil E:Mil	57.0	59.3	—	96.3	12
3	R:Mod E:Sev	27.0	36.8	—	—	—
4	R:Mil E:Mil	41.1	76.9	—	90.6	14
5	R:Sev E:Sev	5.4	13.0	—	53.8	11
6	R:Mod E:Mod	—	45.6	—	71.3	13

TABLE VI.III

CHANGES IN TARGET BEHAVIORS OF PATIENTS AND SPOUSES (FREQUENCY AND PERCENTAGE)

Pat. No.	Target Behaviors—Patient	IRM Pre	IRM Pre %	IRM Post	IRM Post %		HOME Pre	HOME Pre %	HOME Post	HOME Post %	Target Behaviors—Spouses	IRM Pre	IRM Pre %	IRM Post	IRM Post %		HOME Pre	HOME Pre %	HOME Post	HOME Post %
Experimental:																				
1	S+	04	05	25	35	S+	06	55	12	67	P-N+	02	07	08	15	P-N+	01	09	03	27
	U–	42	51	00	00	U–	00	00	00	00	M+	02	07	07	13	M+	00	00	00	00
2	W & P+	55	46	100	5[illegible]	W & P+	10	44	14	58	P-N+	29	18	45	19	P-N+	10	40	13	52
											M+	37	23	101	44	M+	04	16	05	20
											R+	164	—	228	—	R+	25	—	25	—
3	S+	00	00	10	07	S+	00	00	04	20	P-N+	16	18	36	20	P-N+	05	29	09	29
	W & P+	44	94	127	9[illegible]	W & P+	06	75	15	75	M+	22	25	34	18	M+	05	28	08	26
											AQ+	40	45	99	54	AQ+	07	39	14	45
4	S+	43	38	32	27	S+	05	33	07	47	P-N+	03	25	07	77	P-N+	02	50	04	44
	P–	18	16	06	03	P–	04	27	02	13	R+	12	—	09	—	R+	04	—	09	—
5	S+	16	21	26	28	S+	03	27	05	33	P-N+	02	05	04	09	P-N+	01	14	03	27
											M+	02	05	03	07	M+	01	14	02	18
6	S+	40	43	47	53	S+	05	24	10	40	M+	02	04	01	02	M+	00	00	02	11
											R+	45	—	46	—	R+	10	—	18	—
7	W & P+	65	35	94	62	W & P+	09	56	15	88	M+	43	14	67	34	M+	00	00	05	36
	U–	117	63	53	35	U–	07	44	02	12	R–	308	—	193	—	R–	20	—	14	—
8	S+	105	44	102	83	S+	24	62	40	75	P-N+	35	67	59	77	P-N+	06	60	07	15
											R+	52	—	76	—	R+	10	—	46	—
9	S+	21	31	50	33	S+	05	33	09	36	P-N+	46	35	90	52	P-N+	14	44	20	61
	W & P+	26	39	64	42	W & P+	06	40	11	44	M+	15	11	29	17	M+	02	06	04	12
	DA+	37	56	105	70	DA+	—	—	—	—	NS–	17	13	05	03	NS–	05	16	01	03
10	S+	66	39	88	47	S+	32	74	35	51	M+	24	11	35	14	M+	05	08	07	14
	DA+	115	68	169	9[illegible]	DA+	—	—	—	—	AQ+	72	33	82	34	AQ+	37	62	28	56
11	S+	30	17	41	31	S+	07	27	14	44	P-N+	25	22	94	64	P-N+	09	69	17	50
	U–	32	18	17	13	U–	05	19	06	19										
12	S+	58	44	76	54	S+	13	50	20	91	R+	00	—	04	—	R+	03	—	10	—

TABLE VI.III—*Continued*

	Target Behaviors—Patient										*Target Behaviors—Spouses*								
		IRM					*HOME*					*IRM*					*HOME*			
Pat. No.		*Pre*	*Pre %*	*Post*	*Post %*		*Pre*	*Pre %*	*Post*	*Post %*		*Pre*	*Pre %*	*Post*	*Post %*		*Pre*	*Pre %*	*Post*	*Post %*
13	S+	23	23	67	50	S+	22	88	22	73	P-N+	29	20	34	26	P-N+	06	23	02	05
											M–	78	54	17	13	M–	03	12	05	13
14	W & P+	32	54	62	70	W & P+	06	67	14	100	P-N+	07	08	53	29	P-N+	00	00	12	26
	U–	25	42	26	30	U–	03	33	00	00	M–	69	81	69	38	M–	05	18	07	15
15	S+	04	04	25	28	S+	07	32	09	56	P-N+	09	11	15	14	P-N+	02	07	03	11
	U–	19	20	04	04	U–	05	23	02	13	AQ–	62	73	86	78	AQ–	27	93	24	89
16	S+	26	27	39	45	S+	15	60	22	69	AQ–	84	59	64	59	AQ–	38	93	33	87
											R–	143	—	109	—	R–	41	—	38	—
17	S+	55	46	73	54	S+	22	92	24	89	P-N+	00	00	03	12	P-N+	00	00	00	00
											AQ+	12	100	22	88	AQ+	07	100	19	100
											R+	12	—	25	—	R+	07	—	19	—
Control:																				
1	S+	17	30	09	15	S+	06	40	00	00	AQ–	112	81	163	64	AQ–	29	76	30	83
	W & P+	35	62	51	85	W & P+	09	60	08	100										
2	W & P+	13	37	23	64	W & P+	07	78	06	67	P-N+	04	04	11	11	P-N+	02	07	00	00
	U–	21	60	13	36	U–	02	22	03	33	M+	04	04	05	05	M+	00	00	01	04
3	W & P+	28	31	28	29	W & P+	08	21	24	55	P-N+	00	00	00	00	P-N+	00	00	00	00
	U–	61	69	70	71	U–	31	79	10	45	M+	17	28	20	41	M+	00	00	00	00
											R+	60	—	49	—	R+	38	—	40	—
4	W & P+	42	74	44	77	W & P+	22	100	29	100	P-N+	19	16	21	16	P-N+	00	00	01	02
	U–	15	24	13	23	U–	00	00	00	00	AQ–	85	70	87	68	AQ–	42	91	45	85
5	DA+	68	36	27	23	DA+	—	—	—	—	P-N+	35	25	09	12	P-N+	01	02	05	11
											AQ–	92	65	56	75	AQ–	36	84	35	74
6	W & P+	25	24	27	25	W & P+	05	17	06	21	P-N+	22	27	21	26	P-N+	03	12	02	08
	U–	81	76	79	75	U–	24	83	22	79	M+	26	31	22	28	M+	01	04	01	04

Patient Categories:
S—Sentence
U—Unclear
W & P—Words and Phrases
DA—Direct Answers
P—Perseverations

Spouse Categories:
P-N—Positive and Negative Feedback
M—Modeling
AQ—Additional Questions
NS—Negative Subjective
R—Total Responses

+ = Goal is to increase target behavior
– = Goal is to decrease target behavior

TABLE VI.IV
AVERAGE CHANGES PRODUCED IN PATIENT AND SPOUSE TARGET BEHAVIORS

		Experimental					*Control*			
		IRM		*Home*			*IRM*		*Home*	
N	*Patients*	*Freq.*	*%*	*Freq.*	*%*	*N*	*Freq.*	*%*	*Freq.*	*%*
17	Total Target	20.8	14.9	4.6	12.5	6	− 0.8	− 4.4	2.8	5.4
14	Sentences	15.4	13.8	4.8	10.0	1	− 8.0	−15.0	−6.0	−40.0
5	Words & Phrases	3.4	9.6	4.1	16.6	5	6.0	10.4	4.4	13.4
5	Unclear	27.0	22.4	2.0	15.0	4	0.8	6.0	5.5	6.8
2	Direct Answ.	61.0	18.0	—	—	1	41	−13.0	—	—
1	Perseverat.	12.0	13.0	2.0	14.0	0	—	—	—	—
	Spouses									
17	Total Target	17.5	11.6	3.1	3.0	6	−10.8	− 3.0	−1.8	− 2.3
12	Positive and Negative	18.4	14.8	3.0	0.3	5	− 4.4	− 1.4	0.4	− 3.6
10	Modeling	18.5	13.3	1.2	6.7	3	0.0	3.7	0.3	1.3
5	Additional Questions	15.0	0.6	6.0	0.4	3	−29.7	9.7	−1.7	3.7
1	Negative Subjective	12.0	10.0	4.0	13.0	0	—	—	—	—

among subjects in level of verbal functioning and specific deficits, there was considerable variability in frequency and percentage changes among subjects. Although the mean figures aid in assessing general effects, each subject's performance must be viewed individually if one is to gain a more accurate view of change in verbal behavior.

A. General Effects

1. *Changes in verbal output, Functional Communication Profile and percentage of target behaviors.* Table VI.V compares the amount of change in verbal output, Functional Communication scores, and average percentage change in target behaviors in experimental and control group subjects. Median scores are reported because of the wide variability in verbal abilities among subjects and because the number of subjects in several groups was small. Verbal output scores of patients are the total frequency of clear sentences, words, and phrases emitted by subjects during the response periods. Unclear, dysfluent, and perseverative responses are not included in these scores. Average percentage change in target behaviors was obtained by: (1) calculating the percentage of responses in each target category out of the total frequency of emitted responses during pre-treatment baserates and post-treat-

TABLE VI.V

CHANGES IN OUTPUT, FCP AND AVERAGE TARGET IN EXPERIMENTAL AND CONTROL SUBJECTS

N	*Patients*	*IRM Pre Output*	*IRM Post Output*	*Home Pre Output*	*Home Post Output*	*Pre FCP*	*Post FCP*	*Average % Change in Target (IRM)*	*Average % Change in Target (Home)*
17	Experimental—Total Group								
	Median	80	114	15	20	52.4	63.8	10.0	9.0
	Range	164	122	36	54	60.7	55.8	39.5	26.0
6	Experimental—Highest Output Group								
	Median	129	116.5	19.5	26	64.9	80.2	9.8	10.8
	Range	86	76	28	33	33.7	44.3	38	64
6	Experimental—Lowest Output Group								
	Median	45.5	106.5	10	17	44.2	53.6	10.1	12
	Range	37	75	5	6	38.5	33.6	38.5	29.5
6	Control—Total Group								
	Median	35	36	11.5	16	35.1	41.0	1.5	2
	Range	172	96	43	32	42.3	43.0	38.5	45
N	*Spouses*								
16	Experimental—Total Group								
	Median	85	110	18	27	—	—	8.5	3.8
	Range	308	238	57	41	—	—	54	81
6	Control—Total Group								
	Median	107.5	90.5	38	38	—	—	2.5	1.8
	Range	82	167	20	28	—	—	19	13.5

ment baserates, (2) obtaining the change in percentage of each target after treatment, and (3) calculating the mean of these percentage changes for each subject. Percentage changes were used rather than frequency changes in order to have a common basis for comparison between categories which varied widely in response frequency.

a. Total experimental group vs. control group (patients). In comparing all seventeen experimental group subjects with the six control subjects, the experimental subjects' median output increased from eighty to 114 responses in the laboratory and from fifteen to twenty responses at home. Control subject output went from thirty-five responses during pre-treatment baserates at IRM to thirty-six during post-treatment baserates; at home control subject output increased from 11.5 to sixteen. Experimental group FCP's went from 52.4 to 63.8, whereas control FCP's went from 35.1 to 41.0. Average percentage changes in target behaviors of experimental group subjects was 10% in the laboratory and 9% at home; control subjects changed 1.5% in the laboratory and 2% at home.

b. Low output experimental group vs. control group (patients). In viewing pre-treatment output and FCP scores one sees that many experimental group subjects started at a higher functional level than the control subjects. To assess the possibility that gain was a function of the patient's verbal level prior to treatment, the six lowest output experimental subjects were compared with the control subjects. Whereas experimental subjects with the lowest output increased from a median output of 15.5 to 106.5 responses in the laboratory, control subjects went from thirty-five to thirty-six responses. At home, the low group went from ten to seventeen responses, while the control subjects went from 11.5 to sixteen responses. Whereas the low experimental subjects' median FCP increased from 44.2 to 53.6, the control FCP median went from 35.1 to 41.0. The average target percentage change was 10.1% for the low experimental group and 1.5% for the control subjects in the laboratory, and 12% for the low group versus 2% for the control group at home. Whereas every subject in the low output experimental group increased output by at least twenty-eight responses, one subject increasing by ninety-three responses, only one control subject increased output by as many as nine responses. While every low experimental group subject improved by at least 4.8 points on the Functional Communication Profile, only one subject in the control group increased more than 1.3 points on this measure.

c. High output experimental group vs. low output group (patients). In comparing the six highest output patients with the six lowest patients, one must take into account the fact that many of the higher level patients made qualitative gains that are not immediately apparent in viewing the numerical data. The major qualitative change was an increase in sentence output. Since the data consists of frequencies in each response category, one sentence or one word each counts as one response. In the highest output group all subjects increased sentence output, and therefore while their total number of spoken words increased, counting each sentence as one response suggests a decrease in total output responses at IRM. In the laboratory, the low output subjects increased from a median output of 45.5 prior to treatment to 106.5 following treatment; high output patients went from a median of 129 responses to 116.5 responses. At home, both high and low output subjects increased output frequency. Low output subjects increased from ten to seventeen responses during five minute random samples at home; high output subjects went from 19.5 to twenty-six responses. The FCP's of both high and low output subjects improved following the experimental procedures. The median FCP or the low output group went from 44.2 prior to treatment to 53.6 following treatment; the high output subjects made a greater median FCP gain, from 64.9 to 80.2. The median percentage change in target behavior of low output subjects was 10.1% in the laboratory and 12% at home; the median change of high output subjects was 9.8% in the laboratory and 10.8% at home. The data indicates that both the highest and lowest output subjects' functional speech improved following the experimental procedures. Since only two aphasic patients in the Experimental Group had FCP scores of less than 40%, and only one was seen with an FCP over 70%, it is not clear whether the described procedures would be effective with patients at very low or very high functional levels.

d. Experimental group vs. control group (spouses). The output scores of spouses include the total of all verbal responses in all categories. The median verbal output of the seventeen spouses in the experimental group was eighty-five responses in the laboratory and eighteen at home prior to training. Following treatment the median verbal output for this group was 110 in the laboratory and twenty-seven at home. The pretreatment median output of spouses in the control group was 107.5 in the laboratory and thirty-eight at home. Following treatment, the median output for this group was 90.5 in the laboratory and thirty-eight at home. The median of the average percentage change in spouse target behavior was 8.5% in the laboratory and 3.8% at home for experimental subjects. In control subjects the median change was 2.5% in the laboratory and 1.8% at home. The data indicates a greater increase in output for experimental group spouses than control spouses both in the laboratory and at home, and suggests greater change in specified target behavior in experimental subjects.

2. *Change in target behaviors in experimental and control subjects in the laboratory and at home.* Table VI.VI shows significant changes produced in target behavior. Significant changes (.01 level) occurred in patient target behaviors in the laboratory (t=2.45). Changes significant at the .05 level occurred in spouse targets in the laboratory (t=1.89). A Mann-Whitney test indicated

TABLE VI.VI

SIGNIFICANT CHANGES IN TARGET BEHAVIORS FOLLOWING EXPERIMENTAL TREATMENT

	Laboratory	*Home*	*Laboratory vs. Home*
		Experimental Group	
Patient	+‡	+*	0
Spouse	+†	0	+†
Pt. vs. spouse	0	+†	0
		Control Group	
Patient	0	0	0
Spouse	0	0	0
Pt. vs. spouse	0	0	0

* Significant at < .05 level (Mann Whitney test).
† Significant at < .05 level (t test).
‡ Significant at < .01 level (t test).

significant change (z=1.62) in patient target behavior at home following the experimental procedures (.05 level). Although patient changes showed significant generalization to the home, spouse target changes at home were not sufficient to meet the criterion of significance. At home, patients changed more than spouses with regard to target behavior (t=4.11, .05 level). Spouses changed significantly more in the laboratory than at home (2.09, .05 level). Less generalization of training occurred in spouses than in patients.

No significant changes occurred in either patient or spouse target behaviors in the control group. Non-contingent reinforcement was not sufficient to produce significant changes in responding.

Patient target behavior in the laboratory was modified significantly more (.05 level) in the experimental group than in the control group (t=2.18). A Mann-Whitney U test indicated that experimental patient targets were modified significantly more at home, following the experimental procedures, than control target behaviors (.05 level). Significant differences were not obtained between spouses in the experimental and control groups in the laboratory or at home.

Changes produced in patient (Experimental Group) target behaviors at IRM and at home did not differ significantly. A rank order correlation of .58 was obtained between target changes at IRM and at home (.01 level). They improved in both settings. Control patient changes were also not significantly different at IRM and at home. They made slight negative changes in the laboratory and slight positive changes at home. There was little relationship between experimental group spouse changes in the laboratory and at home, and control spouse target changes at IRM showed little correlation with changes at home.

3. *Generalization of effect of treating specific target behaviors on other concurrent response categories.* Table VI.VII indicates increases and decreases in specified patient target behaviors and in other simultaneously recorded response categories. Changes in the desired direction in the laboratory and home are indicated by plus signs (+); undesired changes are indicated by minus signs (−).

Example—The goal (target behavior) for twelve experimental subjects was to increase sentences. In the laboratory, ten of these subjects changed in the desired direction; while two emitted less sentences following the experimental procedures. Although the modification of word and phrase output was not a specified target behavior to be treated, nine of the twelve subjects changed favorably in this response category, two changed in the undesired direction, and one subject remained the same. All five of the twelve subjects in this group who had emitted unclear responses in the initial baserate sessions gave less unclear responses after treatment, even though unclear responses were not directly treated. Sentences, words and phrases, and unclear responses were modified in the desired direction. Of the patients who emitted dysfluency, perseverations, self-corrections and direct answers, however, approximately equivalent numbers increased and decreased in these response categories when *sentences* was the specific target being treated. Table VI.VII also indicates changes in sentences (the target behavior) and the other concurrently recorded categories at home following the experimental procedures (e.g., eleven of the twelve subjects in this group emitted more sentences).

Table VI.VII illustrates changes in all concurrently recorded categories while specific patient targets were being treated. Table VI.VIII shows changes in spouse targets and other concurrently recorded categories, in the same manner. These tables indicate that while both patient and spouse specified target behaviors show most change in the desired direction in the laboratory and at home, several other categories are simultaneously modified in the desired direction.

4. *Comparison of magnitude of target change in patients and spouses.* In the laboratory there was no direct relationship between amount of change in spouses and patients. Spouses who made the greatest positive change did not necessarily produce the greatest change in the patient's speech.

5. *Changes in Functional Communication Profiles (outside criterion).* Functional Communication Profile scores were used as outside criterion measures for assessing changes produced during speech therapy and during the experimental procedures. Whereas the experimental subjects showed a mean gain of 6.5% on the FCP following standard speech therapy, these subjects showed an

TABLE VI.VII

CHANGES IN PATIENT'S TARGET BEHAVIORS AND IN CONCURRENTLY RECORDED RESPONSE CATEGORIES

Experimental: IRM

Goal Sentences

Pat. No.	*1*	*4*	*5*	*6*	*8*	*10*	*11*	*12*	*13*	*15*	*16*	*17*	$\overline{X}$ *Freq. Change*	*N=12*	
S	+21	−11	+10	+07	−03	+22	+11	+18	+44	+21	+13	+18	+14.3	(+10)	(−2)
W&P	+09	−15	−09	+02	+78	00	+41	+16	+07	+10	+22	+05	+13.8	(+ 9)	(−2)
U	+42			+01			+15	+01		+15			+14.8	(+ 5)	
D			+01		+19		−01	−06					+ 3.3	(+ 2)	(−2)
P	−02	+12	−01	+03	+05	+02	−01	−03	−01	+01	+03	−02	+ 1.3	(+ 6)	(−6)
DA	+36	−04	+17	+07	−72	+54	−31	00	−20	+08	−07	−03	− 1.3	(+ 5)	(−6)
SC	+01	00		−07	−13	−05	+02	+02			−01	00	− 2.3	(+ 3)	(−4)

Goal Words and Phrases

Pat. No.	*2*	*7*	*14*	$\overline{X}$ *Freq. Change*	*N=3*	
S	+01	+01	−02	0.0	(+ 2)	(−1)
W&P	+45	+29	+30	+34.7	(+ 3)	
U	−31	+64	−01	+10.7	(+ 1)	(−2)
D						
P	−26	−03	−11	−13.3		(−3)
DA	+16	+21	+16	+17.7	(+ 3)	
SC						

Double Goals

Pat. No.	*3*	*9*	$\overline{X}$ *Freq. Change*	*N=2*	
S	+10	+29	+19.5	(+ 2)	
W&P	+83	+38	+60.5	(+ 2)	
U	+03	−18	− 7.5	(+ 1)	(−1)
D	−03				(−1)
P	−13	+30		(+ 1)	(−1)
DA	+45	+68		(+ 2)	
SC					

Control: IRM

Goal Direct Answers

Pat. No.	*5*	$\overline{X}$ *Freq. Change*	*N=1*	
S	−32	−32.0		(−1)
W&P	+35	+35.0	(+1)	
U				
D	+01	+ 1.0	(+1)	
P				
DA	−41	−41.0		(−1)
SC				

Goal Words and Phrases

Pat. No.	*2*	*3*	*4*	*6*	$\overline{X}$ *Freq. Change*	*N=4*	
S	−01				− 1.0		(−1)
W&P	+10	00	+02	+02	+ 3.5	(+3)	
U	+08	−09	+02	+02	+ 0.8	(+3)	(−1)
D							
P							
DA	+10	+05	+03	+01	+ 4.8	(+4)	
SC							

Double Goals Sentences & Words & Phrases

Pat. No.	*1*	$\overline{X}$ *Freq. Change*	*N=1*	
S	−08	− 8.0		(−1)
W&P	+16	+16.0	(+1)	
U	+04	+ 4.0	(+1)	
D				
P	−03	− 3.0		(−1)
DA	+16	+16.0	(+1)	
SC				

TABLE VI.VII—*Continued*

Experimental: Home

Goal Sentences

Pat. No.	*1*	*4*	*5*	*6*	*8*	*10*	*11*	*12*	*13*	*15*	*16*	*17*	$\overline{X}$ *Freq. Change*		*N=12*
S	+06	+02	+02	+05	+16	+03	+07	+07	00	+02	+07	+02	+ 4.9	(+11)	
W&P	+01	+01	−02	−02	−01	−23	−02	+04	−05	+05	00	−03	− 2.3	(+ 4)	(+7)
U				+02	+04		−01			+03			+ 2.0	(+ 3)	(−1)
D					−01	+01	+04	+07				+02	+ 2.6	(+ 4)	(−1)
P		+02		+01		+01	+01	+01	+01				+ 1.2	(+ 6)	
DA															
SC		−01		−01									− 1.0		(−2)

Goal Words and Phrases

Pat. No.	*2*	*7*	*14*	$\overline{X}$ *Freq. Change*		*N=3*
S	+01			+ 1.0	(+ 1)	
W&P	+04	+06	+08	+ 6.0	(+ 3)	
U	+04	+05	+03	+ 4.0	(+ 3)	
D						
P	+02		−06	− 2.0	(+ 1)	(−1)
DA						
SC						

Double Goals

Pat. No.	*3*	*9*	$\overline{X}$ *Freq. Change*	*N=2*
S	+04	+04	+ 4.0	(+ 2)
W&P	+09	+05	+ 7.0	(– 2)
U	00	00	0.0	
D				
P		+04	+ 4.0	(+ 1)
DA				
SC		+01	+ 1.0	(+ 1)

Control: Home

Goal Words and Phrases

Pat. No.	*2*	*3*	*4*	*6*	$\overline{X}$ *Freq. Change*	*N=4*	
S							
W&P	−01	+16	+07	+01	+ 5.8	(+3)	(−1)
U	−01	+11		+02	+ 4.0	(+2)	(−1)
D							
P							
DA							
SC							

Double Goals Sentences & Words & Phrases

Pat. No.	*1*	$\overline{X}$ *Freq. Change*	*N=1*
S	−06	− 6.0	(−1)
W&P	−01	− 1.0	(−1)
U			
D			
P			
DA			
SC			

Patient Categories:
S—Sentences
W & P—Words and Phrases
U—Unclear

D—Dysfluency
P—Perseverations
DA—Direct Answers
SC—Self Correct

+ = Changes in desired direction
− = Changes in undesired direction
0 = No change in response categories

TABLE VI.VIII

CHANGES IN SPOUSE'S TARGET BEHAVIORS AND IN CONCURRENTLY RECORDED RESPONSE CATEGORIES

Experimental: IRM

Goal Positive and Negative Feedback

Sp. No.	*4*	*8*	*11*	$\overline{X}$ *Freq. Change*	*N=3*	
P	+04	+06	+48	+19.3	(+3)	
N	00	+18	+21	+13.0	(+2)	
NS	+02			+ 2.0	(+1)	
AQ	−05	+03	−37	−13.0	(+1)	(−2)
M		−04	+03	− 0.5	(+1)	(−1)
SW			00	0.0		
FII		−04		− 4.0		(−1)
FIA		−03		− 3.0		(−1)

Goal Additional Questions

Sp. No.	*16*	$\overline{X}$ *Freq. Change*	*N=1*	
P	−08	− 8.0		(−1)
N	−03	− 3.0		(−1)
NS				
AQ	+20	+20.0	(+1)	
M	−05	− 5.0		(−1)
SW	+02	+ 2.0	(+1)	
FII				
FIA				

Goal Modeling

Sp. No.	*6*	*7*	$\overline{X}$ *Freq. Change*	*N=2*	
P	+01	+37	+19.0	(+2)	
N	+01	+04	+ 2.5	(+2)	
NS		−01	− 1.0		(−1)
AQ	−01	+97	+48.0	(+1)	(−1)
M	−01	+24	+11.5	(+1)	(−1)
SW	+01	00	+ 1.0	(+1)	
FII			0.0		
FIA					

Control: IRM

Goal Additional Questions

Sp. No.	*1*	$\overline{X}$ *Freq. Change*	*N=1*	
P	+20	+20.0	(+1)	
N	+02	+ 2.0	(+1)	
NS	+09	+ 9.0	(+1)	
AQ	−51	−51.0		(−1)
M	+08	+ 8.0	(+1)	
SW	+05	+ 5.0	(+1)	
FII				
FIA				

TABLE VI.VIII—*Continued*

Experimental: IRM
Multiple Goals

Sp. No.	*1*	*2*	*3*	*5*	*9*	*10*	*13*	*14*	*15*	*17*	$\overline{X}$ *Freq. Change*	*N=10*	
P	+01	+07	+18	+02	+43	−09	+02	+28	+06	+02	+10.0	(+1)	(−1)
N	+05	+09	+02	00	+01	+17	+03	+18	00	+01	+ 5.6	(+8)	
NS		+01	+08		+12	00	+02	+01	−02		+ 3.1	(+5)	(−1)
AQ	+11	+14	+59	+01	+11	+10	+43	+42	−24	+10	+17.7	(+9)	(−1)
M	+05	+64	+12	+01	+14	+11	+61	00	−07		+17.9	(+7)	(−1)
SW		00	+13		+02	−02	+02	+09			+ 4.0	(+4)	(−1)
FII			−01		−01						− 1.0		(−2)
FIA		−01			+01						0.0	(+1)	(−1)

Experimental: Home
Goal Positive and Negative Feedback

Sp. No.	*4*	*8*	*11*	$\overline{X}$ *Freq. Change*	*N=3*	
P	+01	00	−05	+ 2.0	(+2)	
N	+01	+01	+03	+ 1.7	(+3)	
NS		+01		+ 1.0	(+1)	
AQ	+03	+35	+13	+17.0	(+3)	
M						
SW						
FII		−01		− 1.0		(−1)
FIA						

Goal Additional Questions

Sp. No.	*16*	$\overline{X}$ *Freq. Change*	*N=1*
P	+02	+ 2.0	(+1)
N			
NS			
AQ	+05	+ 5.0	(+1)
M			
SW			
FII			
FIA			

Control: IRM
Multiple Goals

Sp. No.	*2*	*3*	*4*	*5*	*6*	$\overline{X}$ *Freq. Change*	*N=5*	
P	+05		+01	−18	−02	− 3.5	(+2)	(−2)
N	+02		+01	−08	+01	− 1.0	(+3)	(−1)
NS	+03	−01	−01	+03		+ 1.0	(+2)	(−2)
AQ	−02	−14	−02	+36	+02	+ 4.0	(+2)	(−3)
M	+01	+03	+02	−01	−04	+ 0.2	(+3)	(−2)
SW		−01	00	00		− 0.3		(−1)
FII								
FIA				−01		− 1.0		(−1)

Control: Home

Goal Additional Questions

Sp. No.	*1*	$\overline{X}$ *Freq. Change*	*N=1*	
P	−02	− 2.0		(−1)
N	+01	+ 1.0	(+1)	
NS	+02	+ 2.0	(+1)	
AQ	−01	− 1.0		(−1)
M	00			
SW				
FII				
FIA				

TABLE VI.VIII—*Continued*

Experimental: Home
Goal Modeling

Sp. No.	*6*	*7*	$\overline{X}$ *Freq. Change*	*N=2*	
P	+02	+01	+ 1.5	(+2)	
N	+06		+ 6.0	(+1)	
NS					
AQ	−02	+10	+ 4.0	(+1)	(−1)
M	+02	+05	+ 3.5	(+2)	
FII					
FIA					

Multiple Goals

Sp. No.	*1*	*2*	*3*	*5*	*9*	*10*	*13*	*14*	*15*	*17*	$\overline{X}$ *Freq. Change*	*N=10*	
P	+02	+04	+02	+01	+04	−01	−04	+07	+01		+ 1.8	(+7)	(−2)
N		−01	+02	+01	+02	+01	0	+05	0		+ 1.3	(+5)	(−1)
NS		+01	+01		+04	+02					+ 1.5	(+5)	(−1)
AQ	−02	+03	+07	+01	+03	−09	+13	+02	+03	+08	+ 2.9	(+8)	(−2)
M		+01	+03	+01	+02	+02	−02	−02			+ 0.7	(+5)	(−2)
SW					+01			+04			+ 2.5	(+2)	
FII					+01	+01					+ 1.0	(+2)	
FIA													

Multiple Goals

Sp. No.	*2*	*3*	*4*	*5*	*6*	$\overline{X}$ *Freq. Change*	*N=5*	
P			+01	+03	−01	+ 1.0	(+2)	(−1)
N	−02			+01	00	− 0.3	(+1)	(−1)
NS	+02		−02		+01	+ 0.3	(+2)	(−1)
AQ	−01	+03	−03	+01	+01	+ 0.2	(+3)	(−2)
M	+01	−01	+01	+01	00	+ 0.4	(+3)	(−1)
SW								
FII								
FIA								

Spouse Categories:
P—Positive Feedback
N—Negative Feedback
NS—Negative Subjective Feedback
AQ—Additional Questions
M—Modeling
SW—Start Word
FII—Fill in Immediately
FIA—Fill in After Waiting
+ = Changes in desired direction
− = Changes in undesired direction
0 = No change in response categories

additional mean FCP gain of 9.3% following the experimental procedures. The mean FCP score prior to speech therapy was 43.6. Following speech therapy the mean score was 50.8, and following the experimental treatment the mean FCP was 60.4. Nearly all patients had plateaued on the FCP for at least two months when terminated from regular speech therapy classes.

The amount of FCP gain following speech therapy and the additional gain following the experimental procedures were compared using chi square. The FCP scores needed to make this comparison were available for fourteen experimental subjects. Of these fourteen subjects, five subjects who showed high gain (nine or more FCP points) in speech therapy also showed high gain after the experimental procedures; five subjects who showed low gain (eight or less FCP points) in speech therapy also showed low gain after the experimental procedures; three subjects who showed low gain after speech therapy showed high gain following the experimental procedures; and one subject who showed high gain following speech therapy showed low gain after the experimental procedures. The obtained chi square of 1.37 was not significant. For the most part, high or low gain in speech therapy was generally accompanied by a similar amount of gain during the experimental treatment.

Referring to the nurturance scale data, an interesting observation is noted. The three aphasics who showed high gain after the experimental treatment and low gain after speech therapy had spouses who scored high on the nurturance questionnaire (fifteen, fifteen and sixteen). The one subject who showed high gain in speech therapy and low gain after the experimental procedures had a spouse who scored low on the nurturance questionnaire (nine). This finding suggests that one possible major factor in producing high gain in speech therapy is high nurturance.

Although significant improvement in functional speech was indicated in both target behavior and FCP score, a patient's improvement in specific target behaviors did not relate highly with total FCP gain (r=.30). There was also little correlation between the amount of positive change in a spouse and general improvement in an aphasic's functional speech as measured by the FCP.

6. *Prediction of spouses who become effective speech trainers.* To determine whether one could predict a spouse who could be

trained to effectively modify the aphasic's functional speech, two measures were taken prior to training: a) the nurturance score on Katz' adaptation of the Edwards Personal Preference Schedule and b) the difference between the spouse's estimate of the aphasic's functional speech and the speech therapist's FCP prior to the experimental procedures (spouse's FCP under- or over-estimation). These two measures had a significant (.01 level) rank order correlation of .82 with one another. The data suggests a positive relationship between both a) the spouse's over-estimation of her husband's functional speech and her level of nurturance and b) her probability of becoming a good speech trainer. The following correlations were obtained: nurturance score and FCP change during the experimental phase, .42. Spouse's FCP over-estimation and change in patient target behavior, .39. Nurturance score and change in patient target behavior, .42. None of these coefficients are statistically significant.

B. Case Studies

1. *Subject 1.* Mr. A.F. is a seventy-one-year-old right hemiplegic. The onset of his CVA, diagnosed as a possible embolus, was 10/3/66. He was treated for approximately twelve months in speech therapy, and his diagnosis when terminated was: aphasia, receptive-moderate, expressive-severe. His Functional Communication Profile (FCP) Score prior to speech therapy was 52.1. After speech therapy and prior to the experimental treatment his FCP increased to 65.0. At this time his wife evaluated his FCP score as 77.1. After Mr. F. had reached a plateau on the speech therapist's measures, the experimental treatment began. Mr. F. and his wife were seen thirty-two times. Following the experimental treatment sessions Mr. F.'s FCP score increased to 81.3. In filling out the need questionnaire form, Mrs. F. had a nurturance score of fourteen suggesting a high degree of nurturance. The fact that Mrs. F.'s FCP score exceeded the speech therapist's estimate by twelve points, suggests that she considerably over-estimated her husband's functional speech following speech therapy. The target verbal behavior to be modified in Mr. F., suggested by his pre-treatment baserates, was to increase the per-

centage of sentences emitted in his functional speech. The target verbal behaviors to be modified in Mrs. F. were to increase contingent positive and negative feedback and to increase total responses. That is, the goal was to have Mrs. F. talk more to her husband and to give closer feedback as to when he was emitting sentences and when his utterances were not in sentences. In the laboratory, Mr. F.'s sentence output increased from 53% to 87% of his verbal output (after his functional speech had plateaued in speech therapy). At home, his sentence output increased from 77% to 83%. Mrs. F.'s contingent positive and negative feedback, given while the couple was interacting in response to ten questions over a twenty minute period, increased in the laboratory from thirty-five to fifty-nine. The average increase in contingent feedback at home was from six to seven during several five minute samples. In the laboratory, Mrs. F.'s total number of responses increased from fifty-two to seventy-six over the twenty minute baserate period. At home total responses increased from an average of ten to sixteen during five minute random samples.

The following procedure was employed:

a. The experimenter modeled more responses and continuous positive and negative feedback with regard to increasing sentences. Mrs. F. observed through a one-way vision screen. The purpose of this procedure was to demonstrate to Mrs. F. the verbal behaviors that we aimed to increase in her, and to see the response of her husband to this procedure.

b. While in the observation room, the experimenter suggested to Mrs. F. that she respond more and supply continuous positive and negative feedback contingent upon Mr. F.'s emitted sentences. The experimenter continuously reinforced Mrs. F. for increases in responding and increased feedback. The purpose of this procedure was to build Mrs. F.'s target behaviors into her verbal interactions with her husband.

c. The experimenter instructed Mrs. F. to model sentences and words and phrases for Mr. F. and to state whether each of her utterances was in sentence form. Mrs. F. was reinforced by the experimenter for doing this one minute prior to Mr. F.'s responding. When Mr. F. began responding Mrs. F. gave continuous feedback on sentence production. The purpose of this procedure was to aid Mr. F. in discriminating sentences (his target behavior) from other utterances.

d. After each utterance by Mr. F., his wife was instructed to stop him and ask whether his response was a sentence or not. Then, Mrs. F. stated whether his judgment was correct. Mrs. F. was reinforced periodically during each session for carrying out this procedure. The aim was to aid Mr. F. in monitoring his production of sentences, or to become more aware of when his utterances were in sentence form.

Observations

Mr. and Mrs. F. appeared to have a spontaneous, friendly relationship. They were supportive of one another, and were interested and cooperative in the various experimental treatments. Although they both conversed actively with one another and with the experimenter, Mrs. F. frequently dominated the interactions with her husband. She periodically undermined her husband's attempts at functional speech. She stated that in company, when the general conversation was rapid and continuous, few of their friends had the patience to wait for Mr. F. to finish what he had to say. In stating this, she appeared to be more sympathetic and understanding of their friends than of her husband. When Mrs. F. spoke rapidly and continuously to Mr. F. or to the examiner, it had a strong depressant effect on his speech. At such times he spoke less, emitted more dysfluencies, and was more self-critical. Neither Mr. nor Mrs. F. appeared to be overly anxious or depressed about Mr. F.'s aphasia. Mrs. F. seemed to control the anxiety she did have by keeping busy, reading, keeping active in her relationships with friends, going to the theater, etc. Mr. F. controlled his anxiety and depression by denying the permanence of his aphasia, working hard at improving his speech, and keeping busy with friends, reading, etc. Neither Mr. nor Mrs. F. appeared to be overly dependent on one another. Although the reduction of anxiety was not a specific aim of the study, Mr. F. appeared to be increasingly relaxed about his speech as the sessions progressed. The impression is that this is, at least in part, a function of the relaxed, supportive nature of the sessions, with this mode of treatment. In the treatment sessions few real demands are made on the patient and frequent reinforcement is given for emitted responses.

2. *Subject 2.* Mr. J.K. is a fifty-seven-year-old right hemiplegic. The onset of his CVA, diagnosed as occlusion of the left internal carotid, was October 5, 1967. He was treated for 2½ months in speech therapy, and his diagnosis when terminated was: aphasia, receptive-mild, expressive-moderate. His FCP score prior to speech therapy was 63.2. After speech therapy and prior to the experimental procedure his FCP plateaued at 64.7. At this time his wife assessed his FCP as 97.3, a gross over-estimate judging from the speech therapist's estimate. After reaching a plateau on the speech therapist's measures, the experimental procedures began. Mr. and Mrs. K. were seen thirty times. Following the experimental treatment sessions Mr. K.'s FCP score increased to 81.3. On the need questionnaire, Mrs. K. had a nurturance score of fourteen, suggesting a very high degree of nurturance. Mrs. K.'s thirty-three point FCP over-estimate indicates that she evaluated her husband's functional speech as being much better than it actually was at the end of speech therapy. Mr. K.'s target verbal behavior was to increase sentence production. The target behavior to be modified in Mrs. K. was total responses emitted. The goal was to aid Mr. K. in speaking more rapidly, and have Mrs. K. speak more to her husband. In the laboratory, Mr. K.'s sentence output increased from fifty-three to seventy-six during a comparable twenty minute baserate period. At home his sentence production increased from twelve per five minute sample during pre-treatment baserates to twenty per five minute sample during post-treatment baserates. Mrs. K.'s total responses increased from zero during pre-treatment baserates to four during post-treatment baserates in the laboratory. At home, Mrs. K.'s total responses per five minute sample of naturalistic speech increased from two to nine.

The following procedures were employed:

a. The experimenter modeled active responding to Mr. K., periodic suggestions to emit utterances in sentence form, and reinforcement for producing sentences quickly. Mrs. K. observed this procedure through a one-way vision screen. The purpose of this procedure was to demonstrate to Mrs. K. verbal behavior that we wished to increase in her, and to show the effect on her husband's speech.

b. While the experimenter was in the observation room, he gave periodic suggestions that Mrs. K. respond more to her husband's efforts to produce sentences. Because of their long-established relationship in which Mr. K. was the dominant talker, and since he apparently had objections to Mrs. K. playing a strong role as therapist, the experimenter did not push very active responding from Mrs. K.

c. Because of Mr. K.'s high level of anxiety concerning his speech, five sessions were spent on training relaxation with regard to speech. Wolpe's desensitization procedure was employed (Ince, 1968). Relaxation exercises were paired with suggestions of speaking in a variety of situations which had evoked various levels of anxiety.

d. Since Mr. K.'s intellectual level and oral production were high, the topics discussed during treatment sessions were changed frequently. Prior to each session, he prepared at home to discuss a famous person, a city, and a news event. During these sessions as he spoke about the various topics, in addition to interjecting periodic comments, Mrs. K. counted each sentence aloud as Mr. K. emitted it. Counting responses was an effective reinforcer for Mr. K.

e. During four individual sessions, the experimenter instructed Mr. K. to stop after each utterance and state whether the response was in sentence form or not. Then, the experimenter told him if his judgment was correct. The purpose of this procedure was to aid Mr. K. in monitoring his production of sentences. In addition to this procedure, a Differential Reinforcement of Other Responses (DRO) schedule was employed. That is, when Mr. K. not only produced a sentence, but produced it rapidly and with few pauses he was strongly reinforced, verbally, for his behavior.

Observations

Although Mr. and Mrs. K. appeared comfortable while interacting, Mr. K. was clearly the dominant personality. When Mrs. K. attempted to supply a word, her husband discouraged her either verbally or with a glance. Mrs. K. appeared very patient in allowing her husband all the time he wished to emit a statement. She seemed somewhat fearful about offering positive or negative feedback with regard to Mr. K.'s sentence production. Both were most comfortable when she counted each sentence as he emitted them. Counting the number of sentences emitted during a specified time period was an effective reinforcer. It provided motivation for him to exceed previous trials, and he did not object to this kind of feedback. Mr. K. was highly motivated to perform well and he brought pages of unassigned written material relevant to various topics discussed during the sessions. He had a long-established pattern of being very precise in his work, hobbies and speech. During the early sessions he indicated that he was not content to use just any word in expressing an idea. When he was attempting to find a word, he wished to use the precise word he was searching for. One aim in working with Mr. K., was to have him relax more and be more flexible with himself. The desensitization procedure was effective in increasing relaxation. After this training, he appeared to be more relaxed and both Mr. and Mrs. K. stated that he was less anxious and spoke more freely after several weeks of this procedure.

3. *Subject 3.* Mr. E.S. is a sixty-seven-year-old right hemiplegic. The onset of his CVA, etiology unknown, was October 19, 1965. His diagnosis when treatment was terminated after two years of regular speech therapy was aphasia, receptive-moderate, expressive-severe. His FCP score prior to speech therapy was 45.1. After speech therapy and prior to the experimental treatment his FCP increased three points to 48.1. At this time his wife evaluated his FCP at 54.0. The experimental procedures began after Mr. S. had plateaued on the speech therapist's measures. Mr. and Mrs. S. were seen twenty-two times. After the experimental sessions, Mr. S.'s FCP score increased to 55.0. In filling out the need questionnaire, Mrs. S. had a nurturance score of eight suggesting a low degree of nurturance. Mrs. S.'s six point FCP over-estimate suggests that she slightly over-estimated her husband's functional speech following speech therapy. The target verbal behaviors to be modified in Mr. S. were to increase sentences, increase words and phrases and increase percent of relevant utterances. The

target verbal behaviors to be modified in Mrs. S. were to increase contingent positive feedback, increase modeling, and decrease negative subjective feedback. Mrs. S. gave little in the way of encouragement and support for good attempts at functional speech, and gave a considerable amount of person-oriented negative feedback. In the laboratory, Mr. S.'s sentence output increased from twenty to fifty-five, and his production of clear words and phrases increased from twenty-seven to sixty-five during baserate periods of the same duration. Percent of relevant utterances increased from 79% to 94% in the laboratory. At home, his sentence production increased from an average of five to an average of nine per five minute random sample of the tape. Words and phrases at home increased from six to eleven. Mrs. S.'s positive feedback during baserate sessions in the laboratory increased from twenty-five to sixty-eight, modeling increased from fifteen to thirty-one, and negative subjective feedback decreased from sixteen to two. At home, Mrs. S.'s positive feedback increased from an average of eight to twelve per five minute random sample. Modeling at home increased from two to four per sample, and negative subjective feedback decreased from an average of five to one per sample.

The following procedures were employed:

a. The experimenter modeled continuous positive feedback with frequent modeling of appropriate words and sentences while Mrs. S. observed through a one-way vision screen. The experimenter gave no negative subjective feedback, and provided a relaxed highly supportive atmosphere. The purpose of this procedure was to demonstrate to Mrs. S. the verbal behavior we aimed to increase in her, and to observe the response of her husband to this procedure.

b. While the experimenter was in the observation room, he gave suggestions to supply more positive feedback and modeling and less negative subjective feedback. The experimenter continuously reinforced Mrs. S. for her contingent reinforcement and modeling, and gave continuous verbal punishment for negative subjective feedback. The purpose of this procedure was to build Mrs. S.'s target behaviors into her verbal interactions with her husband.

c. The experimenter played back portions of tape of Mr. and

Mrs. S.'s treatment sessions, demonstrating the depressant effect of Mrs. S.'s negative subjective feedback on her husband's speech. The aim of this procedure was to demonstrate the consequence of personal criticism on Mr. S.'s verbal output.

d. The experimenter instructed Mrs. S. to model words, phrases and sentences for Mr. S. and to state after each response whether it was a word, phrase or sentence. Mrs. S. was reinforced for doing this for one complete minute prior to Mr. S.'s responding. When Mr. S. began responding, Mrs. S. gave continuous reinforcement for each response in the target categories. The purpose of this procedure was to aid Mr. S. in increasing his target behaviors and Mrs. S. in being more active and supportive with her husband.

e. The experimenter instructed Mrs. S. to delay before filling in words Mr. S. was apparently searching for. As Mrs. S. began to allow more time (at least five seconds) for her husband to supply the word, the experimenter verbally reinforced this behavior. This procedure was to aid Mr. S. in pushing harder to supply his own words and rely less on his wife.

Observations

Mrs. S. was clearly the dominant personality. While speaking with the experimenter, she had taken the lead and responded to most of the questions directed at Mr. S. She frequently undermined his attempts at speech by smiling and not responding verbally or by telling him that people couldn't understand him and he should try harder. Her negative comments were generally more person oriented than task-oriented. She tended to treat him as a young child, and showed little respect for or understanding of his thoughts and feelings. Mr. S. appeared rather depressed and withdrawn. His appetite was poor and he had difficulty sleeping. He spent most of his time watching television and looking at magazines at home. Mrs. S. gave the impression that she had little sympathy for her husband and felt very upset about her own situation. Mr. S. was very passive when his wife spoke to the experimenter, and he made little effort to express himself in her presence. When the experimenter spoke to the patient individually he was much more verbal, particularly when discussing topics of interest to him such as his work or books he had written when he was younger. Mr. S. was very responsive when encouraged to express himself and given continuous support for his efforts. His wife seemed to serve as a discriminative stimulus for remaining silent. Mrs. S. controlled her anxiety by spending considerable time out of the house, shopping and visiting friends. At the end of treatment, Mrs. S. was much less critical of her husband and more supportive of efforts toward improved functional speech. Mr. S. spoke more frequently and appeared somewhat less anxious.

4. *Subject 4 (control).* Mr. H.L. is a forty-nine-year-old hemiplegic. The onset of his CVA, diagnosed as an embolus, was June 12, 1968. After six months of speech therapy, his diagnosis, when terminated, was: aphasia, receptive-moderate, expressive-severe. After speech therapy and prior to the experimental treatment his FCP was 35.4. At this time, his wife evaluated his FCP score as 49.3. After Mr. L. had reached a plateau on the speech therapist's measures, the experimental control procedure began. Mr. L. was seen fifteen times. Following the control sessions Mr. L.'s FCP score was 36.7, suggesting little change in functional speech following this condition. In filling out the need questionnaire, Mrs. L. had a nurturance score of sixteen, indicating a high degree of nurturance. The fact that Mrs. L.'s FCP score exceeded the speech therapist's estimate by 13.9 points, suggests that she considerably over-estimated her husband's functional speech following speech therapy. The target verbal behavior to be modified if Mr. L. was in the treatment group would have been to increase words and phrases and decrease unclear utterances. The goal with Mrs. L. would have been to increase positive and negative feedback and to increase modeling. That is, the aim would be to have Mrs. L. talk more to her husband, to give more examples of appropriate functional speech, and to supply closer feedback as to when Mr. L. spoke clearly and unclearly. In the laboratory, Mr. L.'s output of clear words and phrases was twenty-eight during the pre-treatment baserates and twenty-eight during the post-treatment baserates. This data suggests little or no change after his control sessions. Unclear responses in the laboratory went from a pre-treatment frequency of sixty-one to a post-treatment frequency of seventy. At home, his output of clear words and phrases changed for eight to twenty-five, and unclear utterances changed from

thirty-one to twenty during random five minute samples. Mrs. L.'s contingent positive and negative feedback, given while the couple was interacting in response to ten questions over a twenty minute period, remained at zero. The frequency of modeling responses in the laboratory went from seventeen to twenty. At home Mrs. L.'s contingent feedback remained at zero, and modeling changed from one to zero during each five minute sample. Neither Mr. nor Mrs. L.'s target responses showed any significant changes during the course of the control sessions.

The following procedure was employed:

The experimenter reinforced Mrs. L.'s responses on a variable ratio schedule. Social reinforcement (e.g., "That was very good." "Fine." "You're doing very well.") was given periodically, but not contingent upon specific target behaviors as in the case of the experimental subjects. The experimenter spoke with Mr. and Mrs. L. for five minutes prior to and following the control procedure each day, and supplied reassurance and answered general questions about aphasia. Other than the non-contingent feedback and lack of specifying target behaviors in Mr. and Mrs. L., the session was conducted in the same manner as with the experimental subjects. No specific suggestions were made as to how to deal with the patient's speech.

Observations

Mr. and Mrs. L. appeared to have a close, friendly relationship. Although Mr. L. emitted very few clear words, and perseverated a great deal on the sound *too,* his wife tried very patiently to understand his communications through inflections and gestures. Mr. L. was extremely anxious about his speech having always been a very social person, and he repeatedly tried to express his frustration to the experimenter and to his wife. He also frequently tried to reassure listeners that while he could not express his thoughts, he was well aware of what others were saying. It seemed to particularly disturb him when he was attempting to emit a common sound or simple word but could not do so. Mrs. L. was very supportive of his efforts, and continuously tried to reassure him that things were going to improve and that he should be more patient with his speech. Frequently Mrs. L. pretended to understand her husband's efforts at speech, and reinforced unclear or perseverative utterances. There was no negative feedback for unclear utterances even though Mr. L. had little awareness of the adequacy of most of his responses. Although Mrs. L. gave few signs of her own anxiety and depression in her husband's presence, in private she indicated to the experimenter that Mr. L.'s frustration and high anxiety were of great concern to her. Mrs. L. was with her husband constantly except for occasional trips to do essential shopping. Mr. L. spent little time outside of the house. At home he attempted to read the newspaper and magazines, and watched a great deal of television. When friends or relatives visited, two or three evenings each week, he made continuous efforts to communicate with them. Mr. and Mrs. L. seemed to enjoy the sessions even though they received no direction or feedback. Other than spending five minutes prior to and following each session in conversation about daily events, the experimenter simply gave periodic non-contingent reinforcement to Mrs. L. for whatever she happened to be doing with her husband.

5. *Subject 5 (control).* Mrs. O.P. is a forty-one-year-old right hemiplegic. The onset of her CVA was August 25, 1967. Her diagnosis when terminated from speech therapy after eighteen months of treatment was: aphasia, receptive-moderate, expressive-moderate. After speech therapy and prior to the experimental procedure her FCP was 63.8. At this time, her husband evaluated her FCP score as 79.2. After Mrs. P. had reached a plateau on the speech therapist's measures, the experimental control procedure began. Mrs. P. was seen fifteen times. Following the control sessions, Mrs. P.'s FCP score was 63.0, suggesting little change in functional speech following this condition. In filling out the need questionnaire, Mr. P. had a nurturance score of eight suggesting a low degree of nurturance. The fact that Mr. P.'s FCP score exceeded the speech therapist's estimate by 15.4 points suggests that he considerably over-estimated his wife's functional speech. The target verbal behavior to be modified if Mrs. P. was in the treatment group would have been to increase direct answers or relevant utterances. The goal with Mr. P. would have been to increase contingent positive and negative feedback and to decrease additional questions. That is, the aim would be to have Mrs. P. stay

more on topics being discussed, and to encourage Mr. P. to ask less questions and give more contingent feedback on his wife's relevant responses. In the laboratory, Mrs. P.'s output of direct answers during pre-treatment baserates was sixty-eight. During post-treatment baserates, direct answers decreased to twenty-seven. Mr. P.'s positive and negative feedback went from thirty-five to nine in the laboratory, and additional questions decreased from ninety-two to sixty-six. At home, Mr. P.'s positive and negative feedback increased from one to five per five minute sample, and additional questions went from thirty-six to thirty-five per sample. Mrs. P.'s direct answers (target behavior) decreased markedly following the control procedure, whereas the aim would have been to increase responses in this category. Although a significant change in the desired direction occurred with Mr. P.'s output of additional questions, positive and negative feedback decreased markedly, the reverse of the desired aim. At home, while Mr. P.'s positive and negative feedback increased somewhat in the desired direction, additional questions remained about the same.

The following procedure was employed:

The experimenter verbally reinforced Mr. P.'s responses on a variable ratio schedule. Social reinforcement (e.g., "That was very good." "Fine." "You're doing very well.") was periodically given but was not contingent upon specific target behaviors as in the case of the experimental subjects. The experimenter spoke with Mr. and Mrs. P. for five minutes prior to and following the control procedure each day, and supplied reassurance and answered general questions about aphasia. Other than the non-contingent feedback and lack of specifying target behaviors in Mr. and Mrs. P., the sessions were conducted in the same manner as with the experimental subjects. No specific suggestions were made as to how to deal with the patient's speech.

Observations

Mr. P. was critical of his wife's speech and of her general behavior. He appeared to be very angry at her. He offered little assistance when she was *searching* for words, and he gave little feedback when she expressed herself clearly and well. Mr. P. dominated their conversations, and Mrs. P. appeared rather fearful of him. When the experimenter asked Mrs. P. questions, her husband generally intervened with lengthy answers, allowing Mrs. P. little opportunity to respond. When the patient was seen individually, she was outgoing and seemed much less self-conscious about her speech than in her husband's presence. During individual sessions, she spoke more fluently, emitted more sentences, and was less critical of herself. Mrs. P. was not overly anxious or depressed about her speech. She was involved in her daily housework and caring for her three children. Mrs. P. was confident that her speech would improve markedly in time. Mr. P. appeared to be embarrassed by his wife's speech. His anxiety was frequently expressed by impatience and by being very demanding with her. Although the patient worked hard at improving her functional speech, frequently talking with friends and family members, and working in a notebook she started on her own, Mr. P. seemed to avoid working on his wife's speech. The couple expressed no dissatisfaction with the control sessions. Other than Mr. and Mrs. P. appearing to be more relaxed with the experimenter, no significant changes were observed at the end of treatment. The quality of their interaction, and Mrs. P.'s speech were essentially unchanged.

IV. DISCUSSION

There are several advantages to training the spouse of an aphasic in methods of improving the patient's functional speech. Since the spouse has much more time with the aphasic than the speech therapist, if she can be trained as a supplemental therapist it would clearly be a valuable addition to regular therapy. Typically, an aphasic patient has no more than two or three half-hour sessions per week with his speech therapist. A second advantage is that families might save a considerable amount of money if family members can learn to carry out some of the responsibilities of speech therapy. This study indicates that the procedures described can help to build in more effective ways of improving functional speech than when the spouse is left to her own resources. Although speech therapists may make suggestions to the spouse as to how she might aid the patient, this procedure offers a way of implementing these suggestions and seeing to it that the suggested procedures are being employed correctly. By including the spouse in the therapy procedures, she acquires the feeling that she is involved and participating in the patient's speech therapy. The results of this study indicate significant gains in functional speech after aphasics had been considered to have reached a plateau in regular speech therapy. Finally, by having regular contacts with spouses of aphasics, one can aid the spouse in understanding the problem, developing realistic expectations, and adapting to the situation.

Several general observations of aphasic patients and their spouses were noted. Nearly every patient and spouse in the treatment group appeared to be more relaxed and more capable of coping with the speech deficit following the treatment procedures. It is believed that this is partly a function of the relaxed, informal, relatively unstructured nature of the sessions and partly due to the highly reinforcing nature of the sessions. Each adequate response is reinforced, and any gains, no matter how gradual, are objectively (numerically) pointed out. Several wives stated that by participating in this program they felt that they were able to do something to aid their husband's speech, whereas formerly they felt quite helpless. They also indicated a liking for the direction and for the opportunity of having a sounding board for expressing their thoughts and feelings. The continuous objective measures of functional speech and the continuous feedback enabled the spouse to be aware of progess and aided her in adapting to the situation.

The spouses' expectations, attitudes, thoughts and feelings had a definite effect on the treatment procedures. These factors could interfere with, slow down, or speed up the process. Some spouses or patients were so angry at, or manipulative of the other that one of the pair refused to continue having sessions with the other. In extreme cases, the long established relationship predating the experimental procedures was so inflexible that little leverage could be gained by experimental intervention. Such cases were exceptions, however. Most of the couples were very involved in and responsive to the various procedures. Many spouses tended to treat the patients like young children, and while some patients went along with this treatment, most clearly resented it. In such situations, efforts were made to have the spouse treat her husband more as an adult. In cases where one marital partner was dominant, although experimental intervention produced some change in the verbal interactions, the basic dominance pattern was not altered. In particular, when the aphasic husband played a strong, dominant role, none of the described procedures caused the spouse to play a very active role in treating the patient.

In addition to the primary results of this study, resulting from the general procedures, there were several secondary findings of interest:

The reliable system of scoring responses into concurrent response categories (Goodkin, 1968) proved to be a useful, easily employed evaluative technique of ongoing verbal output. This procedure can be used to diagnose deficit areas, assess progress in multiple response areas, and evaluate effects of new treatment procedures. When used with a family member and patient or therapist and patient, one can study interactional effects (i.e., the effects that the specific responses of each person has on the other's responses). By evaluating several categories simultaneously, one can determine what effect treatment focused on one target behavior is having on other responses (e.g., as the spouse continually reinforces words and phrases emitted, what happens to the frequency of sentences, or relevant utterances, or unclear responses?). The technique of obtaining concurrent response categories in this way can easily be adapted to evaluating other clinical areas (Catania, 1965). We have obtained Pearson r's of better than .90 between raters independently scoring the concurrent responses of therapists and patients in adult physical therapy ambulation classes and in nursery school classes. In each of these situations both verbal and motor responses of the therapist and patient were scored concurrently.

The use of teleprompting lends itself well to training family members. This procedure enabled the experimenter to have constant communication with the spouse while she was in the process of interacting with the patient. This communication, in the form of suggestions and feedback, enabled the experimenter to build effective training procedures into the spouse's behavioral repertoire with more precision than suggestions following a regular therapy session would. Although it sometimes took two or three sessions for subjects to become accustomed to the headphone, all subjects adapted to the apparatus and made little mention of it after the first few sessions. This procedure would appear to be equally useful as a means of training individuals in other settings. It could be used in on-the-job training of speech therapists, occupational therapists, physical therapists, or psychotherapists. Student therapists could *learn by doing* while *master therapists* (i.e., qualified, experienced therapists) supply suggestions and feedback by means of the headphones. This procedure can also be employed in teaching parents to interact better with their children or to teach their children various skills. Finally, this technique can be used to train family members of disabled individuals to function as auxiliary therapists in other deficit areas (e.g., ambulation, activities of daily living, etc.), This apparatus is simple and can be purchased for under one hundred dollars. The apparatus can be modified so that it can be easily transported in two small suitcases and quickly set up in a patient's home (in less than five minutes). We had employed such portable equipment with six of the subjects in this study.

The home recording device was useful as an outside criterion measure, to determine how the effects of the experimental procedures carried over into the home (naturalistic) environment. This apparatus is compact and is contained in a small suitcase. Since this device was placed in an inconspicuous area (generally not in the room patients and spouses were in), and since the small microphone carried in the patient's pocket was wireless, both patient and spouse adapted quickly to it. Their conversation appeared to be natural and spontaneous. The data obtained was easily and reliably ($r=.93$) scored. Up to twelve hours of running speech were scored on a single one hour spool of tape, since only ongoing speech was recorded and the device automatically turned off during silences. There was generalization from the laboratory to the home in both patient and spouse although changes in patient responses tended to carry over significantly more. This apparatus could be used for other purposes as well. For example, one could compare home, naturalistic speech of aphasics and their spouses with non-aphasic couples of the same age. It might also be used to aid in clinical settings such as examining the naturalistic verbal interactions at home between parents and a child in psychotherapy or between marital partners undergoing marriage counseling. The device could be used to explore how family members respond to a disabled person and to determine how these responses effect the quantity and nature of his responses. Finally, such a device could be employed to obtain periodic reevaluations of home interactions of people undergoing speech therapy, psychotherapy, counseling, etc. In this way one could examine whether the naturalistic, home situation concurs with what the person says about his situation in the laboratory or therapist's office.

Our work has suggested that one very probable reason for the lack of success in several other attempts at programmed instruction with aphasics was due to the lack of empirically determined, workable reinforcers. While the average, non-brain-injured student may profit from a teaching machine or programmed text which uses the correct answer to a stimulus question as a reinforcer, a moderately or severely affected aphasic, who has little awareness of his speech or little ability to comprehend the correct response when presented to him, can make little use of such feedback. Reinforcement to such a subject must be presented in such a way that he can process it (e.g., tokens, repeating the correct response several times, or presenting the correct response through the sensory mode that he can best comprehend). The response category to be treated, the reinforcement employed, and the chosen treatment procedures must be carefully tailored to the individual aphasic subject. Indeed the reinforcement patterns of staff, family and others in social interaction with an aphasic in naturalistic settings would be of great interest.

The question of what constitutes real gain in a complex clinical phenomenon has long been an issue in the literature. It is difficult to measure and state precisely how much a patient has improved in psychotherapy, for example, because of widely differing views of what *improvement* means. That which is regarded as a major improvement for some clinicians may be regarded as having little real importance to others. In speech therapy, while the important dependent variables may be more widely agreed upon and more accessible to measurement than those in psychotherapy, it remains unclear as to whether a measured change is truly significant. In the present study, for example, we have specified response categories, stated target behaviors to be modified, and showed changes in frequency and percent of responses in these categories for each individual and for each experimental group. Yet, the question remains, do these numerical changes in the desired direction constitute major gain? Is the aphasic's functional speech significantly closer to *normal* speech? While statistically significant changes in the prescribed direction occurred and the subjective impression is that several patients had made very noticeable gains, the degree to which the patient's speech now deviates from *normal* speech is not objectively assessed. The reason for this is that there is no normative data on similar parameters of speech obtained from a matched populations of non-brain-injured subjects. Further research in this area is clearly needed. Such normative data could be obtained using the same procedures that were employed in this study. The same stimuli, response categories, and recording techniques could be used with non-brain-injured individuals to obtain normative data. Although it is apparent that individuals will differ widely in their output on these speech parameters, ranges of *normal* speech could be estimated. This data could then be used as a standard against which speed therapists and researchers could compare the speech of their subjects.

Perhaps, at this early stage of aphasia therapy research, the emphasis should be not so much on proving a theory as on empirically assessing the effects of many carefully specified procedures on verbal behavior. Our procedures were most effective when considerable efforts were taken to establish good rapport with subjects. During the pilot research, subjects who perceived the treatment condition as being too mechanical tended to lose interest. The experimenter had to establish and maintain himself as a reinforcer.

Although our data has indicated quantitative improvement in nearly every subject treated, one was constantly reminded that neurological damage posed real limits on what could be expected of a given subject. Whereas some subjects who started the program at a high level of verbal functioning approximated normal speech when the procedures terminated, moderately and severely effected aphasics and apractic subjects made more modest functional gains.

V. SUMMARY

The major purpose of this study was to train spouses of aphasic subjects to serve as supplemental speech therapists. Twenty-three couples were seen. The general plan consisted of obtaining a full day's sample of talking behavior between spouses at home before and after training, obtaining speech samples in a controlled setting, developing a system for analyzing the talking behavior of patient and spouse, teaching the spouse principles and techniques of behavior modification; and evaluating changes in the patient's and spouse's interaction resulting from the training. The home measures were obtained to determine whether training in the laboratory generalized to the home (a naturalistic setting). A small wireless microphone placed in the patient's pocket was used to obtain continuous samples of speech. The tape recorder, kept in an adjoining room, turned off automatically during silences. An average of twenty training sessions were spent with each couple. In addition to explaining the procedures to the spouse, a teleprompting system was employed. The experimenter observed the patient-spouse interactions through a one-way vision screen, and gave suggestions and feedback to the spouse by means of a headphone which was worn over one ear. Patient and spouse target verbal behaviors (to be increased or decreased) were determined on the basis of the initial speech samples (baserates) obtained in the laboratory.

The results of this study indicate significant gains in functional speech after aphasics had been considered to reach a plateau in regular speech therapy. Significant changes in the desired direction were also produced in spouses. The average gain in patient target behaviors was 14.9%; the average gain in spouse targets was 11.6%. Patient changes generalized to the home significantly more than spouse changes. In addition to general outcome data concerning changes in patient and spouse responding, detailed case studies were presented.

Advantages of these procedures, observations of aphasic-spouse interactions, and secondary findings were discussed.

REFERENCES

Bandura, A: Behavioral modification through modeling procedures. In L. Krasner and L. P. Ullman (Eds.): *Research in Behavioral Modification.* New York, Holt, Rinehart and Winston, 1965.

Buxbaum, J.: Nurturance as a factor in wives' judgment of severity of spouses' aphasia. *J. Consult. Psychol.,* June, 1967.

Catania, A. C.: Concurrent operants. In W. K. Honig (Ed.): *Operant Behavior: Areas of Research and Application.* New York, Appleton-Century-Crofts, 1966, 213-270.

Ferster, C. B., and Skinner, B. F.: *Schedules of Reinforcement.* New York, Appleton-Century-Crofts, 1957.

Filby, Y., and Edwards, A.: An application of automated teaching methods to test and teach form discrimination to aphasics. *J. Program. Instr., 1*:25-34, 1963.

Goldiamond, I.: Self-control procedures in personal behavior problems. *Psychol. Rep., 17*:851-868, 1965.

Goldiamond, I.: Perception. In A. J. Bachrach (Ed.): *The Experimental Foundations of Clinical Psychology.* New York, Basic Books, 1962 (b).

Goldstein, K.: *Language and Language Disturbances.* New York, Grune and Stratton, 1948.

Goodglass, H., Quadfassel, F., and Timberlake, W.: Phrase length and type of severity of aphasia. *Cortex, 1*:133-153, 1964.

Goodkin, R.: Case studies in behavioral research in rehabilitation. *Percept. Mot. Skills, 23*:171-182, 1966A.

Goodkin, R.: Improving verbal and motor behavior in hemiplegics through operant conditioning. Paper presented at APA Annual Meeting in New York, in Symposium on *Advances in Rehabilitation of Stroke Patients.* 1966B.

Goodkin, R.: Use of concurrent response categories in evaluating talking behavior in aphasic patients. *Percept. Mot. Skills, 26*:1035-1040, 1968.

Goodkin, R.: A procedure for training spouses to improve the functional speech of aphasic subjects. Paper presented at APA Annual Meeting in Washington, D.C., 1969.

Goodkin, R.: The modification of verbal behavior in aphasic subjects. Paper presented at APA Annual Meeting in Miami, Florida, 1970.

Granick, L.: *Aphasia: A Guide to Retraining.* New York, Grune and Stratton, 1947.

Greenspoon, J.: The reinforcing effect of two spoken sounds on the frequency of two responses. *Amer. J. Psychol., 68*:409-416, 1955.

Greenspoon, J.: Verbal conditioning and clinical psychology. In A. J. Bachrach (Ed.): *The Experimental Foundations of Clinical Psychology.* New York, Basic Books, 1962.

Halpern, H.: Effect of stimulus variables on dysphasic verbal errors. *Percept. Mot. Skills, 21*:291-298, 1965.

Head, H.: *Aphasia and Kindred Disorders of Speech.* New York, Macmillan, 1926.

Holland, A.: The use of programmed instruction with aphasics. Paper presented at The American Congress of Rehabilitation Medicine, Chicago, Feb., 1968.

Honig, W. K.: *Operant Behavior: Areas of Research and Application.* New York, Appleton-Century-Crofts, 1966.

Ince, L. P.: Desensitization with an aphasic patient. *Behavior Research and Therapy, 6*:235-237, 1968.

Jones, L. and Wepman, J.: Dimensions of language performance in aphasia. *J. Speech Hear. Dis., 4*:220-232, 1961.

Kerr, N., Meyerson, L., and Michael, J.: A procedure for shaping vocalizations in a mute child. In L. Ullman, and L. Krasner (Eds.): *Case Studies in Behavior Modification.* New York: Holt, Rinehart and Winston, 1965.

Krasner, L.: Studies in the conditioning of verbal behavior. *Psychol. Bull.,* 1958, *15*:148-171 (a).

Lindsley, O. R.: Free operant conditioning and psychotherapy. In J. H. Masserman (Ed.): *Current Psychiatric Therapies.* New York, Grune and Stratton, 1963.

Mowrer, D. E.: Measurement in speech therapy. *Psychol. Asp. of Disabil., 17*:24-28, 1970.

Salzinger, K.: Experimental manipulation of verbal behavior: A review. *J. Genet. Psychol., 61*:65-95, 1959.

Sands, E., Sarno, M. L., and Shankweiler, D.: Long-term assessment of language function in aphasia due to stroke. *Arch. Phys. Med., 50*:202-206, 1969.

Sarno, M. T.: The functional communication profile manual of directions. *Rehabilitation Monograph, 42*:22-28, New York Institute of Rehabilitation Medicine, 1969.

Schuell, H., Jenkins, J., and Jiminez, P.: *Aphasia in Adults.* New York, Harper and Row, 1964.

Skinner, B. F.: *Verbal Behavior.* New York, Appleton-Century-Crofts, 1957.

Staats, A. W. et. al.: Reinforcement variables in the control of unit reading responses. *J. Exper. Anal. Behav., 7*:139-149, 1964.

Suskin and John: Recording continuous samples of verbal behavior. In R. Barker (Ed.): *The Stream of Behavior.* New York, Harper Brothers, 1963.

Taylor, M. L.: *Understanding Aphasia.* New York, Inst. of Phys. Med. and Rehab. NYU Medical Center, Monograph Pub. #2, 1958.

Taylor, M. L.: A measurement of functional communication in aphasia. *Arch. Phys. Med., 46*:101-107, 1965.

Taylor, M. L., and Sands, E. S.: Reliability measures of the functional communication profile. Presented at the Annual Meeting, Amer. Speech and Hearing Ass., Chicago, 1965.

Terrace, H. S.: Stimulus control. In W. K. Honig (Ed.) : *Operant Behavior: Areas of Research and Application.* New York, Appleton-Century-Crofts, 1966, 271-344.

Tikofsky, R. S., and Reynolds, G.: Preliminary study: Nonverbal learning and aphasia. *J. Speech Hear. Dis., 5*:133-143, 1962.

Travis, L. E.: *Speech Pathology.* New York, Appleton-Century-Crofts, 1931.

Ullman, L. P., and Krasner, L. (Eds.) : *Case Studies in Behavior Modification.* New York, Holt, Rinehart and Winston, 1965.

Vignolo, L.: Evaluation of aphasia and language rehabilitation: A retrospective study. *Cortex, 1*:344-367, 1964.

Wepman, J.: A conceptual model for processes involved in recovery from aphasia. *J. Speech, Hear. Dis., 18*:4-13, 1953.

ACKNOWLEDGMENTS

This study was supported in part under Social and Rehabilitation Service Grant No. RD-2666-P and under the designation of New York University as a Rehabilitation Research and Training Center by Social and Rehabilitation Service, Department of Health, Education, and Welfare (RT-1).

The authors wish to express their appreciation to John E. Sarno and Martha Sarno of the Institute of Rehabilitation Medicine, Diane Erbert and Rosiland Hain of the Kessler Institute of Rehabilitation, and Kathy La Mondo of the DeWitt Nursing Home for their interest, support and cooperation with regard to this study.

CHAPTER VII

MINORITY GROUP LANGUAGES

Benjamin B. Lahey

IN RECENT YEARS, major segments of the American educational system have sought to construct high quality unitary school programs. Following court decisions and research (e.g. Coleman, et al, 1966; Crain, 1971) which concluded that separate educational facilities for cultural minorities could not, by their very nature, be equal, fully integrated schools are now becoming a widespread, although certainly not universal, reality.

While unitary school systems promise a number of advantages for minority group children, the process of integration itself poses certain problems. Blacks, Chicanos, Indians, Puerto Ricans and other American minority cultures have remained quite distinct in many respects in spite of the economic and political dominance of the white culture in America. Bringing these children together in an educational system which is operated according to white rules and standards puts the minority children at a distinct educational disadvantage simply because they are *different.*

This is quite different from saying that the minority children are *educationally disadvantaged* in an absolute sense. It is a relative judgment. If white children were suddenly introduced in a school system operated by black rules and standards, they would be equally disadvantaged because they were different.

But, differences are all too frequently translated into deficiencies by teachers. This results in the problem of *teacher expectations.* Rosenthal and Jacobson (1968) have demonstrated that when teachers are told that children are in some way intellectually inferior, their behavior towards these children will change in subtle ways which will bring about the expected intellectual performance. Children who are labeled as *slow* will achieve slowly, and children who are labeled as *superior* will exhibit superior performance. This is true even when the label that is assigned is selected by the flip of a coin, rather than by a standard test (Rosenthal and Jacobson, 1968).

The treatment of minority children as if they were inferior rather than merely different initiates a self-fulfilling prophecy of academic failure for them. Terms such as *culturally deprived* and *culturally disadvantaged* certainly contribute to this problem. While they avoid the unsupportable notion that minorities have high rates of academic failure because they are genetically inferior to whites, they substitute the implication that it is because they come from an *inferior* culture. This debilitating ethnocentrism can be avoided through the use of terms like *culturally different* or *minority group* which simply acknowledge the existence of differences. Teachers must be convinced that minority children are not culturally inferior so they will stop treating them as such.

Compounding the problem of cultural difference is the fact that most of these children are actually disadvantaged in the economic sense. Most white children have an edge in terms of housing, nutrition, travel, books, movies, the presence of economically successful models, etc. But, while improvements in the economic conditions among minorities would eliminate many of the barriers to academic success, there are many problems based on cultural differences that will still remain and must be dealt with. Seemingly, there are two courses of action that should be followed in dealing with the clash of cultures in the classroom. First, in as many areas as possible, schools must make the shift from white institutions to *multicultural* ones. In most cases, cultural differences can simply be accepted. If cultural differences do not interfere with educational or occupational success in any real way, there is no justification for not accepting them.

In many cases, however, it *appears* necessary to modify some of the behaviors of minority children in order for them to conform with the dominant culture of the school and society at large. This is not a decision that should be made lightly, but should be carefully considered with two facts in mind.

First, the white culture is dominant economically. While there will probably be continued moves towards a more multicultural character for the economic system, as well as towards stronger development of separate minority economic systems, the long-range economic future of minority cultures would seem to rest on full integration into the main business community. While most cultural differences are becoming less important as impediments to this integration (dress, etc.), certain behaviors are essential to full economic parity: among them are reading, mathematical behaviors, etc. Equal economic opportunity will depend on equal facility in these areas.

Secondly, much of the outcry against the modification of the behavior of minority children stems from a misunderstanding of what is meant by the term *modification*. Any educational process modifies the behavior of the child. No one is suggesting that minority children should not be educated, which means that no one is suggesting that the behavior of minority children should not be modified. The real issue is which behaviors should be changed. If the primary guideline is a genuine respect for the cultural heritage as well as for the future of the child, clear choices should be possible.

For example, teaching the black child to read would seem to be a legitimate educational goal as it would contribute to his future well-being in a way that does not interfere with his culture. Teaching him a white-puritanical pattern of emotional behavior, on the other hand, would not necessarily contribute to his future happiness and might violate his cultural heritage. Such decisions, however, should not be unilaterally made by whites.

LANGUAGE DIFFERENCES

One aspect of the behavioral differences of minority group children that has been frequently singled out as a problem area of particular importance is language (Bernstein, 1970; Bereiter and Engelmann, 1966; Deutsch, 1965). The languages of the several American cultures differ in many respects; and because language is almost universally held to be a fundamental skill in academic and vocational achievement, minority children are felt to be at a disadvantage because of their linguistic differences (which, again, most observers translate into *deficits*).

But, while this is a widely held position among educators and other professionals, the supporting data for it leaves much to be desired. Many of the issues involved in the position are still very much up in the air. The two most obvious questions to which no well supported answers can be given are: how do the languages of the several cultures differ? And, which of these differences, if any, are educationally and vocationally important? It is critically important that much of the data that has been recently acquired does not support the traditional heurisms about these questions.

While most of the following studies have focused on black-white langauge differences, the methods, and to some extent the findings, are relevant to the whole question of cultural difference.

Hart (1969), Caselli (1970), Labov (1970), and Houston (1970) have suggested, and in some cases demonstrated, that while Child Black English differs from Child White English in many respects, the differences are not the traditionally suggested ones.

Grammatical Mistakes

These investigators have pointed out that most white teachers feel that black children *make a lot of grammatical mistakes* when they talk. A knowledge of the language patterns of black children shows this notion to be false. The deviations from white English patterns are not random errors, but represent systematic differences in the dialects. When black children are correctly speaking Child Black English, they will produce a lot of sentences that will contain *errors* by the standards of Child White English. The fact that they are correctly speaking a different dialect implies that they are not the *lazy, error prone* speakers their teachers took them to be. They make no more errors in their dialect than white children make in theirs.

The verb form *be* provides a good example of a dialect usage difference which is often interpreted as a *careless grammatical error*. The verb *be* is used in two usage patterns in black English. Because these patterns differ from white English in complex ways, the occurrence of the word often appears *random* to the naive observer.

As the equivalent of will be or would be

In conversational white English, auxiliary verbs are frequently contracted. For example, the sentences

He will be coming later.
He would be coming later.

are usually spoken as

He'll be coming later.
He'd be coming later.

In black English, the contracted suffix is dropped altogether, and the sentences both become

He be coming later.

This is an instance in which black English is grammatically less complex and flexible than white English. The difference in meaning of the *will-would* contrast must be expressed in some way other than the verb phrase. This is also a point on which speakers of the two dialects may fail to communicate. The addition of will or would to the verb phrase carries no meaning to the speaker of black English.

Intrinsic and extrinsic predication

In many languages, a grammatical distinction is made between statements of inherent or usual situations (intrinsic) and adventitious or atypical ones (extrinsic). For example, in Japanese, a predicate postposition is used to distinguish between intrinsic and extrinsic statements.

(a) He - wa is a good man. (Intrinsic)
(b) He - ga is a good man. (Extrinsic)

Sentence (a) states the fact that the man referred to is known to be consistently good. Sentence (b) states that a typically bad man is, for a change, being good (McNeil, 1966).

Black English uses the verb form *be* to make this distinction.

(c) He going to the store. (Intrinsic)
(d) He be going to the store. (Extrinsic)

Sentence (c) would be said about a man who regularly goes to the store (every morning because he works there, for example). Sentence (d) would be said about a man for whom it would be very unusual to go to the store. White English does not contain this grammatical distinction. This is an instance in which white English is grammatically less complex and flexible than black English.

Distinct Language Repertoires

Labov (1970) and Houston (1970) have pointed to another difficulty in assessing black-white language differences. In many segments of the black culture, young black children are often virtually mute in the presence of adults, especially white, high status adults. When they talk at all, it is usually in the form of single-word or short, semigrammatical utterances. This is the view of Child Black English held by most preschool and primary-grade teachers, because this is what they hear.

Labov and Houston argue, however, that this is not a true picture of Child Black English, but is an artifact of the adult-child situation. Although their interpretations of the phenomenon vary, they agree on two essential points: First, black children do not have one but have at least two distinct language repertoires (Houston calls them *registers*): a meager one used in schools, interviews and similar situations, and a complex, sophisticated one used among family and peers. It is only the school repertoire that most teachers hear. Secondly, these authors agree that while difficult, it is possible to produce the nonschool repertoire in school situations. This will be a key point in the discussions of language modification that follow.

Some examples may make the differences between the two repertoires a bit more clear. The following dialogues are excerpts from an interview between a black adult (CR) and two eight-year-old black New York ghetto children taken from Labov (1970, pp. 159-161). The school repertoire is evident in the first two discussions.

CR: What if you saw somebody kickin' somebody else on the ground, or was using a stick, what would you do if you saw that?
Leon: Mmmm.
CR: If it was supposed to be a fair fight—
Leon: I don' know.
CR: You don' know? Would you do anything? . . . huh? I can't hear you.
Leon: No.

CR: Did you ever see somebody get beat up real bad?
Leon: . . . Nope . . .
CR: Well—uh—did you ever get into a fight with a guy?
Leon: Nope.
CR: That was bigger than you?
Leon: Nope . . .
CR: You never been in a fight?
Leon: Nope.
CR: Nobody ever pick on you?
Leon: Nope.
CR: Nobody ever hit you?
Leon: Nope.
CR: How come?
Leon: Ah 'on' know.
CR: Didn't you ever hit somebody?
Leon: Nope.
CR: (incredulously) You never hit nobody?
Leon: Mhm.

Because the topic of fighting is an emotional one, the interviewer switched to a more neutral one, but the school repertoire is still evident.

CR: Well, what's your favorite one? What's your favorite program?
Leon: Superman . .
CR: Yeah? Did you see Superman—ah—yesterday, or day before yesterday? When's the last time you saw Superman?
Leon: Sa-aturday . . .
CR—You rem—you saw it Saturday? What was the story all about? You remember the story?
Leon: M-m.
CR: You don't remember the story of what—that you saw of Superman?
Leon: Nope.
CR: You don't remember what happened, huh?
Leon: Hm-m.
CR: I see—ah—what other stories do you like to watch on TV?
Leon: Mmmm? . . . umm . . . (glottalization)
CR: Hmmm? (four seconds)
Leon: Hh?
CR: What's th' other stories that you like to watch?
Leon: Mi-ighty Mouse . . .
CR: and what else?
Leon: Ummm . . . ahm . . .

Later, when the adult has become a discriminative stimulus for the nonschool repertoire, a marked change can be seen. An explanatory footnote from Labov (1970) accompanies the segment.

CR: What that?
Greg: Black boy! (Leon crunching on potato chips)
Oh that's a *M.B.B.*
CR: *M.B.B.* What's that?
Greg: 'Merican Black Boy.
CR: Ohh . . .
Greg: Anyway, 'Mericans is same like white people, right?
Leon: And they talk about Allah.
CR: Oh yeah?
Greg: Yeah.
CR: What they say about Allah?
Leon: Allah—Allah is God.
Greg: Allah—
CR: And what else?
Leon: I don' know the res'.
Greg: Allah i—Allah is God, Allah is the only God, Allah . . .
Leon: Allah is the *son* of God.
Greg: But can he make magic?
Leon: Nope.
Greg: I know who can make magic.
CR: Who can?
Leon: The God, the *real* one.
CR: Who can make magic?
Greg: The son of po'—(CR: Hm?) I'm sayin' the po'k chop God! He only a po'k chop God!* (Leon chuckles).

If there are at least two languages for every black speaker, how much do we actually know about the language differences of black and white children? Seemingly, most of the previously identified differences are based on studies of the school repertoire only. Their findings are artifacts, in part, of the child-adult interview situation.

---

* The reference to the *pork chop God* condenses several concepts of black nationalism current in the Harlem community. A *pork chop* is a Negro who has not lost the traditional subservient ideology of the South, who has no knowledge of himself in Muslim terms, and the *pork chop God* would be the traditional God of Southern Baptists. He and His followers may be pork chops, but He still holds the power in Leon and Gregory's world.

Some recent data elaborate this point. While suggesting that there probably are some important lexical differences, Houston (1970) makes the following observations about the nonschool repertoire of black children from a rural area of northern Florida:

> In my study I observed fewer than a half-dozen main syntactic divergences between the target language and standard English, although these divergences occur frequently in speech. Other differences between the nonstandard and standard varients of language were phonological (Houston, 1970; p. 954).

A recent investigation by Hart (1969) suggests a similar picture. This study provides the most complete descriptive data to date on black preschool children. The subjects were five female and seven male black preschool children. They all lived within a 1½ mile radius in an urban, low-income area of Kansas City, Kansas. The children were selected on the basis of low family income, large family size and/or problem behaviors.

The children attended the experimental Turner House preschool program directed by Todd Risley of the University of Kansas (Reynolds and Risley, 1968; Hart and Risley, 1968; Risley, 1967). They were in school from 9:30 a.m.-12:30 p.m. for five days per week. Their daily schedule included breakfast, a thirty-minute indoor free-play period, music and rhythms, story reading, a thirty-minute outdoor free-play period, and an indoor group-instruction period. Data was collected during the two free-play periods.

Each day a fifteen-minute language sample was recorded for each child. Everything that each child said during this period was written down by one of three adult recorders. Each recorder observed four children throughout the school year. Observations were rotated systematically so that each child was observed early and late during the play periods, and both indoors and outdoors. In addition to writing down in longhand everything that the child said, each utterance was coded as to whether it was directed to a peer, the teacher, or had no observable direction.

When one of the children was absent, the observer for that child recorded the language of one of the other children. At the end of the observation, the records of the regular and the second observer were compared to assess inter-observer reliability. In all cases, reliability was extremely high.

This procedure was continued for thirty-four school days. It provides, therefore, a very large sample of Child Black English. No comparable sample exists for white children. Comparisons with white English are made with large samples gathered by Templin (1957) and Young (1941) using interview procedures. In these studies, data was gathered in a single interview with an adult who engaged the child in a more or less standard conversation. The sole exception is Smith (1926) who recorded the language of a sample of four-year-olds during one hour of free-play.

Turner House Data

Figure VII.1 shows the total number of words recorded for each child during the thirty-four days of the baseline phase of the Turner House project. The most striking features of these data are the large individual differences. The child for whom the largest number of words was recorded uttered 27,000 words during the approximately eight hours of observation time while the child for whom the smallest was recorded uttered only 2,100. These differences are not out of line, however, with previous studies of middle-income white children. Smith (1926) found the four-year-olds uttered a mean of four hundred words during an hour of free-play with a range from zero (no words recorded at all) to 1,100 words. The findings of Hart (1969) also show that the median child averaged about one hundred words in fifteen minutes.

A great deal can be learned, however, from careful analysis of the individual differences found in Hart (1969). Figure VII.2 shows the total number of *different* words recorded for each subject. Again, the individual differences are striking, but there are some revealing differences between Figure VII.1 (total number of words) and Figure VII.2 (total number of different words). First, note that a greater proportion of the individual differences in Figure VII.1 can be accounted for by differences in the *other* category (adjectives, prepositions, conjunctions, articles, etc.) than in Figure VII.2. This

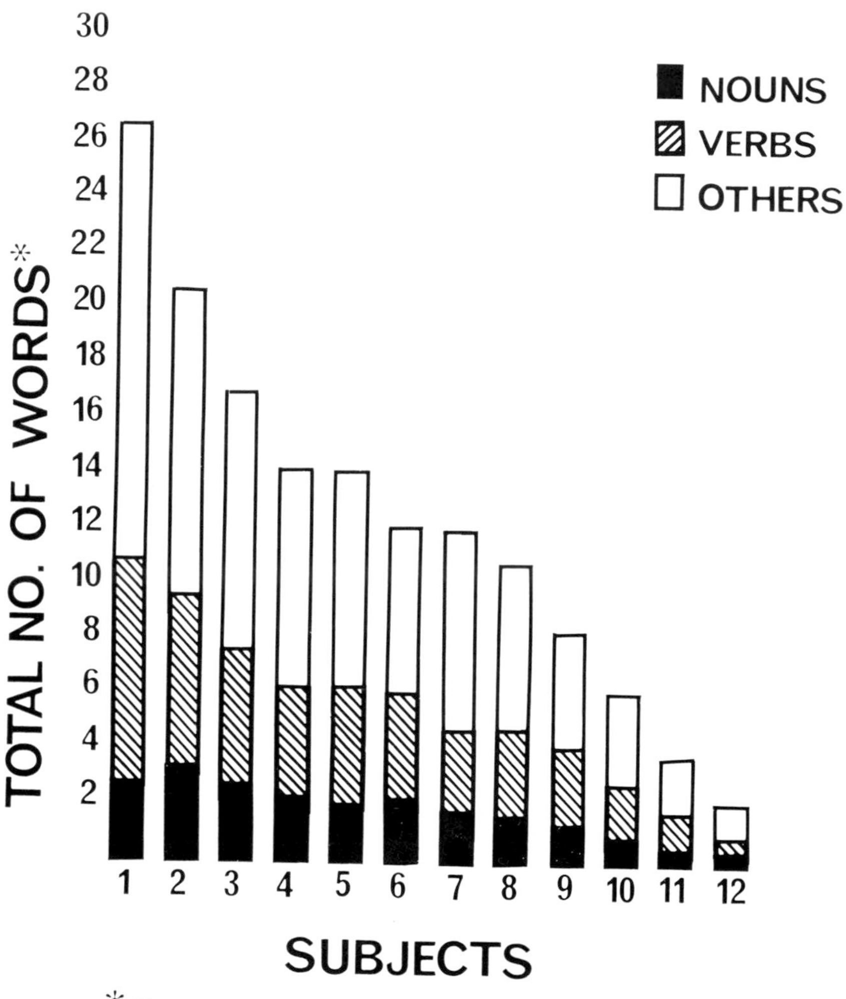

Figure VII.1. Total number of words recorded for each child during the thirty-four days of baseline observation.

indicates that words from the *other* category are frequently repeated by those children who spoke a large number of words, but were infrequently repeated by those children who spoke few words. Since these words are connectives and modifiers, it suggests that the children who used a greater number of words were using

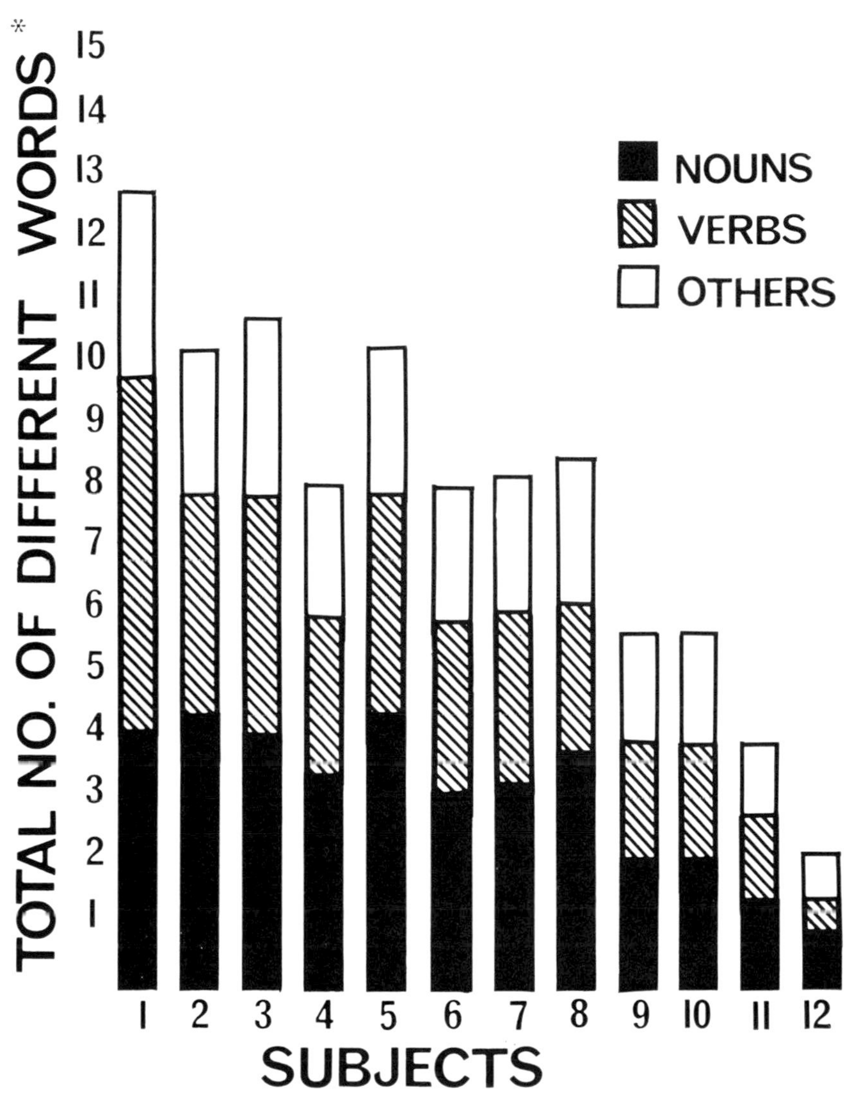

Figure VII.2. Total number of different words recorded for each child during the thirty-four days of baseline observation. Note that the scale for Figure VII.2 is different from that for Figure VII.1.

TABLE VII.I

MEAN LENGTH OF UTTERANCE

Subjects

	1	*2*	*3*	*4*	*5*	*6*	*7*	*8*	*9*	*10*	*11*	*12*
Length of simple utterance:												
1-3 words	3269	2382	1620	1600	1243	1697	1473	1647	1621	651	1747	181
4-6 words	3001	2218	1827	1665	1414	1339	886	1211	958	679	235	254
7-9 words	566	522	435	252	403	242	119	138	54	104	1	8
10+ words	50	51	47	24	64	22	13	13	3	13	0	13
Average words	3.8	3.9	4.1	3.9	4.2	3.7	3.7	3.4	3.1	3.9	2.1	4.0
Length of compound utterance:												
3-6 words	20	17	7	3	9	13	7	2	6	2	0	0
7-9 words	27	21	23	12	35	4	21	12	3	4	1	1
10-12 words	39	40	51	34	50	32	17	24	16	25	1	26
13+ words	16	27	27	15	41	3	0	3	2	10	0	4
Average words	9.5	14.4	10.9	11.0	10.9	9.6	9.8	8.9	9.5	11.5	10.0	11.4
All sentences, average words	3.9	4.0	4.3	4.1	4.5	3.8	4.9	3.6	3.2	4.2	2.8	4.3

them in more complex sentences. This is corroborated by the data on mean length of utterance. Table VII.I shows that the children who spoke the greatest number of words tended also to have the longest mean utterance.

The fact that the rank order of the total number of different works (Figure VII.2) and the mean length of utterance (Table VII.I) differs from that of the total number of words (Figure VII.1) shows that while those subjects who had the highest rate of talking (the greatest total number of words) also tended to use the greatest variety of words and the longest utterances, the relationship was not perfect.

The absence of a direct analysis of the grammar of the recorded utterances by Hart (1969) makes more specific statements impossible, but several comparisons can be made. Templin (1957, p. 79) found that average number of words in the five longest utterances of a four and one-half-year-old lower economic level white children was about ten and was about twelve for upper-economic level children. In Hart (1969), five utterances of thirteen or more words were recorded for six of the twelve children, and a considerable number of simple and compound utterances of ten to twelve words were recorded (Table VII.I). In terms of the occurrence of lengthy utterances, therefore, the children in Hart's study do not appear to differ from middle-income white children.

The comments of Hart suggest that comparisons of *mean* length of utterance tell a different story, however.

> In terms of the mean length of remark, however, the children in the present study fall below the means given in comparison data. The mean length of all remarks (both simple and compound) for the group of twelve children in the present study was 4.0 words, with a range from 2.8 (child 11) to 4.9 words per sentence (see Table VII.I). The average sentence length across all reliability samples for both prime and second observers was 3.7 words (range 2.0 to 4.4 words). In Templin's data (1957, p. 79) the mean number of words per remark for 4½-year-olds of upper socio-economic status was 6.1, and for 4½-year-olds of lower socio-economic status, 5.1 words per remark. Templin found that the sentences from her sample of children were longer than those from McCarthy's (1930) sample; McCarthy found 4.6 words per sentence for [lower-income] children. Young (1941) found that the relief children in her study also used a mean of 4.5 words per sentence, while her [middle-income] children used

> a mean of 5.2 words per sentence. In terms of all of these comparison data, the children of the present study are shown to use in general shorter sentences, shorter even than the sentences used by the [lower-income] children in those studies. This finding may be to some extent the result of differences in sampling: in the present study the children's speech was sampled for a much longer period than in any of the other studies, and the children's verbalizations were recorded when directed both to children and adults. Consequently no firm conclusions concerning a deficit in sentence length can be drawn for the disadvantaged population of the present study, though there are indications of a general abbreviation of sentence for these children as compared to their [middle-income white] peers. Such abbreviation may be related to the lack of elaboration in the speech of [black children], as observed by Hess and Shipman (1965); exactly what is added to his average sentence by a [middle-income white], however, so that it tends to be one to two words longer than the average sentence of a [black] child, remains to be sought in further analysis (Hart, 1969, pp. 74-75).

Because of the differences in procedure, it is difficult to make comparisons between Hart (1969) and the previous studies on the size of vocabulary. It appears, however, that at least some of the children in this population are not deficient in vocabulary. Again, Hart's observations are relevant:

> . . . Forty percent of all the 1,187 different nouns recorded across the group of twelve children, and 40% of all the 248 adjectives recorded across the group, were recorded for only one of the twelve children; about 25% of all the different nouns and adjectives were recorded only once for a single child. These findings concur with those of Uhrbrock (1936) who recorded 24,000 words from a child just prior to her fifth birthday; in his sample, 40% of the total number of different words occurred only once. In the present sample, 83% of all different nouns, 74% of all the different adjectives, and 65% of all the different verbs among the children were recorded for half or less of the twelve children. Only 3% of all the different nouns, 8% of all the different adjectives, and 6% of all the different verbs were recorded for all twelve children. When it is considered that the twelve children in the present study were of a common culture, all of them resident within the same 1½ square mile area, and that their language was sampled within an identical preschool stimulus environment, these small percentages of common vocabulary content imply the existence of much larger total vocabularies (in terms of recognition) among these children. The total vocabulary in usage . . . may be but a very small portion of the total vocabulary potentially available to these

children. More will be said on this point in the discussion of the relation of frequency of sampling to total recorded vocabulary (Hart, 1969, pp. 107-108).

An additional comparison was made by Hart (1969) that is relevant to the question of syntactical complexity. Figure VII.3 shows a comparison of the proportion of several parts of speech for the black preschool children of Hart (1969) and the middle income white children of Templin (1957) and McCarthy (1930). The results show slightly greater proportions of nouns and verbs and slightly smaller proportions of prepositions, pronouns and *other* parts of speech for the black children. The three groups are about equal on the proportion of adjectives. These data suggest that the greater mean length of utterance in middle-income children does reflect greater elaboration and complexity as suggested by Hess and Shipman (1965).

These data should be interpreted with caution, however. Hart (1969) noted that slightly different methods of classifying parts of speech were used by the three investigators, therefore the differ-

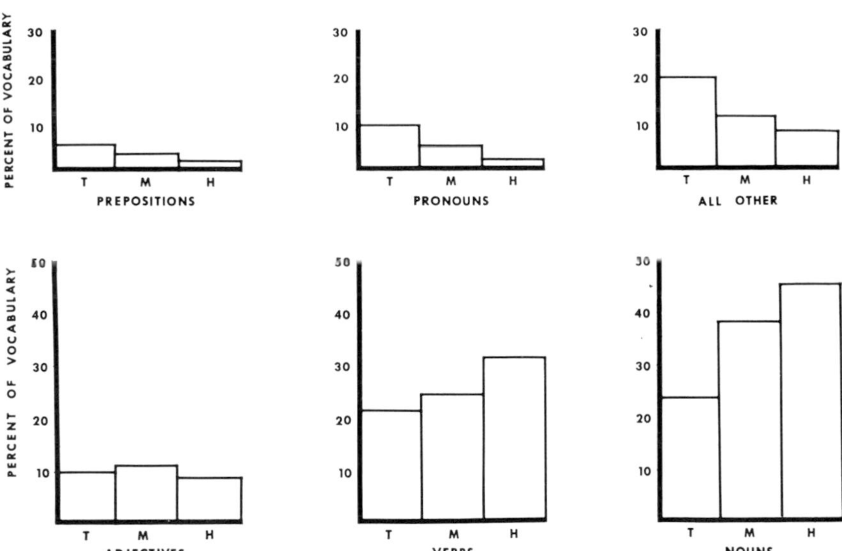

Figure VII.3. Comparison of the proportions of parts of speech found by Templin (1957) for 4½-year-olds, McCarthy (1930) for three to eight-year-olds, and Hart (1970) for preschool age children.

ences in proportions may not be reliable. Secondly, it should be noted that Templin (1957) and McCarthy (1930) differ between themselves almost as much as they do with Hart (1969). Firm conclusions based on these data would be unwarranted.

Finally, Hart (1969) commented on the relationship between language measures, sex, and IQ scores. Young (1941) found a relationship between mean length of utterance and IQ, but no such relationship was found for the Turner House children. Hart (1969) did find a relationship between sex and mean length of utterance as was reported by Templin (1957) and Young (1941). Four of the five girls were recorded as having a mean length of utterance at or above the group average of four words, whereas only three of the seven boys had mean length of utterances of four words or more.

Summary of Turner House Data

Hart (1969) provides data that is inconsistent with the frequently painted picture of the black child as an almost totally nonverbal person, speaking only in short, fragmentary utterances. All of the children in the Turner House sample were observed to use full, grammatical utterances (Hart, 1969, p. 88). Large individual differences were found among these children, but they were no larger than those found among middle-income white children.

As expected, some differences between Black and White Child English were found. The Turner House children spoke utterances that contained, on the average, fewer words, with a higher proportion of nouns and verbs and a lower proportion of pronouns, prepositions, and other parts of speech. No differences were found on any other measured aspect of their language. In spite of these differences, however, it appears that the unobtrusive observational technique used in Turner House was successful in obtaining a measure of the nonschool repertoire of these children.

It should also be noted that these children (who lived in Kansas) represent a relatively mobile segment of black Americans. Larger differences may be found by studying blacks who are more isolated from whites (e.g., those living in inner-city ghettos) or who live in more traditional areas of black concentration (e.g., the Southeast).

Logical Inadequacy

Labov (1970) has also attacked the belief that black English is grammatically inadequate for the expression of logical propositions. This view sees black English as a *simplified* (and therefore less logically flexible) version of white English. In considering this belief two points should be made.

First, most existing studies that suggest the logical inadequacy performed under the assumption that the school repertoire *is* black English (e.g., Bereiter and Engelmann, 1970). The nonschool repertoire is certainly grammatically and logically sparse.

Secondly, most speakers of white English often find it difficult to translate statements in black English (even the nonschool repertoire) into logically equivalent white English forms. The reverse is also frequently true for black speakers. This leads to the conclusion that black English statements are illogical.

While the first point suggests that the reports of logical inadequacy are merely artifacts of the conditions of the studies, the second point deserves more consideration. Are the difficulties of translation and communication due to a basic logical deficiency on the part of black English? In a detailed analysis of sizeable samples of the nonschool repertoire of black children, Labov (1970) provides strong evidence that the two languages are logically equivalent although grammaticaly different. He has concluded that any proposition that can be expressed in white English can be expressed in black English, and vice versa, even though it would be expressed differently in the two languages.

Many of the grammatical differences believed to be logical stumbling blocks in black English are, in fact, also characteristic of many foreign languages. For example, the omission of the present copula *(they mine)* is also characteristic of Russian, Hungarian and Arabic. The use of double negatives *(He don't know nothing)* is also characteristic of Russian, Spanish, French and Hungarian and was characteristic of Anglo-Saxon. Certainly these languages are not logically inadequate. The problems of translation faced by the nonspeaker of black English would appear to be the same as for the nonspeaker of any different language, rather than a difference in logical adequacy.

Furthermore, Labov suggests that much of what passes for the greater logical complexity of white English, may merely be stylistic complexity.

> All too often, standard English is represented by a style that is simultaneously overparticular and vague. The accumulating flow of words buries rather than strikes the target. It is this verbosity which is most easily taught and most easily learned, so that words take the place of thoughts, and nothing can be found behind them (Labov 1970, p. 171).

Far from helping black children to *think better* by giving them a more logical language, white teachers seem to have been imposing on them the cumbersome verbosity of whites. More importantly, however, the assumption of logical inadequacy has probably added to the problems of debilitating teacher expectations (Rosenthal and Jacobson, 1968).

Teaching White English as a Foreign Language

With the growing awareness that black English is an equivalent language to white English rather than an inferior language, has come the point of view that the language of black children (and other cultural minorities) should not be modified in preschool and elementary education. Rather, the education of these children should be carried out in their own language, with white English only being taught to those who wish it during secondary education as a *foreign language* that is a useful economic skill (see for example, Caselli, 1970; Fasold and Shuy, 1970). This view is based on several arguments.

First, traditional methods for changing the language of cultural minorities have not been effective. Teachers have set as one of their main objectives teaching minority children *how to talk,* but they have been conspicuously ineffective (Bailey, 1968; Shuy, 1968).

Second, because schooling is carried out in white English, minority children have to learn a second langauge *and then* acquire the educational fundamentals required of them. White children, on the other hand, need only acquire the latter skills. The early education of black children, this argument runs, would be better carried out in the minority language.

Third, the traditional (and present) approach to changing the language of minority children is to punish non-white usage and to expect white usage as a matter of course (i.e., to not reinforce it; one does not reinforce a child for doing *what he should be doing anyway*). It is small wonder that these methods lead to a suppression of language behavior on the part of the minority child, and probably contribute to a generalized suppression of all academic behavior. Shaming children for ethnocentrically-defined errors is no way to conduct the educational process.

Fourth, there is the possibility that by modifying the language of the young minority child he will be made *different* from his culture, and thus *alienated* from it. While this is largely an unsupported speculation (due to an absence of data), Labov (1970) has noted that the black children who succeed in school are usually the ones who are not accepted by their cultural peers.

The position taken in this chapter is that language modification is needed both in the preschool and the high school. Using behavior modification techniques, educationally important changes can be efficiently made in the preschool. If the other, educationally unimportant, language differences can be accepted in the elementary schools, then integrated education could be carried out without problem. Those minority children who choose to do so, could later learn full white English as a foreign language in high school. It is extremely important to restrict the preschool language changes to only those changes which are essential and will not alienate the child from his family and peers.

Language Modification in the Preschool

Researchers in the area of language modification with minority group children have been pulling themselves up by their own bootstraps. While in the process of gathering descriptive data which would allow sound decisions on which aspects of minority language should be changed, they have simultaneously been developing techniques of language modification. This means that in the beginning, researchers had to select aspects of language to be modified more on the basis of common sense than prior research. We are not much beyond that stage today. Fortunately, most earlier researchers used three critieria for selecting language features for modification: (1) the features appeared to be educationally relevant, but culturally neutral, (2) the features appeared to be ones for which there is an actual cultural difference, and (3) most importantly, the modifications were ones that are educationally desirable independent of the culture of the child, white or minority.

General Aspects of Speaking in the School

While the modification of detailed aspects of the linguistic repertoires of children will occupy most of this section of the chapter, there are several general aspects of speaking in minority children which often must be modified as well. These include such simple, but educationally significant, aspects as polite greetings, discrimination of appropriate occasions for talking in class, etc.

> Some of the behavior we tried to teach the children at first may seem trivial. For example, we spent considerable time teaching them to say *good morning* to their teachers. This may not seem the stuff from which successful scholars are made. However, the child who says *good morning* cheerfully and consistently when he arrives at school will dispose most teachers quite favorably toward him—our own teachers testified to this during the experiment—and the credit he gains may survive a good deal of academic bumbling later in the day. This credit is useful, because it may make the teacher more likely to praise approximations of learning in the child. A similar rationale lay behind several other *social* projects, such as teaching the child to be quiet in some work situations and to converse in others, and to raise his hand and wait to be recognized before speaking in group discussions (Risley, 1967, p. 140).

Instituting appropriate use of *good morning* was one of the goals of the experimental preschool designed and supervised by Todd Risley. Their first step was to take a baseline measure of the frequency of *good mornings*. Three teachers were stationed at the door each morning and greeted each child with a smile and a *good morning*. Initially, the children responded in kind only about twenty percent of the time. The teachers reinforced each of these responses with social praise, and found an increase in the proportion of children responding with *good morning* to seventy to eighty percent.

When it was felt that a stable level of responding had been

reached, the durability of the response was tested by withdrawing the teacher's initiation of the greeting. They continued to stand in the door, and continued to reinforce the children with praise when they said *good morning,* but they no longer said *good morning* themselves. The proportion of children saying, *good morning* dropped immediately, fluctuated for six days, and then dropped to zero. The intent of these teachers was to modify the behavior of the children so that they would say *good morning* even if they were not greeted first, so a more potent reinforcer was introduced.

In addition to social praise, each teacher gave the child an M&M each time he greeted her appropriately. The proportion of children saying *good morning* rose immediately to 100 percent and remained there. The question of durability still remains, however:

> The public school, of course, does not offer M&Ms for desirable behavior. However, our results indicate the need for something more powerful than friendly approval to establish durable behavior in the children, especially if the behavior is to remain despite minimal stimulus support. Had we not run out of time, we would have begun shifting the behavior maintained by candy to the control of social approval only, a process that requires consistent social reinforcement combined with a gradual cutback on the distribution of candy (Risley, 1967, p. 141).

Other examples of the need to modify these general aspects of speaking can be drawn from the author's personal experience. One case involved a four-year-old black male enrolled in a Head Start program who did not talk at all in the classroom. Conferences with his parents and his playmates indicated that he spoke normally away from school and had never before been mute in any other situation, except for normal *shyness* when meeting new people.

It was felt that some aspect of the classroom situation was producing his silence. During a day of observing the child, it was noticed that the teachers were trying very hard to, as they explained it, *to make the child feel welcome.* Every few minutes, one of them would go over to the table where the child spent each day and read a story to him, give him an extra cookie, etc., all with accompanying warm smiles.

It was suggested to the teachers that it might be their efforts to help the child that were holding him back. Perhaps his relatively normal silence during the first days of school was reinforced and maintained by their attention. Rather than trying to deal with what they imputed the child's *feelings* to be, the teachers were convinced to remove their social reinforcement of the child's silence and ignore him completely until he began speaking in class. The child began moving about the classroom following the teachers and aides on the second day of the program, spoke his first word on the third day (which was reinforced by social attention), and was speaking normally by the fifth day.

A second example also comes from a Head Start classroom. One deficiency in children's speaking in the classroom that seems both widespread and widely ignored is the failure of many children to learn to speak in groups. In this particular Head Start class, the children were divided daily in small groups of six to eight for sessions which involved group recitation of short poems and songs, group labeling of pictures, etc. Almost invariably these groups contain one or two children who rarely or never joined in with the others. Instead they stared about or busied themselves with their own activities. These are frequently the same children who do not know the answer when called upon individually.

Because the ability to speak in group situations is essential to the educational process, a proceduce was initiated to institute group speaking in one of these children. While a volunteer took over the rest of her group, an aide began working individually with the child who participated least well in the group activity. The child was individually taught to perform the verbal tasks used in the group by the aide through prompting and reinforcement. He quickly acquired these behaviors in a one-on-one situation, and after about ten days the second phase of the procedure was begun. Another child who participated well in the group was introduced into the one-on-one situation. This produced a transient disruption in the first child's verbal behavior, but he was quickly back to complete participation. During the ensuing three weeks, the five remaining children were introduced one at a time, several days apart, without disruption to the first child's performance. At the end of this period, the aide had all of her group back, all of whom now participated.

These techniques could, of course, be applied to many other

general aspects of speaking. The techniques mentioned serve only as examples.

Training Parents to Modify Their Children's Language Behavior

With recent advances in techniques of behavior modification, time and personnel seem to be the major obstacles to effective remedial programs. Knowing what needs to be done and how to do it is useless if the personnel to carry out the program are not available. Limited availability of funds makes this frequently the case. The training of parents to carry out modification programs on their own children is one solution to this problem.

In parent-training programs the time of professionally trained personnel can often be put to much better use than in working with children on an individual basis. Usually a large number of parents can be trained to effectively carry out simple programs in a short period of time. In addition, modifying the home environment can be expected to have a more lasting effect than a program that is only carried out in the school. Risley (1967) used such a parent-training program in one of his experimental preschool programs.

Several contingencies were placed on the behavior of the parents. First, although the parents of thirty, four-year-old children volunteered for the program, their attendance was reinforced with a set of dishes, dispensed one dish per week. More importantly, the parents received praise from the teachers for appropriate teaching behaviors, but did not when they reverted to their typical teaching behaviors.

During an initial observation period, the parents were observed to have many maladaptive teaching behaviors.

> At first, the mothers were poor teachers. They used almost no praise or approval, and they showed very little grasp of the technique of attacking a complex problem starting with its simplest form. Their usual pattern was to present a difficult problem and then to punish errors or silence with nagging or threats. They told the child to sit up, to pay attention; they informed him that they knew he knew the answer, so he had better say it (Risley, 1967, p. 145).

That is, the parents did not use shaping and positive reinforcement of appropriate behavior, but relied on the unproductive strategy of punishing inappropriate behavior.

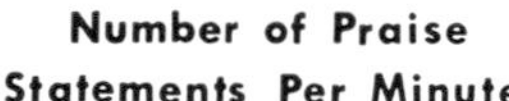
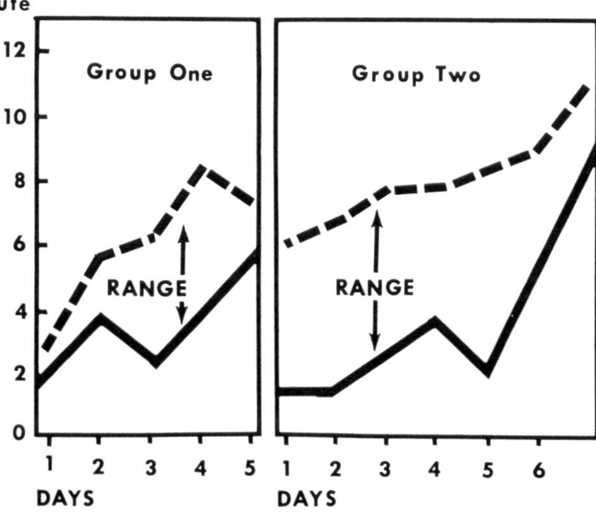

Figure VII.4. Change in frequency of mothers' use of praise in teaching their children in the preschool.

The parents were then asked to participate in a series of lessons with a child (initially a child other than their own) and were given detailed instructions on how to teach. Early lessons included object naming. The parents were instructed to:

> Hold up an object in front of the child. Say "Can you tell me what this is?" Praise him by saying "Good for you!" if he names it right (Risley, 1967, p. 145).

In addition, a teacher was stationed behind the child in sight of the mother. Whenever the mother reinforced appropriately she was in turn reinforced by a light flashing by the teacher. Figure VII.4 shows the results of this program. The frequency of appropriate social reinforcement increased markedly in a short period of time for all of the mothers.

Producing the Nonschool Repertoire in the Classroom

A major portion of the introductory sections of this chapter were devoted to the observation that black children frequently use a much more extensive language outside of the classroom (the nonschool repertoire) than they do in it. Few investigations, however, have sought ways to produce the nonschool repertoire in the classroom. One part of the Risley preschool experiments is relevant to this problem, though.

Although it was not known to what extent the school and nonschool repertoires differed for the Turner House children, a child who was very non-verbal was chosen as the subject for an experimental technique (Risley, 1967). Their prior observations, and the results of the procedure, suggest that this child had an especially large discrepancy between his school and nonschool repertoires.

The procedure developed to bring the nonschool repertoire into use was a combination of prompting and reinforcement. A baseline measure of the child's language was taken before the start of the procedure. Over a period of thirteen days, the child was repeatedly asked five questions, such as, "Who do you like to play with?" The total number of words, total number of different words, and the mean length of utterances used by the child were recorded during baseline. The latter measure turned out to be a meager 1.5 words per answer.

Then training was begun by the teacher:

> Then the teacher began training. She asked, "What did you see on the way to school?" When she prompted the boy's answers with "What else," he simply repeated one- and two-word answers, alternating between the two responses, "A doggie" and "TV," and repeating the pair over and over.
>
> When it had become clear that this pattern was not likely to change by itself, the teacher provided a more logical prompt: "What kind of doggie?" The boy replied that it was a German shepherd, and the teacher praised him and gave him a bit of snack. Then she asked again what he saw on the way to school. He answered, "A doggie." At this point, the teacher raised her eyebrows, cocked her head, and waited. Presently the child amended his answer: "A German shepherd doggie," and was praised and fed.
>
> When the original question was asked again, with the reply "A German shepherd doggie," the child was given a second prompt: the teacher asked what the doggie was doing. In this way the training proceeded, with the teacher prompting each logical step, waiting for all previous steps to be chained together in reasonable sequence, and reinforcing only increasingly long and meaningfully connected se-

quences. The child's average answer to this first question eventually rose to about 200 words per ten-minute sessions, which amounted to about fifty words per session if duplications were eliminated.

When the teacher asked a new question, "What do you do when you go home from school?" The child's answer showed that he had profited from the training on the first question; therefore, the teacher reduced her logical prompts and asked simply, "what else" or "what then," while continuing to dispense praise and snacks only for more and more elaborate phrases (Risley, 1967, pp. 142-143).

In all, five questions were used in the prompting and reinforcement training procedure. After each of the questions, five new questions were asked on which the child had not received training. These were answered in full, meaningful discourse, with an average length of over 7.5 words, more than five times greater than given to the questions asked in baseline.

Although marked improvements occurred in this child's school language, there was doubt as to the accuracy of the answers in some cases. Improperly applied, this technique could produce elaborate lying. To counter this possibility, the last of the five questions was chosen so that a check could easily be made on the accuracy of the answers. The child was asked, "What have you been doing at school today?" Only accurate elaborations were reinforced during this phase. Answers continued to grow longer and progressively more accurate.

Modification of Specific Linguistic Forms

The most complete and detailed study of the modification of specific aspects of minority-group langauge was also carried out in the Turner House experimental preschool. This study was the second phase of the program reported by Hart (1969). The normative data gathered by Hart, which was discussed earlier, was drawn from her extended baseline period.

During baseline, three aspects of the child's language were selected for modification: the use of nouns, adjective-noun combinations, and compound sentences. The procedures used by Hart and the Turner House staff were used on all twelve of the children in the program simultaneously. The procedures were selected, therefore, to be ones that would be compatible with the daily preschool program and would not require individual sessions.

Except for the observers who recorded the data, no personnel were required beyond the normal preschool complement.

The procedure required a general reorganization of some aspects of the preschool. During baseline, the typical kinds of blocks, toys, paints, trikes, etc. were freely available to the children. During the training phase, however, most materials were available to the children only upon request. Toys were placed in glass-fronted cabinets, paints and brushes were kept on the *teacher's* counter, and trikes, wagons, sand toys, and other outdoor materials were kept in a storage shed. Only a few manipulative toys were freely available to the children during the training phase, and outdoors, swings, etc. were freely available. The children could use the restricted materials only by asking for them. Other than prompting requests and request form, and delivering requested materials, the behavior of the teachers remained basically the same as in baseline. They continued to praise appropriate use of materials and the children's talking to them, to other children or to other teachers.

Training Phase

The modification of the selected aspects of the children's language was divided into three parts based on the part of speech to be modified.

Use of Nouns. During part one, the children were required to include the name of each object in their requests for materials. Instead of pointing or just saying "that," the child would have to at least say "paint" in his request. When necessary, the teacher prompted the child to ask for the materials, and prompted the child to use the materials' name when this was absent.

> A child who stood in an area saying nothing was asked by the teacher in the area, "What do you want?" If the child made a general statement, such as "To paint," the teacher in the first two weeks of the procedure specified for him the materials he must then ask for, by saying, "Then you need to ask for an apron, and brushes, and paint." After the second week, teachers responded to such statements by children simply by asking, "What do you need?" and then providing the materials as asked for by the child. To a child who merely pointed to an object, or who requested it with an indefinite such as "it," "that," or "one of those," the teacher asked, "What is that called?" If the child then named the material, he was simultaneously

> given the object and praised by the teacher for naming it. A complete sentence was not required. If the child did not respond to the teacher's question, answered incorrectly, or said that he did not know, the teacher named the material, and when the child repeated the name, praised him and handed him the object. Often the teacher prompted by asking another child to supply the requesting child with the name of the material and then praising him for doing so (Hart, 1969, pp. 8-10).

New materials were frequently introduced, some of which the children were unfamiliar with, so the prompting procedure never fully dropped, although it was rarely necessary after the first week. All children were reliably naming all of the materials at the end of thirty days, so the second part of the training phase was begun.

ADJECTIVE-NOUN COMBINATIONS. On the sixty-sixth day of school, the contingency was modified so that materials could be obtained only through the appropriate use of an adjective-noun combination. The child was required to both name and qualify the object with some appropriate descriptive adjective, such as color, number or size.

Children who did not ask for materials with an adjective-noun combination were prompted for the correct response, but in no case did the teacher supply a descriptive adjective in her prompt.

> Initially, teachers prompted only the form of the request. A child who requested a material using only a noun, was asked: "What kind of a . . . do you want?" Since the observer data had shown that all of the children had exhibited some adjectives, teachers prompted adjective use not by supplying the child with a specific response but by offering him alternatives, such as, "I have big cars and little cars, red cars and blue cars, old cars and new cars, what kind of a car do you want?" If the child responded with an adjective, but no noun, as "A red one," the teacher prompted, "A red what?" and asked the child to, "Say the whole thing, 'a red car.' " When the child emitted an adjective-noun combination, he was praised, his request was repeated by the teacher, and he was handed the material he had specified.
>
> Whatever adjective a child used, he was given a material which corresponded to his description. If no material of his description was available, the teacher told him this, and described the materials which were available (as, "I don't have any green boats, all I have are red boats and yellow boats"). (In thus naming materials for chil-

> dren, teachers always used an adjective-noun combination.) In addition, descriptions of materials were supplied in response to children's requests: a child who had already asked for and received, big blocks and little blocks, for example, might ask a teacher (or another child), "What kind of a block is that?," be told "A round block," and receive it after repeating the phrase. A child who had asked for yellow paint, for instance, might, on receiving it, say that he had not wanted that color, he had wanted "that color" (pointing to orange). If necessary, the teacher told him the name of "that color"; if possible, she pointed out another item of the same color, the color of which the child had already named, and, for example, said, "It is the same color as your apron, what color is that?," holding the paint next to his apron (Hart, 1969, pp. 11-12).

This phase was continued for thirty-one school days after this period, a test of color names was carried out. In this test, the child was presented with a sheet of paper containing nine pure-color paper swatches. The child was first asked to point to each swatch and name it; then the teacher pointed to each swatch and asked the child to name it; and finally the teacher named the swatches and asked the child to point to them. At this time, seven of the twelve children appropriately named five or fewer of the colors on two or more trials, only five children appropriately on all three trials.

It was decided, therefore, to work only on color adjectives for awhile. Materials were then made contingent on requests containing a noun and the correct color adjective.

> Teachers asked children, "What color of a . . .?" rather than "What kind of a . . .?" material they wanted, and they supplied descriptions by naming alternatives between colors only (as, "I have red dough and blue dough"). When necessary, color names were supplied by the teacher in the manner described previously. In practice, the three children who had demonstrated knowledge of all nine colors were not strictly held to the color-adjective-noun contingency; also, a color-description was not required of any child for a material of no definite color, such as water. However, an adjective-noun combination was still always required (as, *hot, cold, clean,* or *dirty* water).
>
> This procedure was continued for twenty-seven days (Hart, 1969, p. 13).

Compound Sentences. Beginning on the 125th day of the program, an attempt was made to increase the complexity of the sentences that the children spontaneously used. Materials were, therefore, made contingent on the making of a request in the form of a compound (two verb phrases joined by a conjunction).

> When a child requested a material, the teacher asked him, "Why?," or "What for?"; if he responded with a simple phrase such as, "So I can play with it," the teacher asked him to "Say the whole thing"; if he hesitated, she then prompted him with as much of the terminal behavior as necessary. For example, she said, "I want a block so I can . . ." and then waited for the child to repeat, "I want a block so I can . . . play with it."
>
> Prompting of the response by having a child repeat after the teacher was discontinued for an individual child as soon as he began responding to the earlier teacher statements ("Why?" or "Say the whole thing"); for a few children, however, additional prompts were necessary in order to elicit clear enunciation of a conjunction. When having a child repeat after her, a teacher presented as simple a form of the behavior as possible in order to emphasize the compounding; i.e., sentences which did not contain adjective-noun combinations. Adjective-noun combinations were never required as part of a compound sentence. However, when a teacher repeated a child's request while delivering the corresponding material, she always repeated the two clauses in the same form the child had said them, i.e., she used an adjective-noun combination if the child had done so in his initial statement, otherwise she did not (Hart, 1969, pp. 13-14).

At first, the teacher repeated the compound sentence, gave praise and dispensed the materials for any *reason* given by the child. When the child was reliably using compound sentences, however, the appropriate sense of the reason was also prompted. Reasons such as, "I want a shovel because I don't have one," were replied to with, "Very good, but why do you really want it?" ("So I can dig with it.") (Hart, 1969, pp. 14-15). This phase was continued until the end of school (twenty-three days).

RESULTS. As can be seen in Figure VII.5, marked increases in the appropriate linguistic characteristics were produced in each of the three parts of the procedure. It should be noted that these data came from spontaneous speech, not just from the student's requests from the teacher. The effects are generalized, therefore. As would be expected, the increased frequency of nouns was maintained in the two succeeding conditions. More importantly, adjective-noun combinations were maintained in frequency during

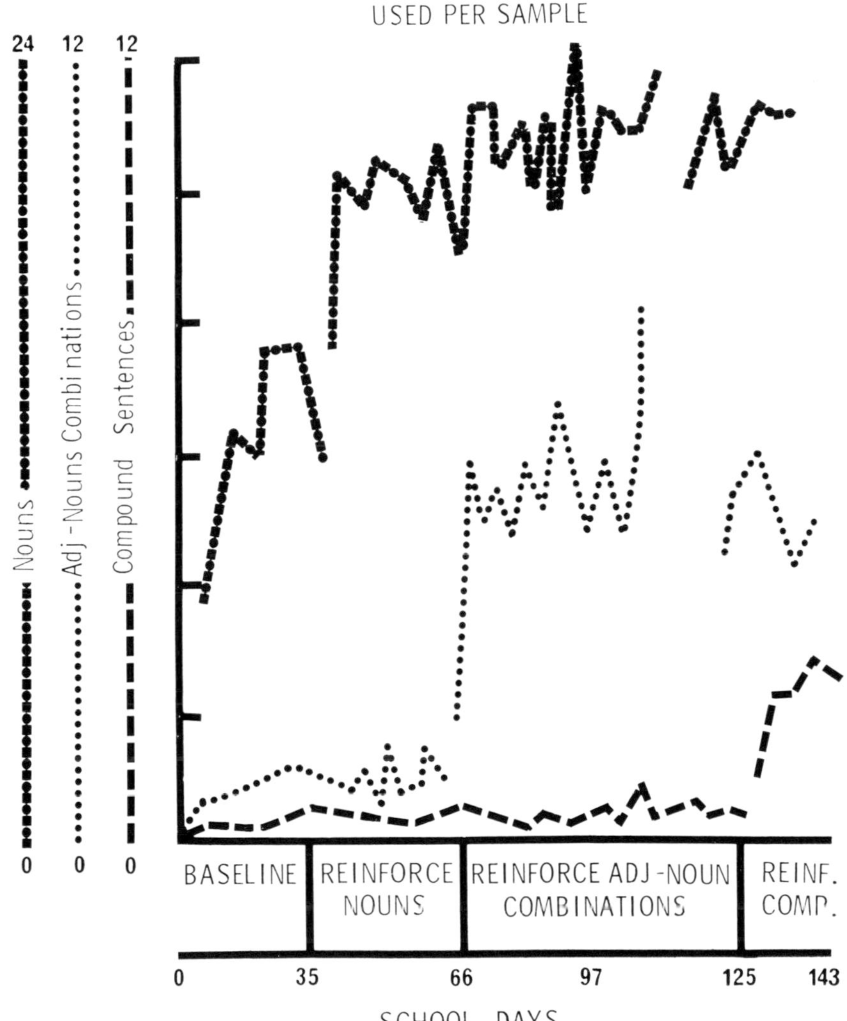

Figure VII.5. Change in frequency of selected parts of speech in the spontaneous speech of preschool children.

the compound-sentence segment, even though their occurrence as part of the compound sentence was not required in the contingency.

Results-Color Names. The change in the requirements of the adjective-noun combinations to an emphasis on color names, pro-

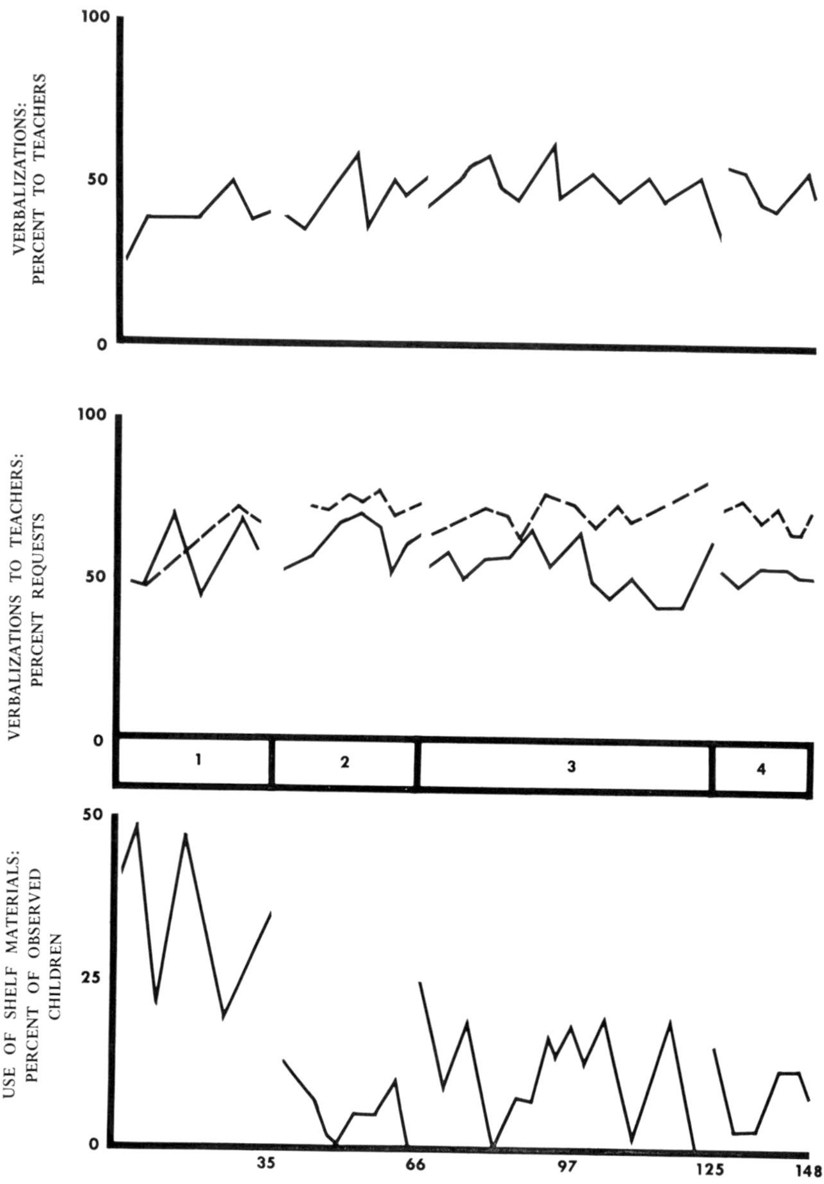

Figure VII.6. Patterns of verbalization and play with free materials during the phases of the Turner House project.

duced changes in their appropriate use by the children. At the end of the program, the color test was readministered. This time eleven of twelve children used five or more of the color names appropriately on two out of three trials, and nine of twelve children used seven or more of the color names appropriately.

Results-Side Effects. In spite of the fact that the modifications reported above concerned some very specific aspects of child language, the procedures themselves required some major alterations of the physical and verbal environments of the children. For this reason it was decided to monitor several aspects of the children's interactions with social and physical objects in order to detect possible unanticipated collateral changes.

Figure VII.6 shows the results of these observations. Frequency of verbalizations to teachers was not seen to change in any of the experimental conditions in spite of the several changes in the contingencies placed upon such verbalizations. Percentage of children using *free* materials was seen to decrease during those times in which some of the materials were used as reinforcers (If they were worth playing with, they wouldn't be free!).

Instituting Appropriate Verb Usage

Clark, Sherman and Kelly (1971) have developed a technique based on modeling and reinforcement for the modification of verb forms in poverty-level minority children. A major goal of their investigation was the establishment of generative usage of verb inflections in children who did not previously exhibit them. Specifically, this means getting children to use appropriate inflections both for verbs on which they have received training, and for new verbs on which they have not received training. This is a key point. The sheer number of verbs in a normal repertoire makes it educationally impossible to provide specific training on each member of the class. Instead, it is this kind of generalized use of verb endings which must be achieved. This is, of course, true for many other aspects of language as well.

The subjects for this experiment were eight retarded and four poverty-level children. This fact provides an excellent footnote to the concept of *etiology-independence* mentioned in the Introduction section of this book. Even though the two sets of subjects were from different populations with different histories, they all showed the same linguistic deficit and they all responded to the training program in the same way. This fact multiplies the significance of the chapter in this book many times. This is not meant to imply that minority children are retarded. It also does not mean that any credence is being given to the term *retardation*. It does mean that the same behavior can be altered with the same technique regardless of what theoretical label has been given to the subject population.

The children in this study showed relatively normal articulation and demonstrated good verbal imitation at the start of the program. None of the children, however, used white English noun suffixes or present, past and future verb inflections. The children were in the training program five days per week for thirty minute sessions in individual experimental rooms.

To establish a baseline frequency of the appropriate use of verb inflections, the experimenter asked a series of questions, each preceded by a related statement. For example, "He is a *baker*. What did he do yesterday?" A different stimulus item was included in each statement, but the form of the statement-question remained the same for each trial. In the present example, *"baker"* is the stimulus item and "yesterday he *baked*" would be the correct response.

During the later stages of the training procedure (which is discussed below), test questions were presented. These included both stimulus items on which the subject had received training and new stimulus items on which the subject had not received training. Subjects were reinforced for correct answers to previously trained stimulus items during the testing periods (social praise and snacks), but were not reinforced for responses to the untrained or generative stimulus items. Correct responses to the untrained items would indicate the acquisition of a generalized or generative pattern of behavior, rather than specific behaviors.

Statement-questions were also used for present, imperfect, future and past tense constructions. All nouns used as stimulus items take a phonemic [t] inflection to form the past tense verb form, *is* plus *ing* to form the present imperfect, and *will* plus the third-person singular present form to form the future tense.

TRAINING PROCEDURES. During the initial phase of the training, the experimenter modeled each word of the answer one at a time. The child was to repeat each word after the experimenter said it and was reinforced if he imitated each word in the sentence. For example:

E: "yesterday"
S: (Repeating "yesterday" produced reinforcement)
E: "he"
S: (Repeating "he" produced reinforcement)
E: "baked"
S: (Repeating "baked" produced reinforcement)

When the subject failed to respond within five seconds, or responded incorrectly, the experimenter said "no" and diverted his attention from the subject for five seconds. When the subject was reliably imitating sequences of individual words, the modeling was changed to larger groups of words. This was carried out by adding one word to the size of the group of words each step until the full sentence was modeled. Requirement for reinforcement at this stage was imitation of the full sentence. This was continued until the subject was reliably imitating one answer in the form of a full sentence. This procedure is a variant of shaping called *graduated modeling*. The statement-questions were not said by the experimenter during this phase, only the answers.

The second phase of training was begun when the subject was reliably imitating the one answer as a full sentence. In this phase the experimenter modeled the full correct answer as before, but in addition the modeled answer was preceded by the appropriate statement-question, such as, "He is a *baker*. What did he do yesterday? Yesterday he *baked*." To insure that the subjects would not also imitate the statement and question, they were spoken very softly at first and then gradually spoken with greater volume on successive trials. As in the previous stage, the subject was reinforced for correct imitations of the answer.

During the third and final phase of training the modeling of the correct answer by the experimenter was faded out. This was accomplished by progressively modeling the correct answer more softly and by deleting parts of the answer (beginning with the last parts of the answer) until it was not modeled at all. This phase was accomplished without disrupting the correct answers of the subject. At its completion, the subject was reliably giving the correct answer to one statement-question. Following this, question-answering was trained for additional stimulus items using the same three phases.

After the subjects had been trained to give correct verb-form answers to a series of different statement-questions, they were periodically presented with items on which they had not received any direct training (*probe* trials). These items were used to determine if the subjects had developed a generalized or generative pattern of answering behavior for this form of question. Correct answers were given about 85% of the time to the *trained* stimulus items, but the concern of this study was with the frequency of correct answers to the *untrained* stimulus items.

The subjects were trained on three different forms of statement-questions, one at a time, in the following order: past, future, present participle. During each probe trial, thirty questions were asked involving answers on which the subject was receiving training mixed with eighteen questions involving untrained answers (six each for the three forms of statement-questions). No reinforcement was given for answers to these untrained items.

RESULTS. Prior to the training phases for answers, three baseline trials were run. No correct answers were given by any of the subjects to any of these statement-questions. After training on the past-tense form, all subjects showed near 100% correct responding to the past-tense probe items, but responding to future and present-tense probe items remained at zero.

Following training on the second form (future tense), the subjects showed near 100% correct responding on the future-tense probe items. Correct responding on present-tense probe items remained at zero, while responding on past-tense probe items (the first tense to be trained) fell sharply below 100%. The previous level of correct responding was reestablished, however, following mixed training on both the past and future tense forms.

Correct responding on present tense probe items rose to near 100% following training on that form. Again, responding on both previously established forms fell below 100%, but reestablished following mixed training on all three forms. The interference with previously established discriminations produced by new discrimination training resembles a similar finding by Lovaas in the language training of autistic children (Lovaas, 1968).

Modifying Language Through Modeling

The behavior modification techniques discussed thus far have been built primarily around positive reinforcement. Modeling has been used in many of these procedures, but only as a prompt—only as a technique to produce the desired bit of behavior so that it could be reinforced. Recent research, however, has suggested that modeling can be used alone to modify selected linguistic features (Lahey, 1970; Risley and Reynolds, 1970). This research is important in pointing out the fact that teachers influence the language behavior of their pupils through the language they use in addition to the language of the children that they reinforce. They influence their pupils language behavior through what they practice as well as what they preach. Some modeling techniques for producing specific changes are discussed below.

In an experiment with children enrolled in a Head Start program, Lahey (1970) demonstrated a technique through which the frequency of descriptive adjectives could be modified through modeling without reinforcement. The procedure centered around teaching situations in which the children were asked to describe sets of objects.

Ten children were randomly divided into two groups and were taken individually into a room by the experimenter. They were asked if they would like to play a tape recorder game and were shown a table covered with open boxes. Each box contained a number of simple, easily identified monochromatic toys (red planes, green cars, etc.). After each child was allowed to say his name into the tape recorder, he was given the following instructions: "Now, I want you to tell me what you see in this box. Tell me all about what you see. Then it will be my turn and I'll tell you what I see in this box. Then it will be your turn again. Okay, tell me what you see in this box." On a few occasions, the child did not name each object in the box and was asked, "Anything else?"

Each box contained several toys arranged in two groups of two or three identical toys and two single toys. A complete description of the contents of the box (in terms of descriptive adjectives), therefore, would contain four nouns and six adjectives, four adjectives of color and two of number, or 1.5 adjectives per noun. The first description of the contents of a box was made by the child and was taken as his baseline frequency of descriptive adjectives.

After the baseline trial, the children in the two groups received slightly different treatment. The second box of toys was described by the experimenter. For the children in the adjective group (ADJ), the experimenter gave a full description of the contents of the box (1.5 descriptive adjectives per noun). For the no adjective group (NA), the experimenter used no descriptive adjectives at all in his description of the contents of the box (e.g., "I see a plane and some cars and a dog and some Indians."). The child then made the next description in both groups, followed by the experimenter in alternation until the experimenter had made three descriptions and the child had made three descriptions after baseline. After each description the experimenter said only, "Now it's my turn" or "Now it's your turn." Nothing was said or done contingent on the child's use or failure to use descriptive adjectives in his descriptions.

Results. The data for individual subjects in both groups are presented in Figure VII.7. The baseline data shows an extremely low frequency of descriptive adjective usage. Only one of the ten subjects used a significant number of descriptive adjectives during baseline. After the model's descriptions, however, the children in the ADJ group, showed a marked increase in descriptive adjectives, whereas the NA group did not.

These results clearly demonstrate that modeling alone can produce strong and immediate changes in children's language. It would appear to be an especially useful technique in situations like the above (which might be thought of as *science readiness*

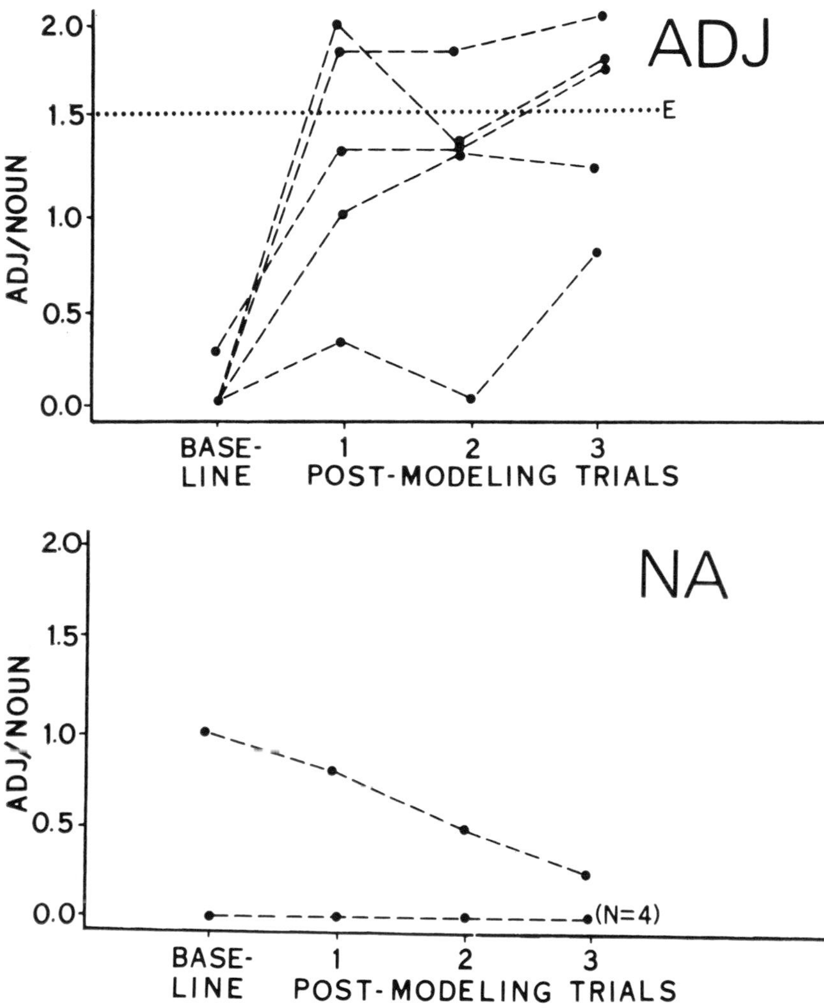

Figure VII.7. Change in the frequency of descriptive adjectives in the speech of minority children during modeling of descriptive adjectives (ADJ) or modeling of no adjectives (NA).

exercises or the like), but modeling can be used in other ways as well.

Facilitating Imitative Change

It is not always possible to effect significant changes in language behavior through modeling alone. Many children do not have well-developed imitative repertoires. It is for this reason that Risley and others have developed techniques to facilitate imitative learning (Risley and Wolf, 1967; Sherman, 1965). It is important to discuss this topic following the discussion of modeling without reinforcement to avoid a potential misunderstanding. Modeling can profitably be used alone as a behavior modification technique, but modeling and reinforcement are not alternative techniques. In many cases, the most effective strategy involves a combination of the two procedures. In this section, a procedure for increasing the frequency of verbal-imitation through the use of reinforcement is discussed.

Reinforcement of Imitation

Risley (1967) noted that many of the Turner House children imitated the language of their teachers infrequently. A program was undertaken, therefore, to train imitation. Because verbal behavior is rather complex, imitation training was begun on gross motor behaviors.

A teacher worked with three children one at a time in a group. She began by simply taking a snack from a bowl that sat in front of them, and prompted the children to imitate her. Then snacks were presented only for the imitation of simple behaviors, such as leaning to one side, raising the arms, etc. Training then progressed to more detailed motor behaviors, then to simple speech behaviors, and finally to complicated speech behaviors. Reinforcement was given only after each appropriate imitation of the teacher. This led to an increase in the frequency of imitation of both motor and verbal behaviors.

In order to demonstrate the importance of reinforcing the children for imitating, the contingency was reversed for fifteen days. When the children were reinforced for not imitating, the frequency of appropriate imitations fell off sharply. When the original contingency was reintroduced, frequency of imitation rose again to its previous level. These data are shown in Figure VII.8.

This technique is apparently an effective tool for increasing verbal imitation. It should be pointed out, however, that there is a danger in this procedure. If applied too broadly, it would produce a generalized tendency to imitate; this might result in the

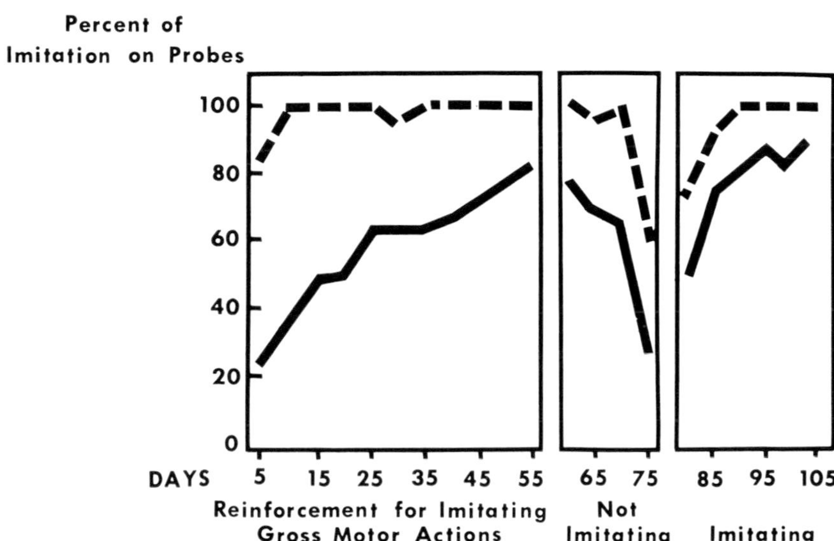

Figure VII.8. Change in frequency of imitation of adult model by preschool children when reinforced for imitating and when reinforced for not imitating.

modification of aspects of Child Black English that were not intended by the teacher. This might be easily avoided, however, by using discriminated imitation training. If reinforcement for imitating were limited to a specific classroom situation (e.g., an oral language period), increases in imitation should occur only, or mostly, in that situation. This would allow the teacher to carefully choose what she will model in that situation.

Stress as a Prompt for Verbal Imitation

Another technique for increasing the effectiveness of language modeling was developed by Risley and Reynolds (1970). Minority group children were individually asked to repeat several sentences one at a time. After each imitation, the child was given a snack, regardless of the accuracy of the imitation.

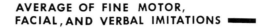

As the experimenter read the sentences, she emphasized one or more of the words through an increase in voice volume. Throughout the series, different proportions of words are emphasized. As would be expected, stressed words were imitated considerably more frequently than unstressed words. In addition, it was found that all of the words in the phrase containing the stressed word were more repeated more frequently, and that there was an inverse relationship between the number of stressed words and the increase in frequency of repetition. While these results are not surprising, they do suggest an effective way to facilitate imitative language change.

Bereiter and Engelmann Preschool Programs

Any discussion of preschool langauge programs would be incomplete without mention of the work of Bereiter and Engelmann (Bereiter and Engelmann, 1966; Engelmann, 1970). Their work has not been excluded thus far due to any question about the effectiveness of the techniques that they advocate. On the contrary, they are based on the same principles as those suggested in this text and are apparently quite effective. But, while their techniques are not in question, two of their basic assumptions are.

First, Bereiter and Engelmann appear to be unaware of the existence of Nonschool Repertoires. They treat the language spoken in the preschool as *the* language of minority children.

> The child of poverty has language problems. These are problems far more crippling than mere dialect problems. Too frequently, a four-year-old child of poverty does not understand the meaning of such words as *long, full, animal, red, under, first, before, or, if, all* and *not*. Too frequently, he cannot repeat a simple statement, such as, "The bread is under the oven," even after he has been given four trials (Englemann, 1967a). Too frequently, he cannot succeed on a task in which he is presented with a picture of two boys and two girls and is asked to "Find the right ones: He is big. . . . She is not standing on the floor. . . . She is next to a chair" and so on (Engelmann 1967a). In brief, the child of poverty has not been taught as much about the meaning of language as a middle-class child of the same age (Engelmann, 1970, p. 102).

Secondly, it is clear from the goals of their program that white English is the only language that they believe to be appropriate for the classroom: "Through education, we would like to be able to teach disadvantaged Negro children the same set of skills we require for middle-class white children" (Engelmann, 1970, p. 104).

SUMMARY AND CONCLUSIONS

Several conceptions and misconceptions about the language of minority children were discussed. The limited descriptive data which is available was summarized and the gaps in it pointed out. Several behavior modification techniques for altering the language of minority children in the preschool were discussed, based on the following set of assumptions: (1) language is a key factor in educational and occupational achievement; (2) minority group children speak languages that are different in many ways from white English, but they cannot in any sense be said to speak inferior or deficient languages; (3) still, because of the dominance of the white culture, some changes in the language of minority children should be made in the preschool; (4) these changes must not violate their cultural heritage and ostracize them from their family and peers; and (5) most importantly, the decision on whether to modify and what to modify should be made by an informed, representative, multicultural body, rather than by the white-dominated school system alone.

REFERENCES

Bailey, Beryl L.: Some aspects of the impact of linguistics on language teaching. *Elementary English, 45*:570-578, 1968.

Bereiter, C. and Engelmann, S.: *Teaching Disadvantaged Children in the Preschool.* Englewood Cliffs, Prentice-Hall, 1966.

Bernstein, B.: A sociolinguistic approach to socialization. With some reference to educability. In F. Williams (Ed.) : *Language and Poverty.* Chicago, Markham, 1970, pp. 25-61.

Caselli, R.: Keys to standard English. *The Elementary School Journal, 5*:86-89, 1970.

Clark, H. B., Sherman, J. A. and Kelly, Karen K.: Use of modeling and reinforcement to train generative sentence usage. Paper presented to American Psychological Association, Washington, D. C., 1971.

Coleman, J. S., et al.: *Equality of Educational Opportunity.* Washington, D. C.: U. S. Government Printing Office, 1966.

Crain, R. L.: School integration and the academic achievement of Negroes. *Sociology of Education, 44*:1-26, 1971.

Deutsch, M.: The role of social class in language and cognitive development. *American Journal of Orthopsychiatry, 35*:78-88, 1965.

Engelmann, S.: *The Basic Concept Inventory*. Chicago, Follet, 1967.

Engelmann, S.: How to construct effective language programs for the poverty child. In F. Williams (Ed.) : *Language and Poverty*. Chicago, Markham, 1970, 102-122.

Fasold, R. W. and Shuy, R. W. (Eds.) : *Teaching Standard English in the Inner City*. Washington, D. C.: Center for Applied Linguistics, 1970.

Hart, B. M.: Investigations of the language of disadvantaged preschool children. Unpublished Doctoral dissertation, University of Kansas, 1969.

Hart, Betty M. and Risley, T. R.: Establishing the use of descriptive adjectives in the spontaneous speech of disadvantaged preschool children. *Journal of Applied Behavior Analysis, 1*:109-120, 1968.

Hess, R. D. and Shipman, Virginia C.: Early experience and the socialization of cognitive modes in children. *Child Development, 36*:869-886, 1965.

Houston, Susan H.: A reexamination of some assumptions about the language of the disadvantaged child. *Child Development, 41*:947-963, 1970.

Labov, W.: The logic of nonstandard English. In Fredrick Williams (Ed.) : *Language and Poverty*. Chicago, Markham, 1970, 153-189.

Lahey, B. B.: Modification of the frequency of descriptive adjectives in the speech of Head Start children through modeling without reinforcement. *Journal of Applied Behavior Analysis, 4*:19-22, 1971.

Lovaas, O. I.: *Behavior Modification* (Film), New York, Appleton-Century-Crofts, 1968.

McCarthy, D.: *The Language Development of the Preschool Child,* Minneapolis, University of Minnesota Press, 1930.

McNeil, D.: *The Acquisition of Language*. New York, Harper and Row, 1970.

Reynolds, Nancy J. and Risley, T. R.: The role of social and material reinforcers in increasing talking of a disadvantaged preschool child. *Journal of Applied Behavior Analysis, 1*:253-262, 1968.

Risley, T. R.: Learning and lollipops. In Phebe Cramer (Ed.) : *Readings in Developmental Psychology Today*. Del Mar, CRM Books, 1967.

Risley, T. R. and Wolf, M. M.: Establishing functional speech in echololic children. *Behavior Research and Therapy, 5*:73-88, 1967.

Risley, T. R. and Reynolds, Nancy J.: Emphasis as a prompt for verbal imitation. *Journal of Applied Behavior Analysis, 3*:185-190, 1970.

Rosenthal, R. and Jacobson, Lenore: *Pygmalion in the Classroom: Teacher Expectation and Pupil's Intellectual Development*. New York, Holt, Rinehart and Winston, 1968.

Sherman, J. A.: Use of reinforcement and imitation to reinstate verbal behavior in adult psychotics. *Journal of Abnormal Psychology, 70*:155-164, 1965.

Shuy, R. W.: Detroit speech: Careless, awkward, and inconsistent or systematic, graceful, and regular? *Elementary English, 45*:565-569, 1968.

Smith, M. E.: An investigation of the development of the sentence and the extent of vocabulary in young children. *University of Iowa Studies in Child Welfare, 3*:No. 5, 1926.

Templin, M. C.: *Certain Language Skills in Children.* Minneapolis, Univer-versity of Minnesota Press, 1957.

Uhrbrock, R. S.: Words most frequently used by a five-year-old girl. *Journal of Educational Psychology, 27*:155-158, 1936.

Young, F. M.: An analysis of certain variables in a developmental study of language. *Genetic Psychology Monographs, 23*:3-141, 1941.

NAME INDEX

Adams, M. R., 99-100, 127
Anderson, V. A., 181, 216
Andrews, G., 118, 122, 127-128
Ansberry, M., 179, 217
Arnold, G. E., 179-180, 183-184, 193, 195, 200, 216-217
Azrin, N. H., 91-93, 127-128

Baer, D. M., 6, 8, 10, 28, 39, 44, 55, 57-59, 85, 88
Bailey, B. L., 288, 313
Baker, L., 213, 217
Baker, R., 163, 177
Bandura, A., 219, 267
Bar, A., 107, 127
Becker, K. P., 180, 182, 184, 216
Beebe, H. A., 202, 216
Bellugi, U., 23, 57
Berberich, J., 62, 89
Bereiter, C., 272, 287, 312-313
Berndt, L. A., 99, 104, 128
Bernstein, B., 272, 313
Berko, J., 8, 57
Berry, M. F., 181, 216
Biggs, B., 102, 127
Bijou, S. W., xviii, xix
Blake, P., 71, 78, 88
Blind, J. J., 117-118, 127
Bradbury, B., 8, 58
Bradley, P., 199, 202, 217
Brady, J., 201, 212, 216
Bricker, D. D., 7, 57
Bricker, W. A., 7, 57
Brown, P., 213, 217
Brown, R., 23, 57
Browning, R. M., 107, 127
Buxbaum, J., 223, 226, 267

Cady, B. B., 101, 104, 127
Carrier, J., 163, 176
Carroll, J. B., 8, 57
Caselli, R., 273, 288, 313
Catania, A. C., 219, 262, 267
Cattell, R. B., 123, 127, 129
Chess, S., 81, 90
Chomsky, N., 9, 23, 57
Clark, A. W., 106, 128
Clark, H. B., 303, 313
Coleman, J. S., 270, 313
Cooper, E. B., 95, 99, 101, 104, 127
Crain, R. L., 270, 313
Cunningham, M. A., 64-65, 88
Curlee, R. F., 104, 108, 120-121, 127

Daly, D. A., 95, 99, 104, 127
Darley, F. L., 123, 128
Dehn, J. K., 72, 88
Deutsch, M., 272, 313
Dickerson, D. J., 39, 57
Dokecki, P., 72, 88

Edwards, A., 248, 267
Egolf, D. B., 99, 117-118, 127, 129
Eisenberg, L., 63-64, 88
Eisenson, J., ix, xix, 181, 216
Engelmann, S., 272, 287, 312-314
Eysenck, H. J., 123, 127
Eysenck, S. B. G., 123, 127

Fasold, R. W., 288, 314
Ferster, C. B., 65, 71, 88, 219, 267
Filby, Y., 267
Fitch, J., 153-161, 166, 176
Flanagan, B., 91-93, 95, 127, 128
Fraser, C., 23, 57
Freund, H., 197, 216
Frick, J. V., 104, 127
Froeschels, 200, 201

Garrett, E., 162-163, 176
Giddan, J. J., 65, 83, 90
Girardeau, F. L., 39, 57
Gleason, H. A., 57, 60
Goldiamond, I., 80, 88, 91-94, 104, 127-128, 201, 212, 216, 219, 267

Goldstein, K., 74, 88, 220, 267
Goodglass, H., 220, 267
Goodkin, R., 219-220, 223, 226-227, 262, 267
Granick, L., 220, 267
Greenspoon, J., 219, 267
Grundmann, K., 180, 182, 184, 216
Guess, D., 10, 15-16, 22-24, 27-28, 31, 39, 44, 55, 57-58

Hall, J., 68, 89
Hamilton, J., 39, 57
Halpern, H., 220, 268
Halvorson, J. A., 100-101, 128
Haroldson, S. K., 97-98, 102-103, 105, 108, 128
Harrelson, A., 27-28, 39, 58
Harris, M., 105, 118, 127
Hart, B. M., 273, 278-279, 283-286, 296, 298-300, 314
Hartung, J. R., 80-82, 88
Hawkins, N., 86, 89
Head, H., 220, 268
Hess, R. D., 285, 314
Hewett, F., 67, 78, 80, 88
Holland, A., 161, 176, 219, 268
Holloway, C., 212, 216
Honig, W. K., 219, 268
Hoshiko, M., 212, 216
Houston, S. H., 273, 275, 278, 314
Hull, H., 72, 88

Ince, L. P., 252, 268
Ingham, R. J., 118, 122, 128
Isaacs, W., 80, 88

Jacobson, L., 270-271, 288, 314
Jenkins, J., 268
Jiminez, P., 268
John, 223, 268
Johnson, W., 123, 128
Jones, L., 220, 268

Kanner, L., 61-63, 65, 88, 89
Kantor, J. R., ix, xix
Kelly, K. K., 303, 313
Kerr, N., 219, 268
Kingery, M., 199, 202, 217
Knott, M., 166, 176
Koegel, R., 62, 89
Kozloff, M. A., 89
Krasner, L., 219, 268-269
Kuhl, 108

Labov, W., 273, 275, 277, 287-289, 314
Lahey, B. B., 307, 308, 314
Langova, J., 183-184, 190, 212, 214, 216
Leach, E., 107, 128
Lenneberg, E. H., 9, 23, 58
Lenske, J., 213, 217
Leonard, L., 162, 176
Lindsley, O. R., 219, 268
Lovaas, O. I., 8, 58, 62-63, 66, 68, 77-78, 82, 89, 307, 314
Lovell, K., 8, 58
Luchsinger, R., 179-180, 183, 193, 195, 200, 217

MacDonald, E., 162, 165, 177
McCauley, B., 7, 58, 199, 217
McCarthy, D., 3, 23, 58, 283, 285-286, 314
McDearborn, J., 213, 217
McDermott, L. D., 108, 128
McNeal, S., 86, 89
McNeil, D., 274, 314
Mann, R., 39, 58
Marshall, R. C., 213, 217
Martin, R. R., 94-99, 102-105, 108, 128
Matthews, J., 161, 176
Mees, H., 66, 90
Meisel, J., 83, 90
Metz, J. R., 71, 73, 75, 89
Meyerson, L., 219, 268
Myerson, M. J., 219, 268
Milstead, J., 68, 71-72, 89
Moore, J., 147-152, 177
Moss, T., 74, 78, 88
Moravek, M., 183-184, 190, 212, 214, 216
Mowrer, D., 163-165, 177, 213, 217, 219, 268
Mundy, M. B., 105, 128
Myklebust, H. R., 23, 58

Palermo, D., 4, 58
Patterson, B. R., 86, 89
Perkins, W. H., 104, 108, 120-121, 127
Perloff, B., 62, 89
Peterson, R., 8, 73-74, 85, 88-89
Phelps, R., 86, 89
Piaget, J., 66, 89

Popelka, G., 99-100, 127
Powers, M., 180-181, 217
Preisler, L., 39, 59
Pronovost, W., 77, 89
Provence, S., 66, 89

Quadfessel, F., 220, 267
Quist, R. W., 96, 128

Rehm, R., 62, 89
Reynolds, G., 269
Reynolds, N. J., 278, 307, 311, 314
Rhodes, R. C., 117, 129
Rickard, H. C., 105, 128
Rimland, B., 62-64, 71, 89
Risley, T. R., 8, 58, 66, 68, 70-71, 73-74, 76, 80, 82, 87, 89-90, 278, 290-291, 293-296, 307, 310-311, 314
Ritvo, S., 66, 89
Robbins, C. J., 101, 104, 127
Roll, J., 130-147, 177
Rosenthal, R., 270-271, 288, 314
Russell, J. C., 106, 128
Rutherford, G., 10, 57-58
Ryan, B. P., 114-116, 128

Sailor, W., 10, 16, 24, 31, 39, 57-59
Salzinger, K., 9, 58, 219, 268
Sands, E., 268
Sarno, M. L., 268
Sarno, M. T., 268-269
Schaeffer, B., 62, 89
Scheier, I. H., 123, 129
Schell, R. E., 65, 76-77, 85, 90
Schreibman, L., 62, 89
Schuell, H., 220, 268
Schutz, R., 163, 177, 213, 217
Seeman, M., 189, 193, 217
Seltzer, H. N., 99, 127
Shankweiler, D., 268
Shames, G. H., 99, 116-118, 127, 129
Sheehan, J. G., 91, 102, 127, 129
Sherman, J. A., 8, 55, 58, 71, 77, 79, 85, 88, 90, 303, 310, 313-314
Shipman, V. C., 285, 314
Shumaker, J., 55, 58
Shuy, R. W., 288, 314
Sidman, M., 58-59, 219
Siegel, G. M., 94-96, 128, 213, 217
Simkins, L., 199, 202-203, 212, 217
Skinner, B. F., ix, xix, 4, 9, 23, 58, 219, 267-268
Sloane, H. N., 7, 58, 199, 217
Smith, M. E., 279, 314
Spradlin, J. E., 7, 39, 57-58
Spriestersbach, D. C., 123, 128
Staats, A. W., 4, 58, 219, 268
Staats, C. K., 4, 58
Stark, J., 65, 83, 90
Starr, C. D., 97, 128
Stimbert, V. E., 86, 90
Strait, R., 86, 90
Stumphauzer, J., 212, 217
Suskin, 268

Taylor, D., 68, 89
Taylor, M. L., 219, 221, 226, 268
Templin, M. C., 279, 283, 285-286, 315
Terrace, H. S., 219, 269
Thomas, J., 80, 88
Tikofsky, R. S., 220, 269
Timberlake, W., 220, 267
Tramontana, J., 86, 90
Travis, L. E., 220, 269
Turner, R., 62, 68, 70, 72, 87, 90

Uhrbrock, R. S., 284, 315
Ullmann, L. P., 219, 269

Van Riper, C., 162, 177, 179, 181, 197, 214-215, 217
van Sommers, P., 106, 128
Vignolo, L., 219, 223, 269

Wakstein, J. J., 89
Wakstein, M. P., 89
Wepman, J., 220, 268-269
Webb, C., 162, 177
Weiss, D., 179-180, 182-183, 186-188, 190, 195, 200-203, 207, 214, 217
West, W. R., 179, 217
Wingate, M. E., 93, 129
Winitz, H., 39, 59, 162, 177
Wolf, M. M., 8, 58, 66, 68, 80-82, 89-90, 310
Wolff, S., 81, 90
Wolpe, 230
Wyllie, J., 179, 217

Young, F. M., 279, 286, 315

SUBJECT INDEX

A

ABAB design, xvi
Adjectival inflections, 44
Adjectives, 298, 307
Avoidance conditioning, xiii

B

Bandwidth, 132, 177
Baseline, xvii
Behavior modification, ix
Between groups design, xvii
Blocks, 107

C

CRF, xiv
CVA, 221
Central language imbalance, 191
Comparative adjectives, 44
Compound sentences, 299
Continuous reinforcement, xiv
Control group, xvii

D

Desensitization, 230
Diagnostic categories, xviii
Discriminative stimulus, xiv

E

Echolalia, 79
Edwards personal preference schedule, 226
Escape conditioning, xiii
Etiology, xviii
Expectancy effects, 270
Expectation, 104
Extinction, xv
Extrinsic predication, 274

F

Fading, xvi, 230
Filters, 131, 177
Fixed interval, xiv
Fixed ratio, xiv, 72
Functional communication profiles, 226

G

Generative property of language, x, 9
Generative response class, x, 39, 44
Generalized response class, x, 39, 44
Graded delayed auditory feedback, 120ff
Grammar, xi, 7

H

Hereditary influence, 193
Herz unit, 132, 177

I

Imitation, 66, 74, 76, 310
Imitative learning, xv, 91
Inter-observer reliability, 59, 114
Intrinsic prediction, 274

L

Language, ix, 3, 55
Learning principles, xii
Logical inadequacy, 287

M

Mean length of utterance, 282
Method of successive approximations, xiii
Mind, ix
Model, xv
Modeling, xv, 307
Modeling and reinforcement, xv, 310
Morpheme, xi
Morphological grammar, 7, 10, 39
Motor conditioning, 74
Musicality, 184

N

Negative reinforcement, xiii
Neurological deficit, 194
Noun suffixes, 39

O

Observer, xv
Operant learning, xii, 91

P

Parents as therapists, 86, 293ff
Phonation, 181
Phoneme, xi, 77ff, 166ff
Pitch, 130, 181
Plural morpheme, 10
Positive reinforcement, xiii, 101, 105
Post check, xvii
Probe, 23, 29, 47, 53
Productive language, x, 22
Prompt, xvi, 74, 75
Punishment, xv, 70, 101, 108

R

Rate of speech, 181
Receptive language, x, 22
Reliability, 59, 114
Response cost, 100
Restraint, release from, 68
Reversal, xvii
Rhythm, 181, 184

S

Shaping, xiii
Social reinforcer, 71
Stimulus control, xiv
Stuttering vs. cluttering, 195
Successive approximations, xiii
Superlative adjectives, 44
Syntax, xi

T

Thematic content modification program, 117
Time out from positive reinforcement, xv, 68, 97
Token economy, xiii
Token reinforcers, xiii, 24, 29, 40, 47
Traditional speech therapy, 116, 118

U

Unintelligible speech, 178

V

Variable interval, xiv
Variable ratio, xiv, 16, 24, 30, 47, 72
Verbal conditioning, 219
Verbal imitation, 76
Verb inflections, 303
Vocal fundamental frequency, 130, 177
Vocal responses, 77

W

Within-subjects design, xvi